Atlas of Anatomic Pathology

Series Editor
Liang Cheng

For further volumes:
http://www.springer.com/series/10144

Scott R. Owens • Henry D. Appelman

Atlas of Esophagus and Stomach Pathology

Springer

Scott R. Owens, MD
Department of Pathology
University of Michigan
Ann Arbor
Michigan
USA

Henry D. Appelman, MD
Department of Pathology
University of Michigan
Ann Arbor
Michigan
USA

Series Editor
Liang Cheng, MD
Department of Pathology
and Laboratory Medicine
Indiana University School of Medicine
Indianapolis, IN
USA

ISBN 978-1-4939-4285-5 ISBN 978-1-4614-8084-6 (eBook)
DOI 10.1007/978-1-4614-8084-6
Springer New York Heidelberg Dordrecht London

Printed on acid-free paper

Springer is part of Springer Science+Business Media (www.springer.com)

Series Preface

"One Picture is Worth Ten Thousand Words"

– Frederick Barnard, 1927

Remarkable progress has been made in anatomic and surgical pathology during the last ten years. The ability of surgical pathologists to reach a definite diagnosis is now enhanced by immunohistochemical and molecular techniques. Many new clinically important histopathologic entities and variants have been described using these techniques. Established diagnostic entities are more fully defined for virtually every organ system. The emergence of personalized medicine has also created a paradigm shift in surgical pathology. Both promptness and precision are required of modern pathologists. Newer diagnostic tests in anatomic pathology, however, cannot benefit the patient unless the pathologist recognizes the lesion and requests the necessary special studies. An up-to-date Atlas encompassing the full spectrum of benign and malignant lesions, their variants, and evidence-based diagnostic criteria for each organ system is needed. This Atlas is not intended as a comprehensive source of detailed clinical information concerning the entities shown. Clinical and therapeutic guidelines are served admirably by a large number of excellent textbooks. This Atlas, however, is intended as a "first knowledge base" in the quest for definitive and efficient diagnosis of both usual and unusual diseases.

The *Atlas of Anatomic Pathology* is presented to the reader as a quick reference guide for diagnosis and classification of benign, congenital, inflammatory, nonneoplastic, and neoplastic lesions organized by organ systems. Normal and variations of "normal" histology are illustrated for each organ. The Atlas focuses on visual diagnostic criteria and differential diagnosis. The organization is intended to provide quick access to images and confirmatory tests for each specific organ or site. The Atlas adopts the well-known and widely accepted terminology, nomenclature, classification schemes, and staging algorithms.

This book Series is intended chiefly for use by pathologists in training and practicing surgical pathologists in their daily practice. It is also a useful resource for medical students, cytotechnologists, pathologist assistants, and other medical professionals with special interest in anatomic pathology. We hope that our trainees, students, and readers at all levels of expertise will learn, understand, and gain insight into the pathophysiology of disease processes through this comprehensive resource. Macroscopic and histological images are aesthetically pleasing in many ways. We hope that the new Series will serve as a virtual pathology museum for the edification of our readers.

Liang Cheng, MD
Series Editor

Preface

Some readers may wonder why another gastrointestinal pathology textbook is needed, especially one that is basically nothing more than a picture book. We have found that the current textbooks contain photographs that are ideal examples of what is described in the text. The images are invariably of perfectly oriented specimens, exquisitely stained and artefact free. In contrast, pathologists who deal with such specimens daily have to handle poorly oriented specimens cut in various biases. The stains often vary dramatically from day to day, depending on the peculiarities of the reagents and the automatic stainers. Artefacts of cutting, including folds, chattering, shredding, and variable thicknesses are extraordinarily common. We felt that it was time for a reality check on textbook visual perfection, so we have tailored many of our images to reflect the technical problems that we face daily. We also decided to deal almost exclusively with biopsies, since biopsies are the bread and butter of modern gastrointestinal pathology practice.

This atlas is limited to the esophagus and the stomach, common targets for endoscopic biopsies. The range of normal microscopic anatomy is stressed. Not every disease or change is included, but all the common ones and a few rare ones are covered. We have also included some biopsies that have diseases without names and without literature to indicate to the reader that not everything we see has a specific diagnosis. In order to offer some additional insights about biopsy handling and interpretation, we have included a number of statements to the figure legends covering our personal experiences, and what we know and what we don't about certain cases. Very few references are listed, because exhaustive reference lists are found in all the other textbooks, so we thought it would be a waste of time and print to repeat them. We hope that this atlas will be useful for the general surgical pathology practitioners who are the ones who deal with most such biopsies by far. The specialist does not need it, but is welcome to look at it and give us feedback of any type.

It is customary to express appreciation in these prefaces. Our mentors and family members really had nothing to do with this atlas, but we have been privileged to know and love them regardless. However, Lee Klein from Springer was a huge help. He tried valiantly to keep us on some kind of schedule, and he kept us focused on the final product. It is up to the reader to decide if he and we succeeded.

Scott R. Owens, MD
Henry D. Appelman, MD

Contents

Part I

Esophagus

Normal Histologic Anatomy and Common Variations

1

This first chapter illustrates the components of the normal esophagus as seen in biopsies. In addition, we have been impressed with a wide range of changes in these normal structures that keep appearing and reappearing in biopsies, and these changes or variations from the norm do not seem to indicate specific diseases. In our practice, our most common diagnosis for biopsies from all gastrointestinal (GI) sites is "no significant abnormality," which indicates that there may be some minor, clinically unimportant change but no namable disease. The variations on normal in these chapters ultimately fall into this group of "no significant abnormality."

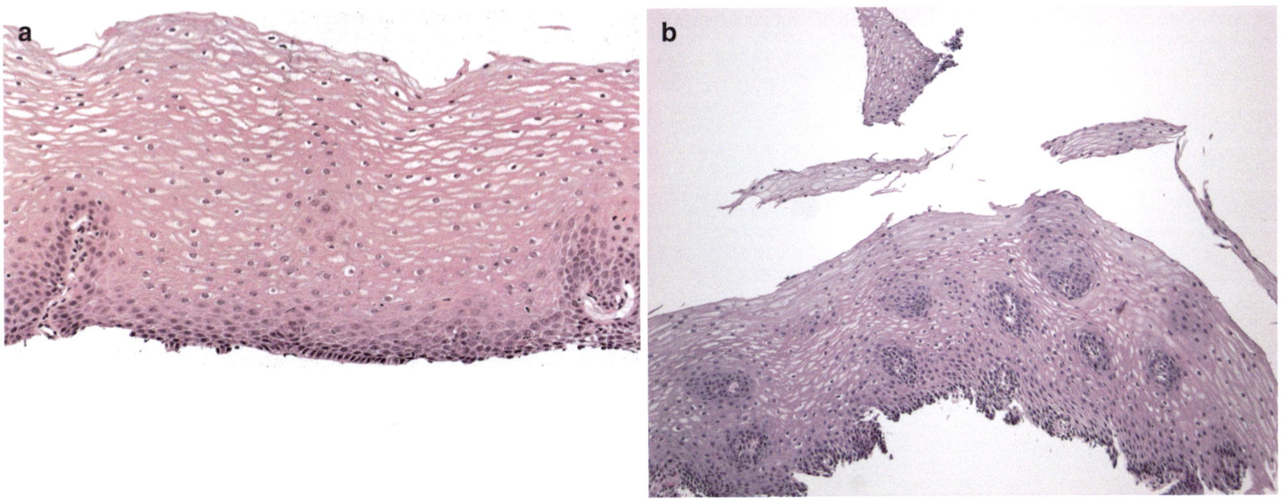

Fig. 1.1 Normal squamous epithelium. (**a**) In a perfectly oriented cut, the normal epithelium is nonkeratinizing, has a basal proliferative zone about one sixth or less of the total thickness, and has short papillae-containing cores of lamina propria with tiny vessels surrounded by a few layers of basal cells. (**b**) In typical biopsies, such well-oriented areas as in **a** are less common than areas like this with papillae in cross-section that extend higher in the epithelium than one sixth of the total thickness. The basal layer has been cut across, so it appears to be incomplete, and there are detached squamous fragments at the top

S.R. Owens, H.D. Appelman, *Atlas of Esophagus and Stomach Pathology*, Atlas of Anatomic Pathology,
DOI 10.1007/978-1-4614-8084-6_1, © Springer Science+Business Media New York 2014

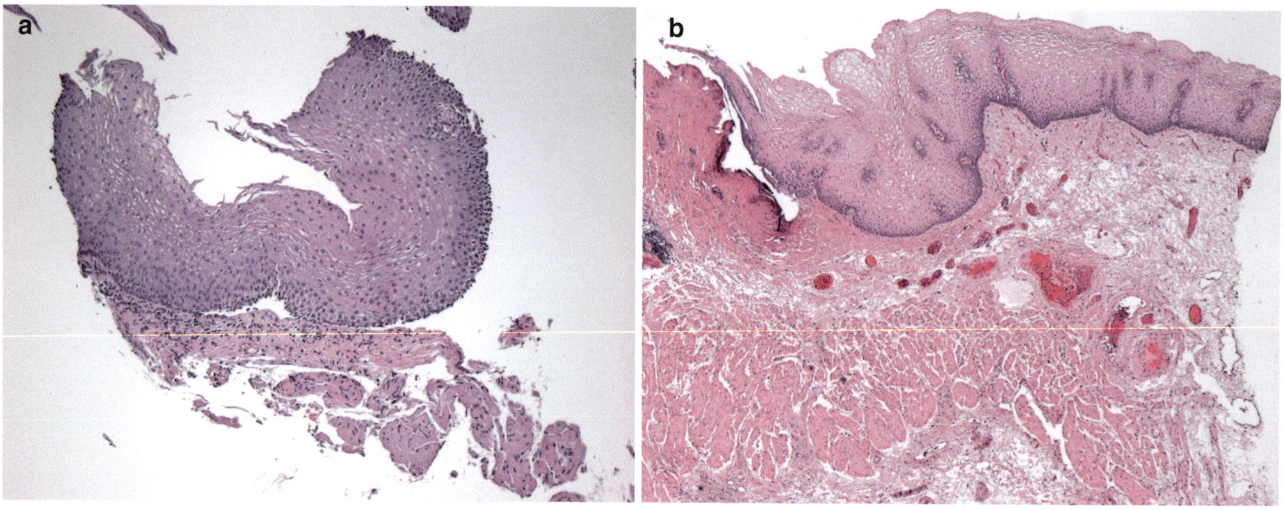

Fig. 1.2 Normal lamina propria, muscularis mucosae, and superficial submucosa. The esophagus and the anus are the only sites in the gut where the epithelium is squamous, and the epithelium and the lamina propria form separate layers. Everywhere else, the epithelium is columnar and mixed with the lamina propria. Most adult esophageal biopsies do not capture lamina propria but only the squamous epithelium. Compared to adult biopsies, routine esophageal biopsies in small children are more likely to include lamina propria. (**a**) In this unusually deep forceps biopsy, the full lamina propria appears as a thin layer beneath the squamous epithelium that contains small blood and lymphatic vessels and scattered lymphocytes. Beneath the lamina propria is the superficial part of the muscularis mucosae, which has discrete bundles of smooth muscle. (**b**) A specimen from an endoscopic mucosal resection (EMR) almost always captures the full thickness of the lamina propria, the muscularis mucosae, and usually some of the superficial submucosa. In this image, the lamina propria is a discrete layer of loose collagen, blood vessels, and lymphatics right beneath the squamous epithelium. The lamina propria also looks edematous but the fluid is an artifact of the procedure. For EMRs, fluid is generally injected beneath the resection site to lift it so it can be more easily removed. Some fluid is often trapped in the lamina propria. Beneath this layer is the thick muscularis mucosae composed of discrete bundles of smooth muscle. Beneath this is another layer of collagen and vessels, the superficial submucosa

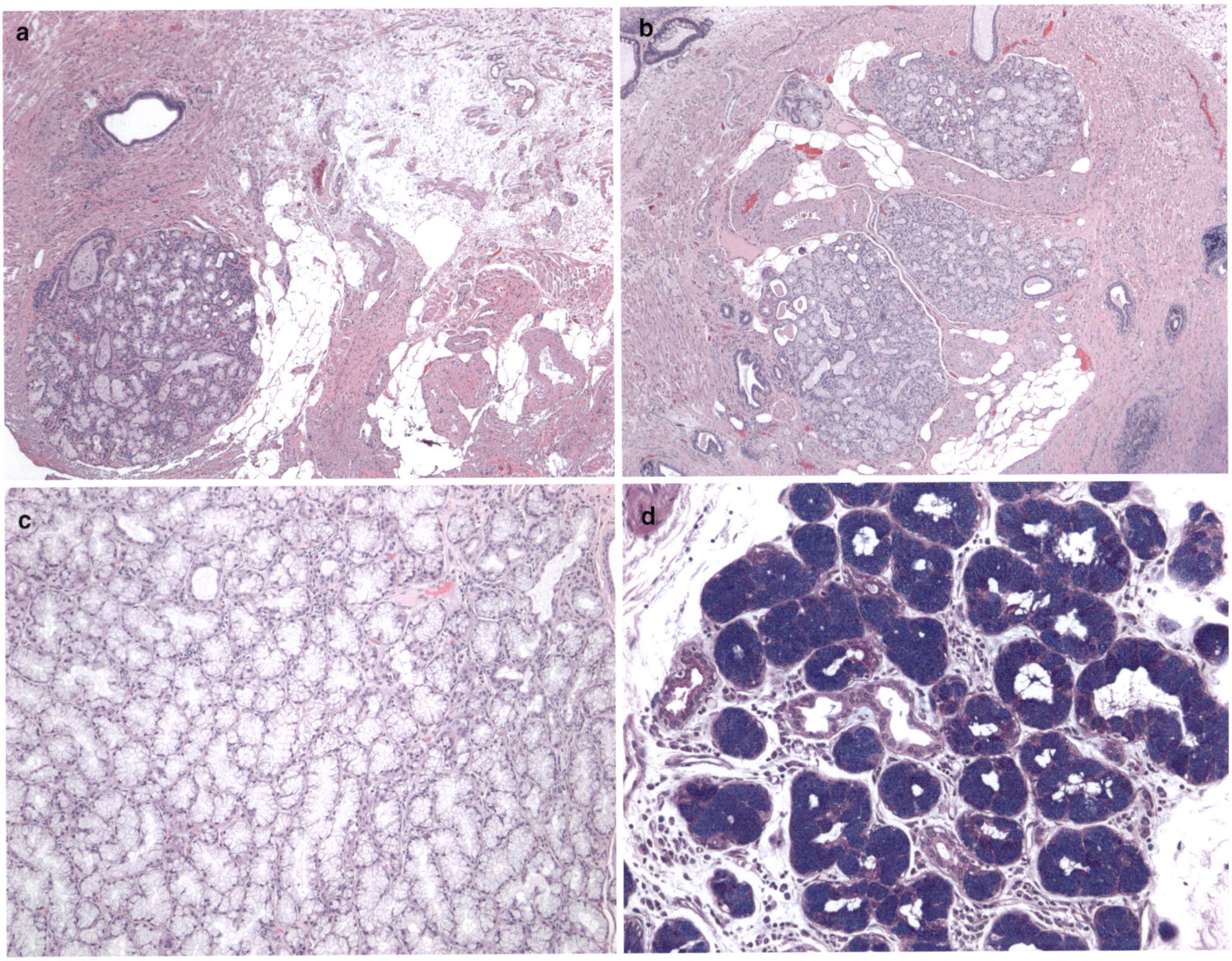

Fig. 1.3 Submucosal glands. Throughout the esophageal submucosa, especially distally, often plastered to the bottom of the muscularis mucosae, there are lobulated glands composed of uniform clusters of mucus-containing cells and a draining duct. Because they are so deep, these glands are less often encountered in biopsies than ever-increasing endoscopic mucosal resection specimens, which usually contain submucosa. The number and density of these glands varies from person to person. (**a**) A typical solitary gland. (**b**) A cluster of glands. (**c**) Higher magnification of the uniform mucus cells in the acini. (**d**) In an Alcian blue/periodic acid-Schiff (PAS) stain, the glands stain intensely blue, indicating that they contain acid mucins. In contrast, the superficially located cardiac glands contain neutral mucins. (**e**) The submucosa glands may undergo a variety of changes. Often they contain small dense lymphocytic collections. (**f**) They are commonly inflamed with scattered foci of lymphocytes and a few plasma cells, similar to what occurs in minor salivary glands. (**g**) Also common is oncocytic cellular change, presumably a metaplasia

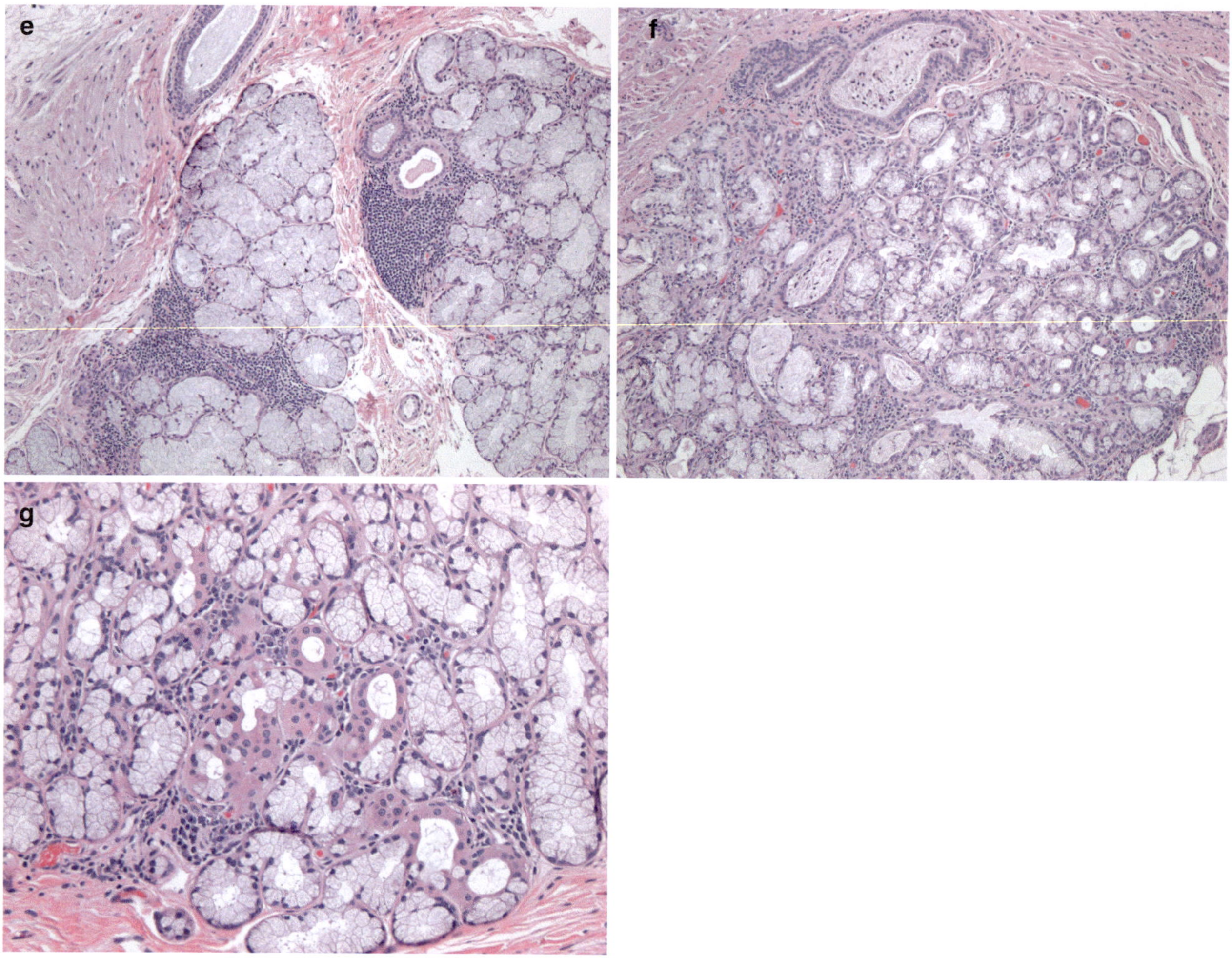

Fig. 1.3 (continued)

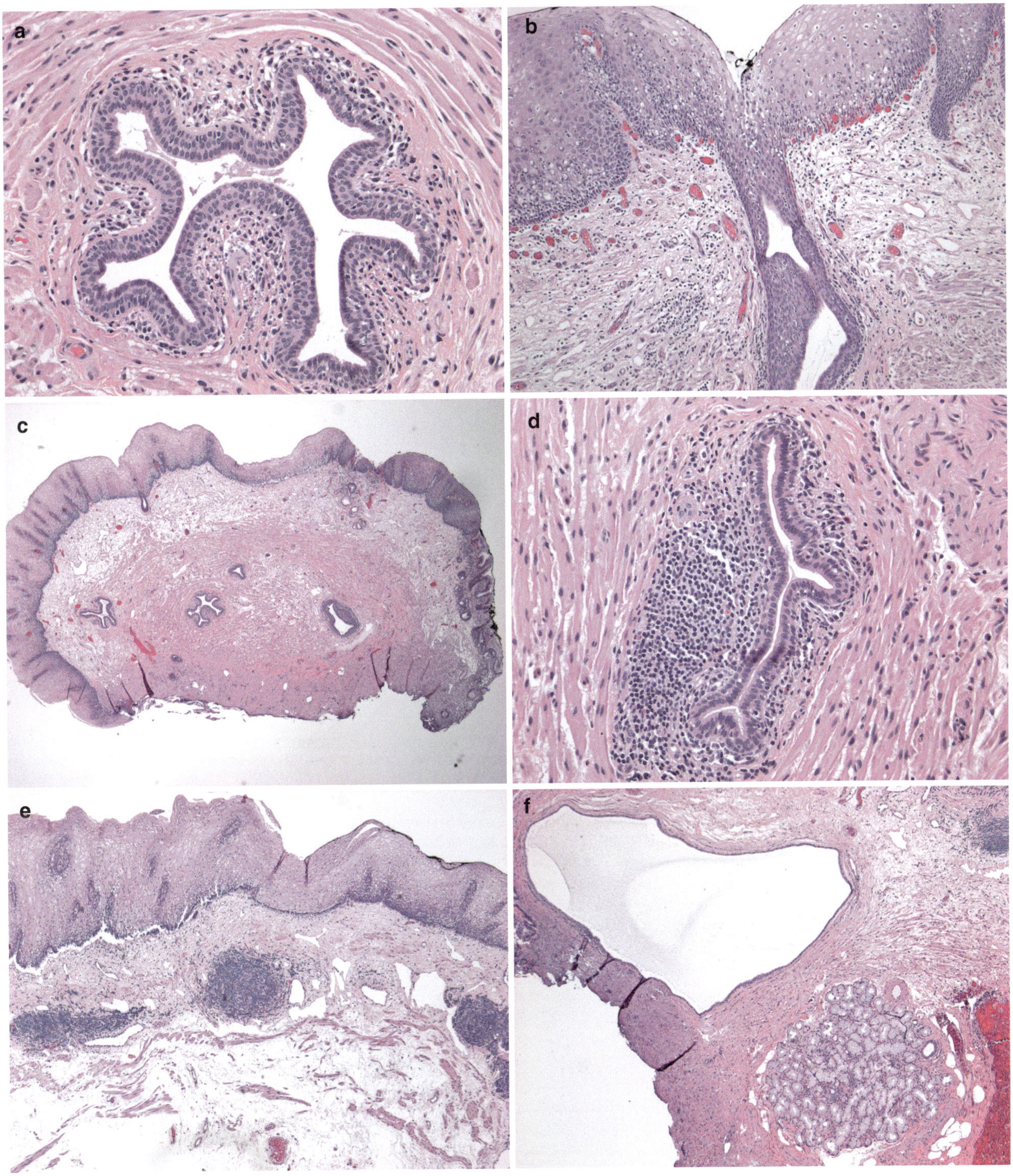

Fig. 1.4 Submucosal gland ducts. (**a**) The ducts from the submucosal gland are lined by thin layers of cuboidal epithelium. They are commonly surrounded by a loose rim of inflammatory cells, mainly lymphocytes. They extend toward the mucosa, penetrating the muscularis mucosae and lamina propria. (**b**) They enter the squamous epithelium and extend to the surface, and if the section is just right, the lumen can be seen surrounded by the squamous cells. (**c**) Some ducts have simple cross-sectional contours but others are complex and appear to branch or bud. (**d**) The periductal inflammation varies from mild as in *A* to intense as in this image. We have no idea why this occurs. (**e**) It is not unusual to encounter dense lymphocyte aggregates right below the muscularis mucosae where ducts usually are found. We suspect that these lymphocytic collections mark the spots of obliterated ducts. (**f**) Occasional ducts become cystic, presumably the result of obstruction closer to the surface. It is thought that these are the precursors of the intramural dissecting squamous cysts that characterize the unusual condition known as "pseudodiverticulosis"

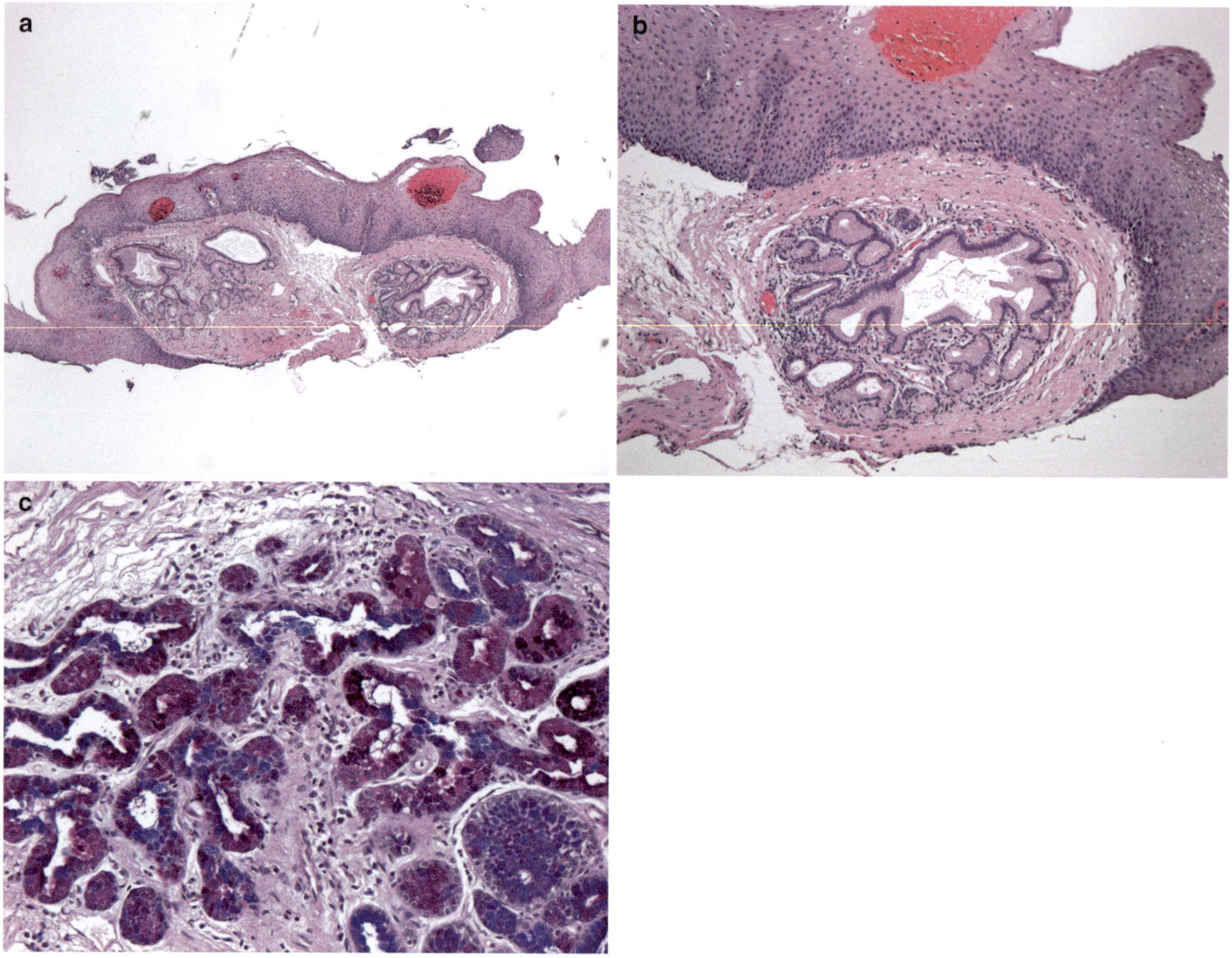

Fig. 1.5 Cardiac glands. (**a**) Beneath the squamous epithelium, in the deep lamina propria, there are two clusters of mucus glands known as cardiac glands, because they are identical to those in the proximal stomach, the cardia. They are normal in the esophagus, especially distally, and they should not be confused with metaplastic cardiac mucosa. Because of their superficial location, finding them in biopsies is common. (**b**) They often have a central dilated branching duct-like structure and small glands peripherally. (**c**) In the Alcian blue/PAS stain, the mucus in these glands mainly takes the PAS stain, indicating neutral mucin, identical to that in the glands in the cardia and antrum of the stomach. A few cells also pick up the Alcian blue, indicating they contain acid mucins

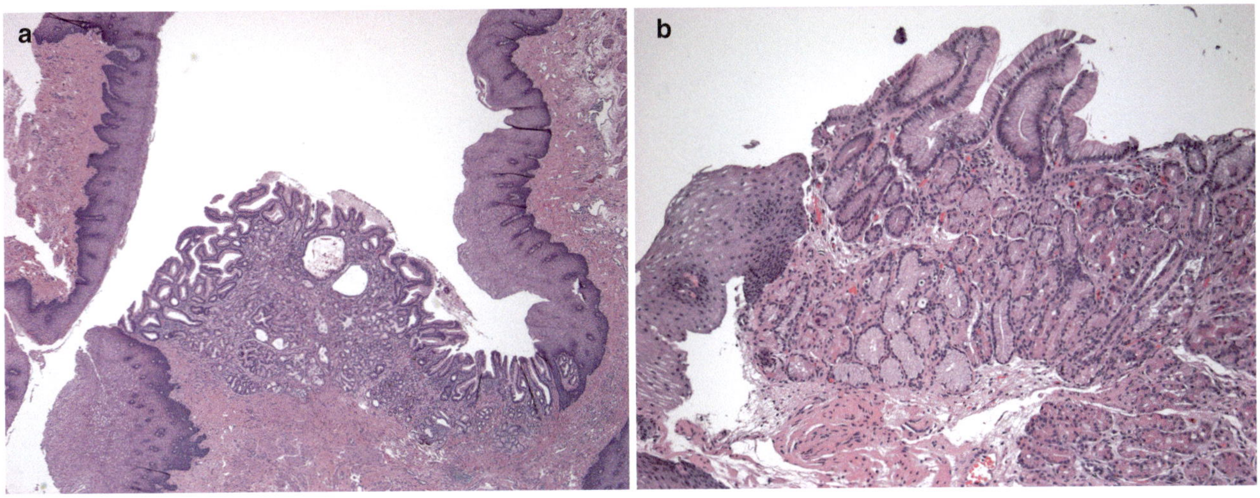

Fig. 1.6 Inlet patch. (**a**) An inlet patch is a focus of ectopic or heterotopic gastric mucosa in the proximal esophagus, just behind the cricoid cartilage. It derives its name because of its position at the esophageal inlet. These patches are so common that they may be considered normal variants. Experienced endoscopists are likely not to even biopsy them because they are so typical endoscopically. There are a few case reports of symptomatic patches but almost all are asymptomatic. In this example, normal squamous epithelium surrounds the patch of columnar mucosa, which is almost entirely cardiac with pits and mucus glands of about equal thickness. (**b**) This inlet patch has a mixture of cardiac mucus glands next to the squamous epithelium on the left and oxyntic glands with parietal and chief cells toward the center and right

Suggested Reading

Normal esophageal microscopic anatomy is covered adequately or even well in the usual textbooks of anatomy and gastrointestinal pathology. The most detailed discussion is in the Esophagus chapter In: Mills SE, editor. Histology for pathologists. 4th ed. Philadelphia: Wolters Kluwer Health; 2012.

2 General Microscopic Changes

This chapter covers a collection of microscopic changes that lack diagnostic specificity but occur in different specific diseases, as will become apparent in subsequent chapters. Almost all of these changes are responses to injury, generally involving the squamous epithelium and the lamina propria.

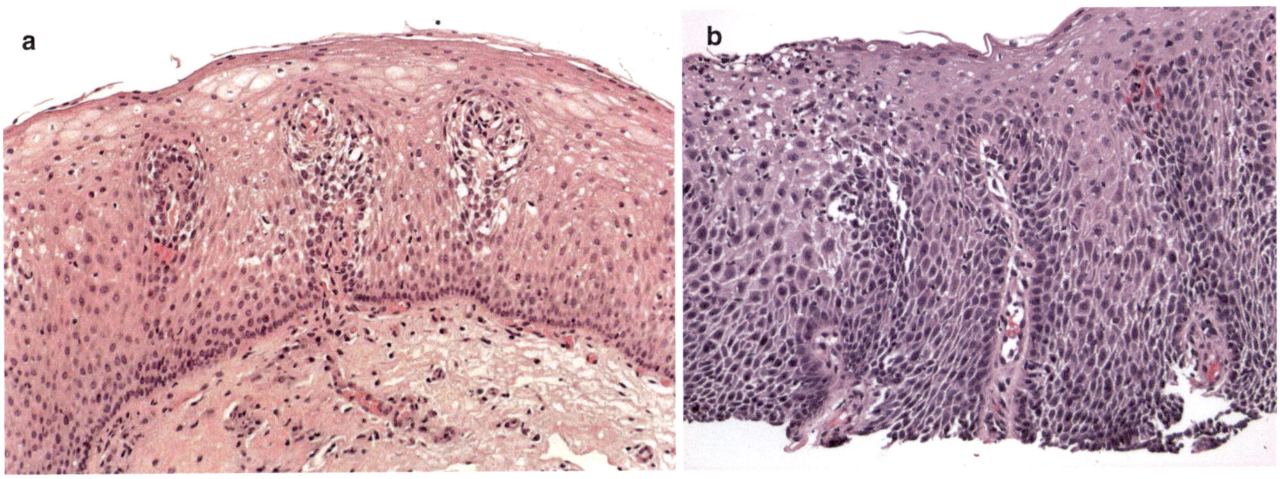

Fig. 2.1 Papillomatosis, basal cell hyperplasia, and spongiosis. (**a**) In contrast to normal squamous mucosa in which the papillae of lamina propria are limited to the basal fifth, in this squamous epithelium the papillae extend close to the surface. Each of these papillae is surrounded by several layers of basal cells; in other words, there is an expansion of the proliferative zone, also known as basal cell hyperplasia, which is a common reaction to injury in all squamous surfaces including both skin and mucous membranes. Since the most common injury to the squamous esophagus is gastroesophageal reflux, chances are that reflux is the culprit whenever this is found in a distal esophageal biopsy. Infections and direct toxic injury produce the same response, however, so it lacks specificity. (**b**) This is a more advanced example with much longer papillae that extend nearly three quarters or more of the way to the surface. The layers of basal cells around the papillae are thicker. In addition, the basal cells and squamous cells are separated so intercellular bridges are easily seen. This is the result of intraepithelial edema or spongiosis. In the esophagus, it is also referred to as dilated intercellular spaces

S.R. Owens, H.D. Appelman, *Atlas of Esophagus and Stomach Pathology*, Atlas of Anatomic Pathology, DOI 10.1007/978-1-4614-8084-6_2, © Springer Science+Business Media New York 2014

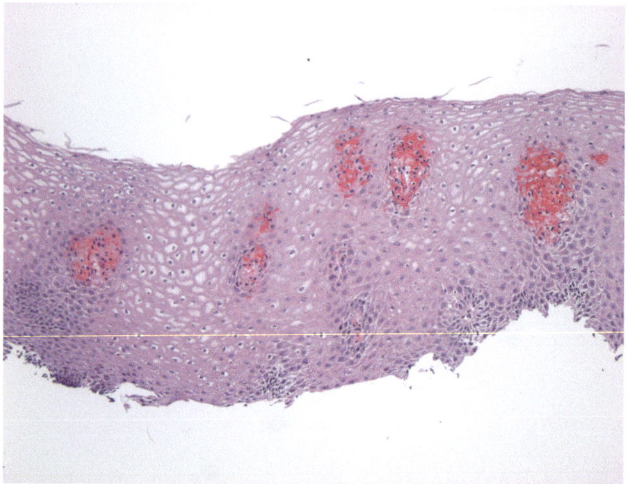

Fig. 2.2 Acute papillary hemorrhage. All the fibrovascular papillae that extend into the squamous epithelium from the lamina propria are filled with extravasated blood (*ie*, acute hemorrhage). This may be due to trauma from the biopsy procedure but in some cases it may be due to in vivo injuries, reflux being one. In fact, in the past, it was touted as one of the characteristic reflux-associated changes

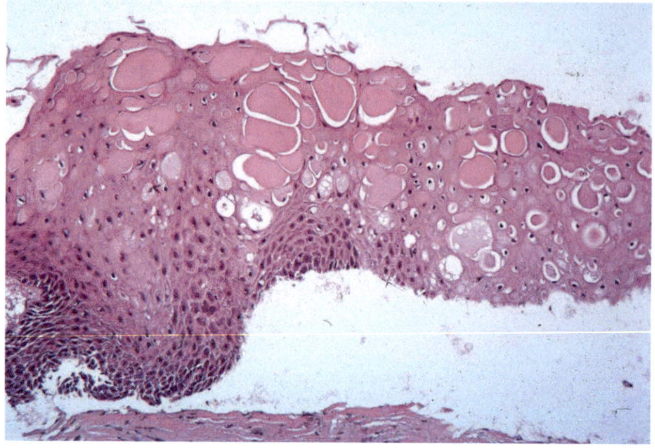

Fig. 2.3 Balloon cell change. Within the squamous epithelium, several cells have no nuclei but instead have large smooth proteinaceous inclusions filling the cytoplasm referred to as balloon cell change. This is a response to surface injury in squamous mucosae in different sites, and, in the esophagus, the most common injury inducing this change is reflux. The inclusions are plasma proteins and fluid that presumably have leaked into damaged squamous cells

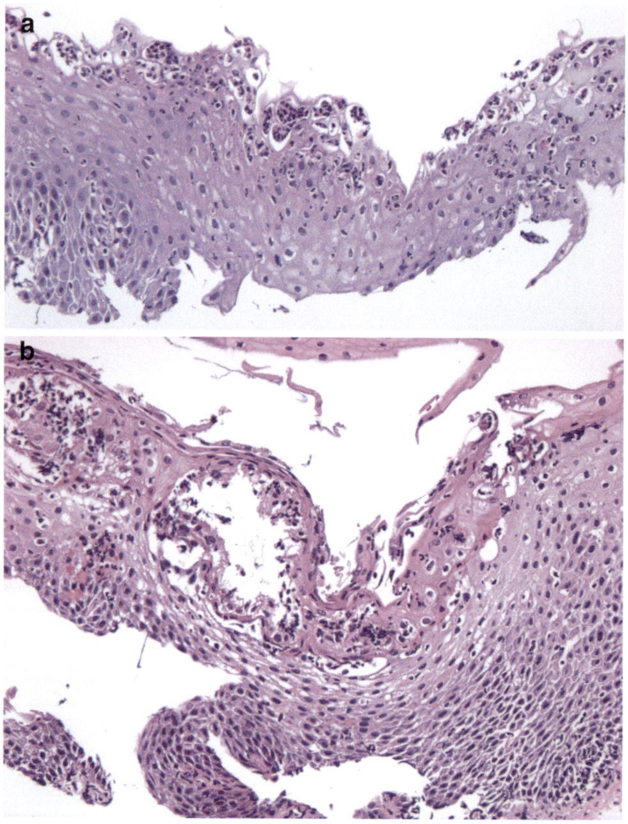

Fig. 2.4 Generic acute inflammation with microabscesses. (**a**) In this field, there is a row of tiny abscesses, also known as microabscesses, in the superficial squamous epithelium. Below this row, the squamous cells appear relatively normal. (**b**) This is a more intense variant with larger intraepithelial abscesses. This pattern of acute injury usually leads to a search of the slide for an infectious cause, the most common being *Candida*. However, all too often, no cause is found. In fact, in many cases, a cause may never be identified. We have seen a couple of cases of pill-induced injury with similar acute inflammation. We have virtually no follow-up biopsies to give us a clue as to the natural history of these changes

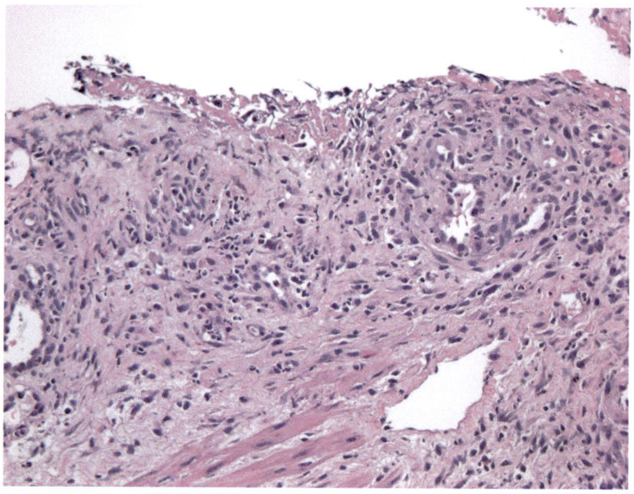

Fig. 2.5 Generic ulcer bed. There is no epithelium on the surface. Instead, the mucosa consists entirely of lamina propria, which contains small vessels with hypertrophied endothelial cells, probably capillaries and venules. The lamina propria also contains spindle cells, presumably myofibroblasts, and scattered inflammatory cells including polymorphonuclear leukocytes (PMNs). On the surface are a few strands of fibrin mixed with some of these spindle cells, evidence of organization. This is the bed of an acute superficial ulcer. It lacks chronicity changes, such as plasma cells. The changes have no specificity in terms of defining the injury that caused the ulcer. Most of these are in the distal esophagus where reflux is by far the most common cause

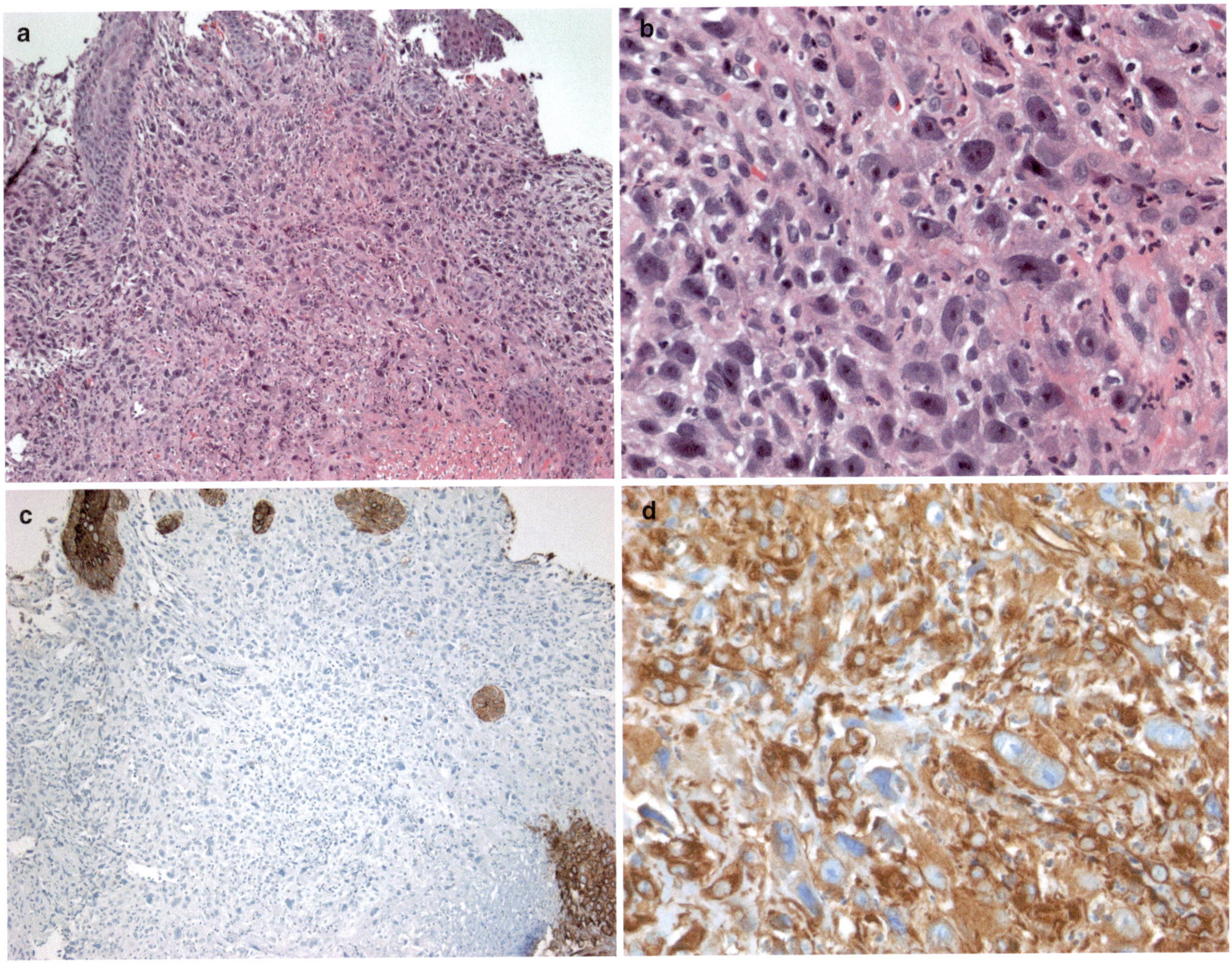

Fig. 2.6 Hypertrophied myofibroblasts in the bed of an ulcer (ulcerocytes). (**a**) This is the base of an ulcer with prongs of regenerating squamous cells at the surface. There are numerous large plump spindle cells with large, hyperchromatic, and pleomorphic nuclei in the ulcer bed. (**b**) At high power, the nuclear changes are striking and the resemblance of these cells to some kind of spindle cell malignancy is obvious. (**c**) With the keratin stain, the cells are negative whereas the prongs of primitive squamous cells at the ulcer edge are strongly positive. (**d**) In contrast, in the Vimentin stain, the spindle cells are strongly and diffusely positive. These cells have the ultrastructural features of myofibroblasts and fibroblasts. We refer to them as "ulcerocytes." For some odd reason, they are more common in the base of esophageal ulcers than anywhere else in the gut. Because the pleomorphism makes them look like a type of spindle cell malignancy, they are a real diagnostic pitfall. We emphasize that these cells should never be called malignant

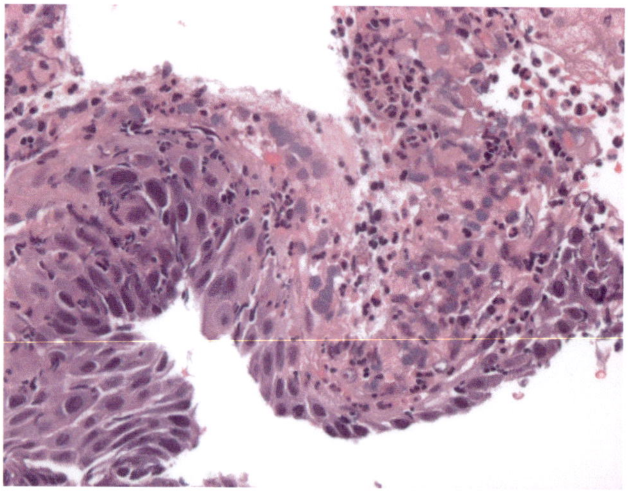

Fig. 2.7 Healing ulcer in squamous mucosa. Extending from the thin squamous mucosa with large hyperchromatic nuclei and little cytoplasm on the left, a thinner layer of squamous cells grows beneath some exudate on the right. Because this is typical of changes in squamous mucosa right at the edges of ulcers of all causes, this has no specificity other than to identify the biopsy site as an ulcer edge. The next step in ulcer healing is the extension of the long squamous prongs from this regenerating layer of squamous cells into the stroma. Such prongs are in Fig. 2.8

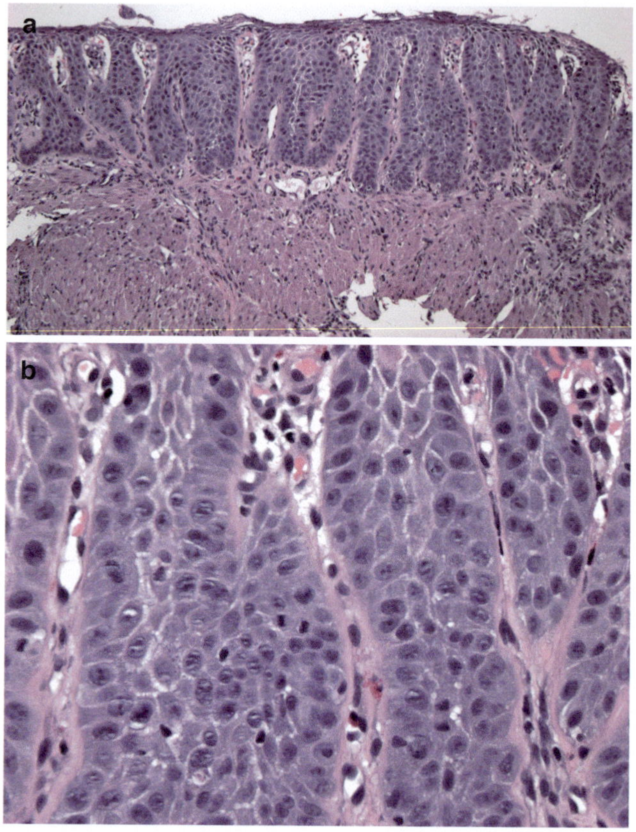

Fig. 2.8 Ulcer edge changes in squamous mucosa. (**a**) This mucosa has a thin layer of superficial squamous cells from the base of which project prongs of dark squamous cells which project into the hypervascular lamina propria almost to the inner fibers of the muscularis mucosae. We refer to this locally as "long-prong disease." (**b**) In the higher-power image, the cells in these prongs have a high N:C ratio and frequent mitoses. There is little cytoplasmic differentiation, but there is some spongiosis toward the top. This pattern of regeneration is typical of what happens at the edges and eventually at the bases of ulcers in squamous mucosae. With time, these prongs become thicker and more differentiated and the superficial layer also becomes thicker, thus reconstituting the normal squamous epithelium

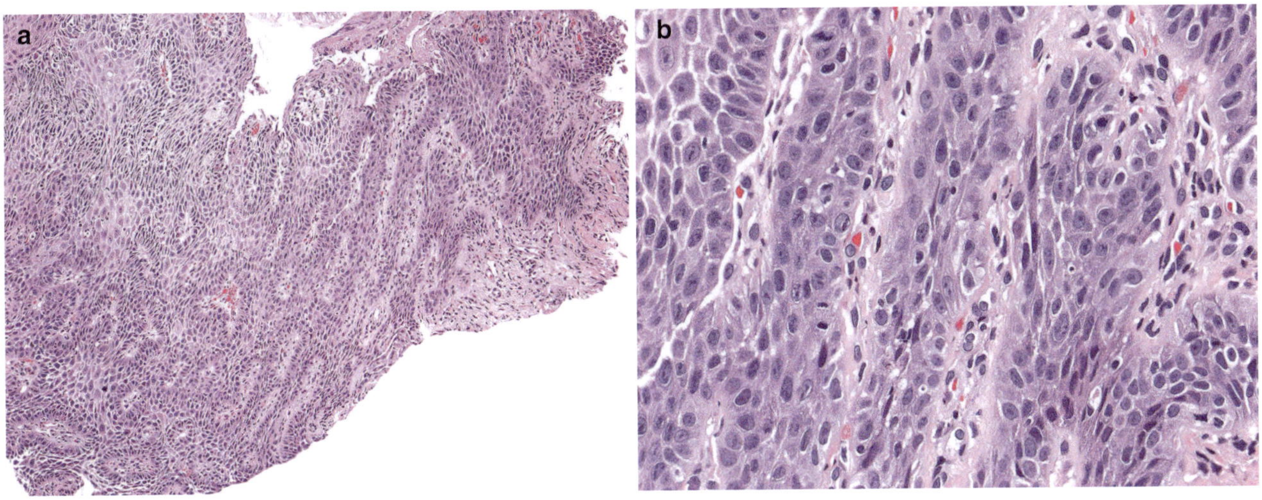

Fig. 2.9 Florid ulcer edge changes, mimicking squamous cell carcinoma. (**a**), In this example, the prongs of regenerating squamous epithelium are very long and thin, and they have extensive interconnections. (**b**), At higher magnification, the poor differentiation of the cells in these prongs is evident. There is considerable nuclear pleomorphism and many nuclei have prominent nuclei. Mitoses are also present. Because of the complex architecture and the primitive appearance to the cells, it may be tempting to diagnose this as squamous cell carcinoma. It is basically a form of pseudoepitheliomatous hyperplasia

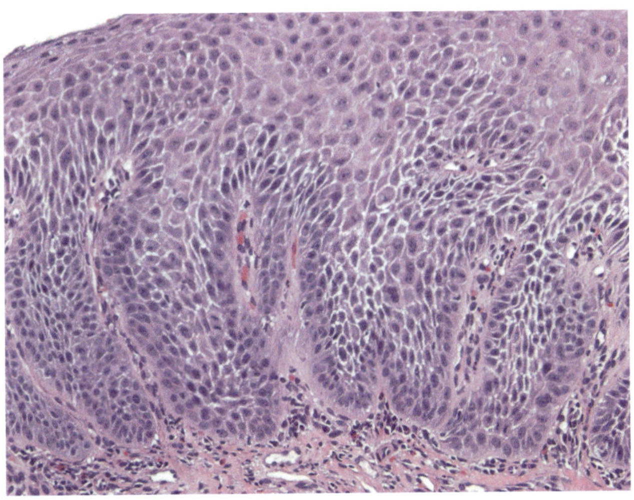

Fig. 2.10 Maturing ulcer edge changes. In comparison with Figs. 2.8 and 2.9, the superficial layers of squamous cells and basal prongs are thicker and the squamous cells are more mature. This squamous epithelium is much closer to normal

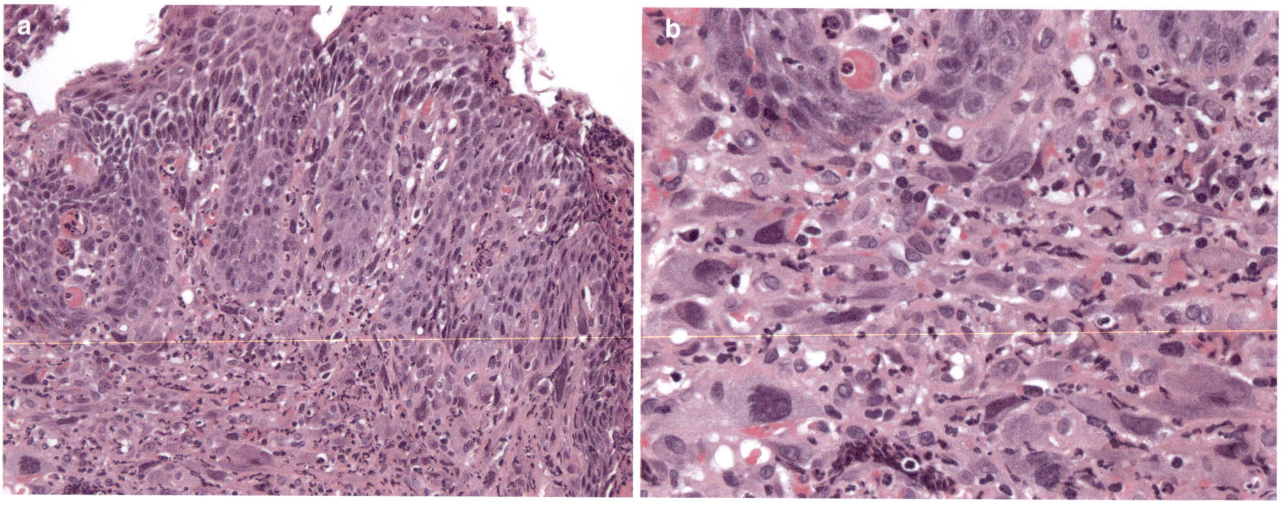

Fig. 2.11 Long prong and ulcerocytes in a single biopsy, a great temptation for a malignant diagnosis. (**a**), From the thinned surface, the typical long prongs of regenerating primitive squamous epithelium extend into the lamina propria, which contains many atypical stromal cells with atypical nuclei characteristic of the weird myofibroblasts in ulcer beds described in Fig. 2.5. (**b**) This can be seen in better detail in higher magnification. Based on these changes, one must resist the temptation to call this spindle cell squamous carcinoma when it is nothing more than the edge of an ulcer in the squamous esophagus

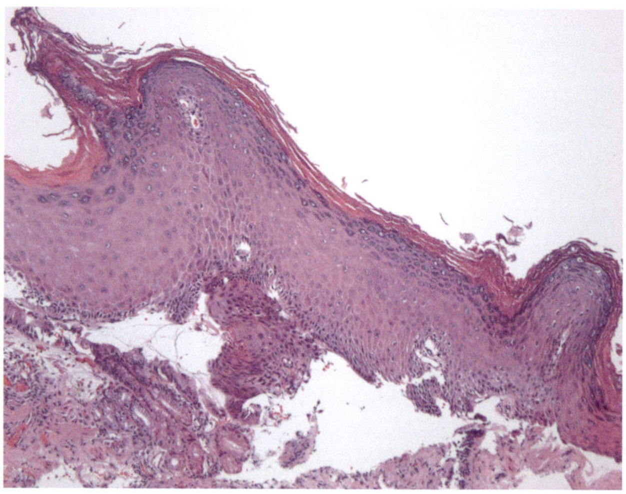

Fig. 2.12 Keratinizing surface epithelial metaplasia, also referred to as hyperkeratosis. The normal esophagus has no granular layer or surface keratin; because both are present in these images, the epithelium resembles hyperkeratotic epidermis. The cause is not well defined but presumably is a response to surface injury. Surprisingly, there is very little published information about this change, either in the literature or in the textbooks. Yet, in a busy biopsy service, this appears periodically. Sometimes the endoscopist will recognize it as a white area or plaque

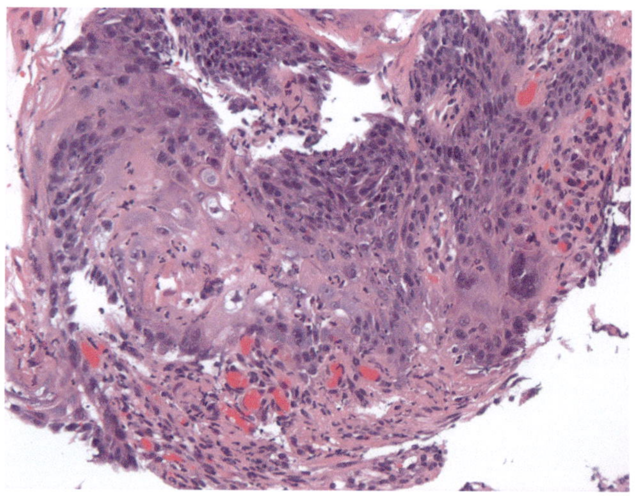

Fig. 2.13 Atypical regenerative changes in squamous epithelium with multinucleation and nuclear pleomorphism. This is hyperplastic squamous epithelium at the edge of an ulcer. Many of the nuclei in the deeper cells are enlarged and hyperchromatic. Toward the right, there is a collection of such cells with more pleomorphic nuclei, and some of these cells are even multinucleated. This is a well-recognized pattern of squamous repair or regeneration that can be seen in a number of situations including following radiation or after the use of several drugs that are toxic for esophageal squamous epithelium. The key in separating this pattern from squamous dysplasia is that this epithelium matures normally. Further, the cells with the atypical nuclei have abundant cytoplasm, so although it looks frighteningly bizarre there is little change in the N:C ratio

3 Noninfectious Inflammatory Conditions

This chapter includes the most common esophageal diseases—more common than all the neoplasms combined, more common than Barrett's mucosa, which is more of a headline grabber. All of these inflammations are due to something other than infection, similar to what happens in the skin, except that most are uniquely esophageal. Reflux-induced inflammation and ulcer complications are included, as is the "trendy" eosinophilic esophagitis. There are even some recently described conditions such as lymphocytic and sloughing esophagitis, which we see fairly often in our practice. We even include a severe destructive inflammation with no record in the literature; we figured it was about time it had a reference.

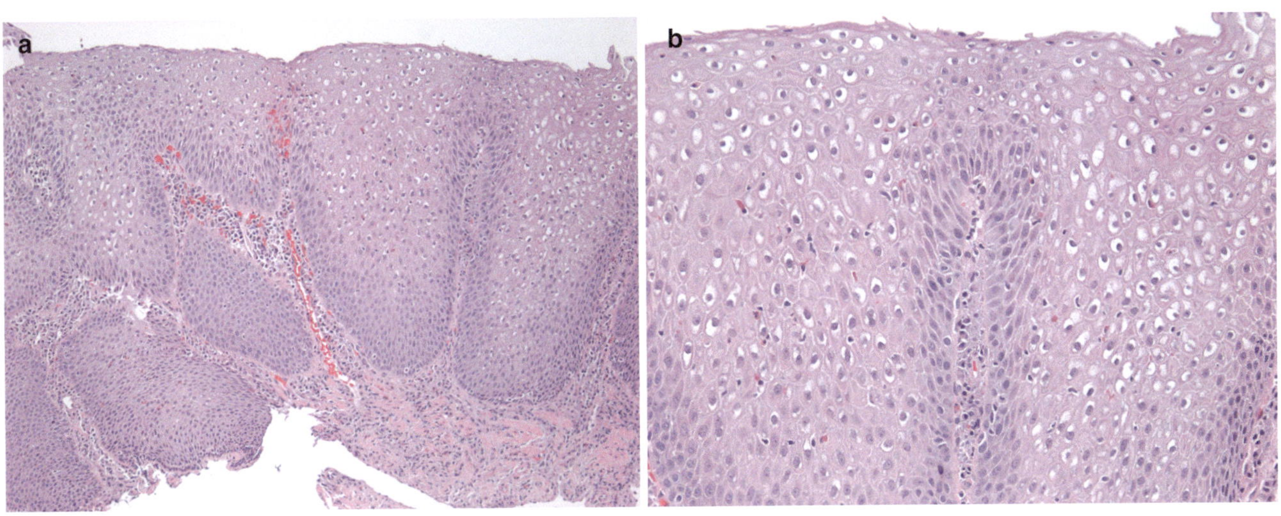

Fig. 3.1 Reflux-type esophagitis. (**a**) The squamous epithelium is thicker than normal with expansion of the proliferative zone characterized by two changes: (1) hyperplasia of the basal cell zone, which normally is about one sixth of the thickness, and (2) papillomatosis. Normal lamina propria papillae, which contain small vessels, normally extend only about one fifth into the squamous epithelium. In this field, basal cells now account for about a third of the entire squamous thickness, and the lamina propria papillae are more numerous than normal and extend close to the surface. (**b**) In the higher magnification, scattered eosinophils and lymphocytes are present within the squamous epithelium. Changes in papillae and basal cells, as well as low- grade inflammation such as this, are common to many surface esophageal injuries and therefore lack specificity. Reflux can only be diagnosed with confidence when it is proven to occur by clinical studies such as those measuring lower esophageal pH and motility at the gastroesophageal (GE) junction

S.R. Owens, H.D. Appelman, *Atlas of Esophagus and Stomach Pathology*, Atlas of Anatomic Pathology,
DOI 10.1007/978-1-4614-8084-6_3, © Springer Science+Business Media New York 2014

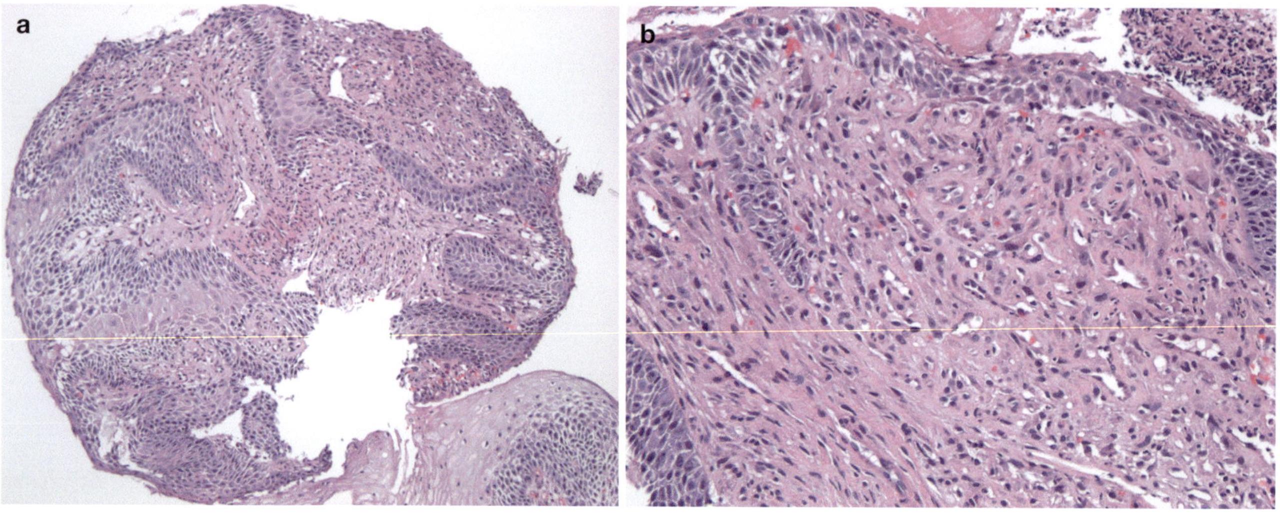

Fig. 3.2 Healing reflux ulcer. This biopsy came from the expanded edge of an ulcer in the distal esophagus in a patient with terrible heartburn. (**a**), At lower magnification, the granulation tissue from the ulcer is partly covered by flattened squamous epithelium when compared to normal. Extending the granulation tissue from that thin or atrophic layer are several long prongs of poorly differentiated squamous cells best seen at higher magnification (**b**). These are most prominent on the upper right of **a**. Following the surface from right to left, the surface squamous epithelium becomes more differentiated and the prongs thicken and differentiate. This is the typical set of squamous reparative changes at the bases and edges of ulcers; in the distal esophagus, the most common cause of these ulcers by far is reflux

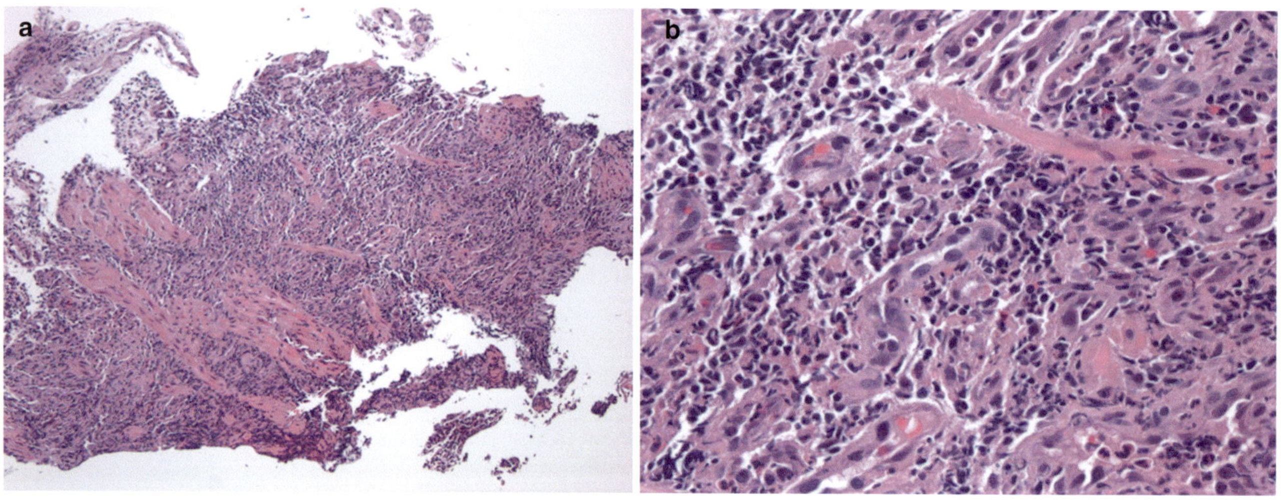

Fig. 3.3 Pill-induced ulcer. (**a**) This biopsy contains an ulcer, the bed of which straddles the muscularis mucosae, separating the fibers. (**b**) At high magnification, the ulcer bed is composed of granulation tissue with numerous capillaries and a mixed low-grade inflammation that contains neutrophils and lymphocytes but no plasma cells, indicating that the ulcer is recent. There is nothing about this biopsy to indicate that it was caused by a pill. However, from a clinical standpoint, there were some clues, one of which was the location in the midesophagus. Pill ulcers often occur in the midesophagus near where the aorta indents it slightly, possibly creating a point for potential injury. However, any part of the esophagus is actually at risk. This was also a small circumscribed ulcer, another expression of a very localized but very intense surface injury such as by a pill. Another hint is the type of medication that the patient is taking. In this case, the culprit was doxycycline, a pill that has been known to cause such ulcers. The mechanisms by which drugs induce such damage are numerous and are discussed in all good clinical gastrointestinal textbooks

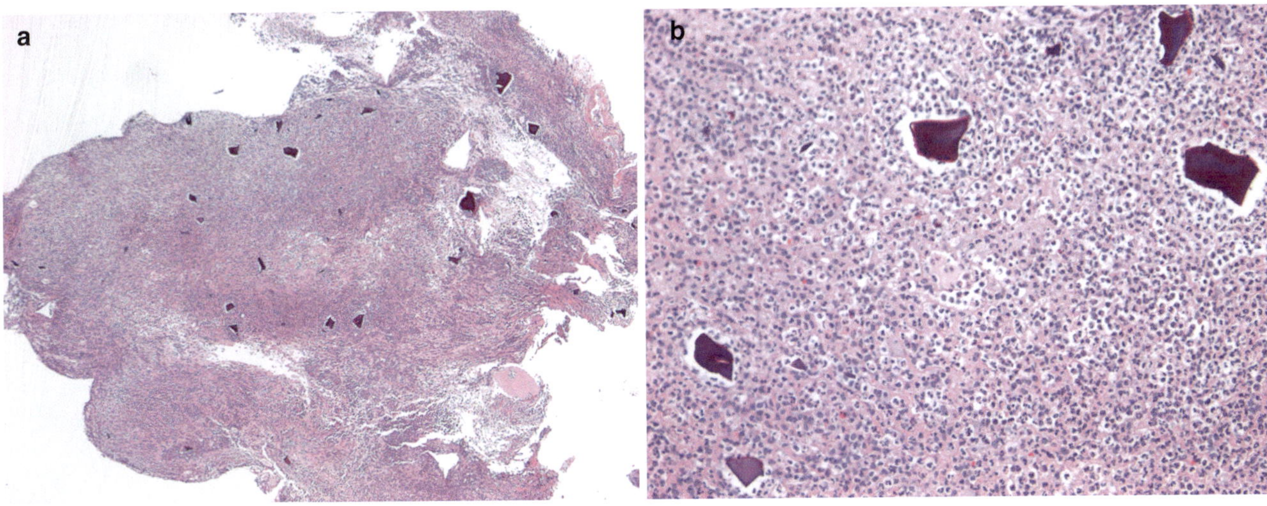

Fig. 3.4 Kayexalate-induced ulcer. (**a**) Low-power view of a biopsy of an ulcer of the distal esophagus, just above the GE junction. The biopsy is mainly a thick layer of pus from the surface of the ulcer in which purple Kayexalate crystals are trapped. (**b**) High-power view of the sheet of neutrophils and the characteristic rhomboid-shaped Kayexalate crystals with the sharply pointed ends. These crystals are also periodic acid-Schiff (PAS) positive and they are acid fast. Kayexalate (sodium polystyrene sulfonate) is used to bind potassium in the lumen of the gut in patients with hyperkalemia, usually patients in renal failure. It is often combined with sorbitol, It can damage any site in the gut, usually the colon, but upper gut damage has been described. The pattern of damage is sometimes identical to that caused by acute ischemic injury. Actually, it is not the Kayexalate itself that does the damage but the accompanying sorbitol. Without the characteristic crystals, there would be nothing about this biopsy to suggest an etiology for the ulcer

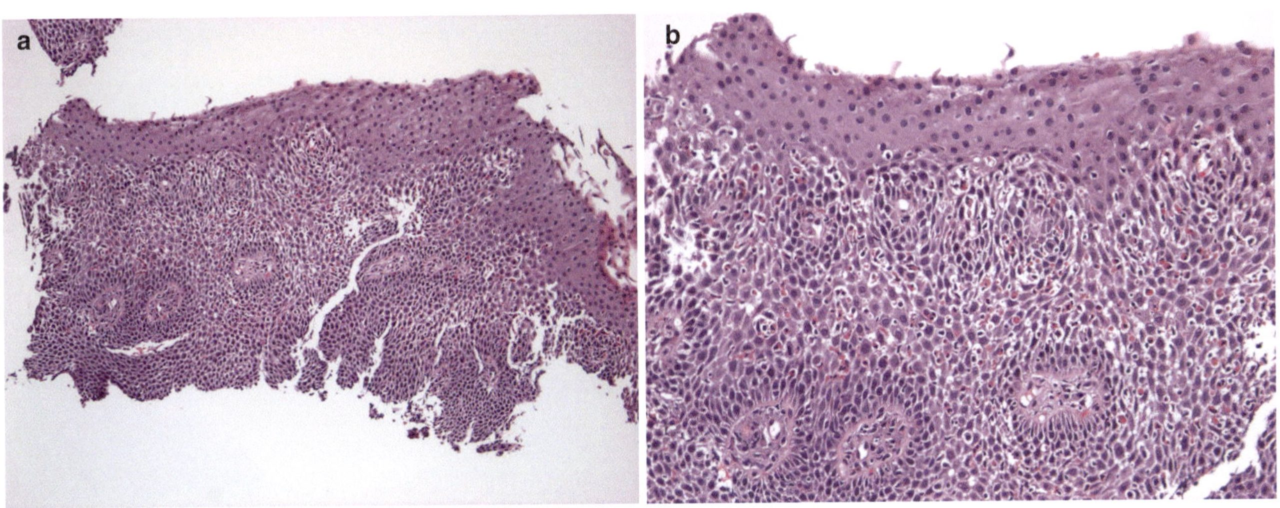

Fig. 3.5 Eosinophilic esophagitis (EE). (**a**) At low magnification, the squamous epithelium of full-blown EE looks dark because of the expansion of the basal cell zone—basal cell hyperplasia and the eosinophils can be seen in the epithelium. (**b**) At higher magnification, it becomes obvious that spongiosis is also present and intense. Eosinophils are now easy to identify

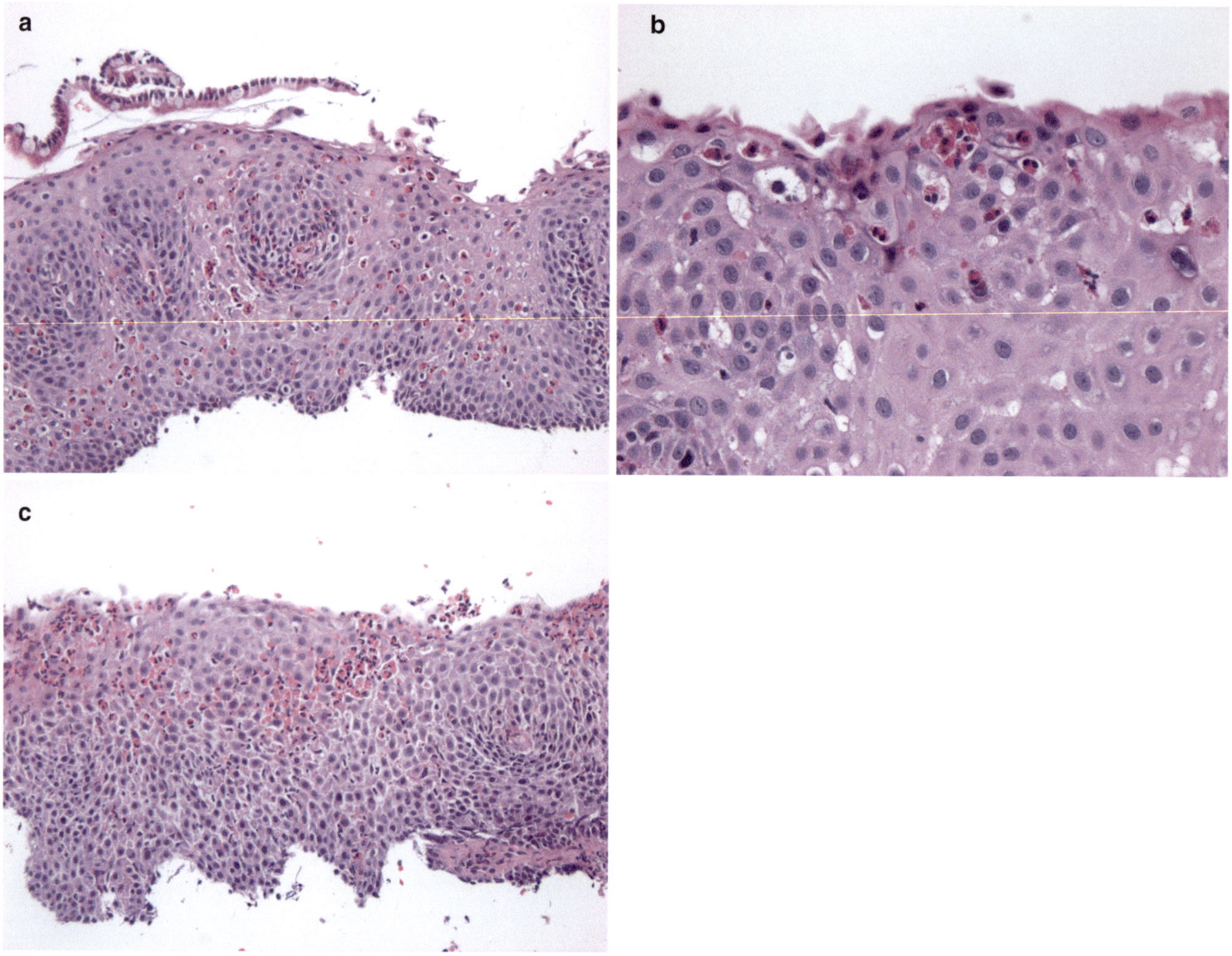

Fig. 3.6 (**a**) Eosinophils may be diffusely distributed as in this view. The current guidelines state that for a case to qualify as EE, there must be at least 15 eosinophils in one high-power field, but there are also clinical and endoscopic diagnostic requirements for the disease. (**b**) In intense cases, eosinophils aggregate to form intraepithelial abscesses, often close to the surface. (**c**) Sometimes the eosinophil aggregates are huge, as in this view

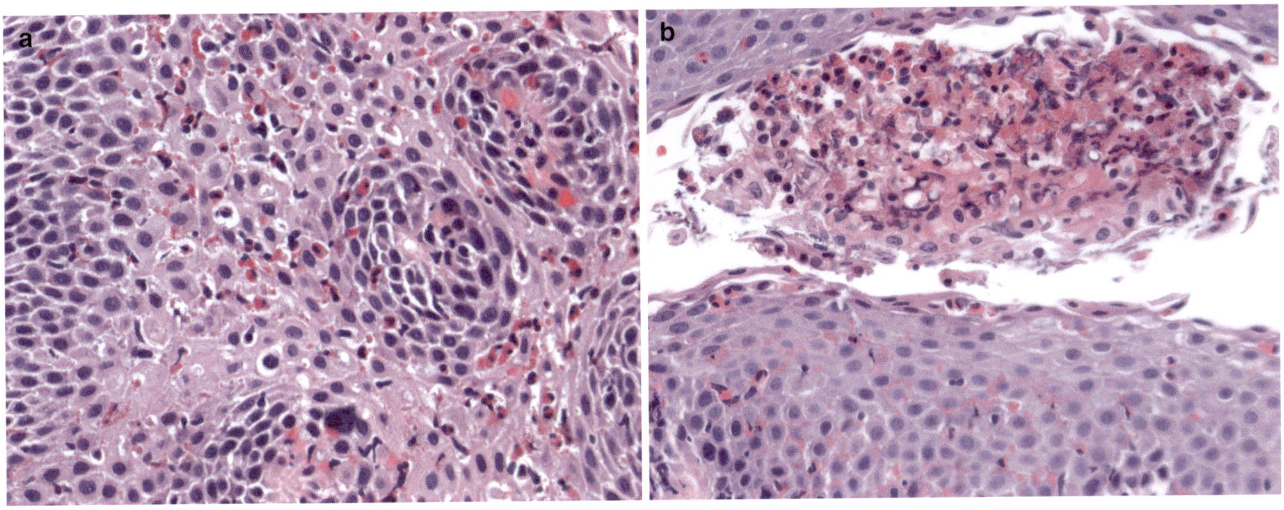

Fig. 3.7 (**a**) Eosinophil granules are often prominent. Unfortunately, we cannot include them in the total count, but they generally only occur in cases with high eosinophil counts. (**b**) In some cases, small exudates composed of eosinophils and squamous debris are found on the surface. Some larger exudates can be seen endoscopically

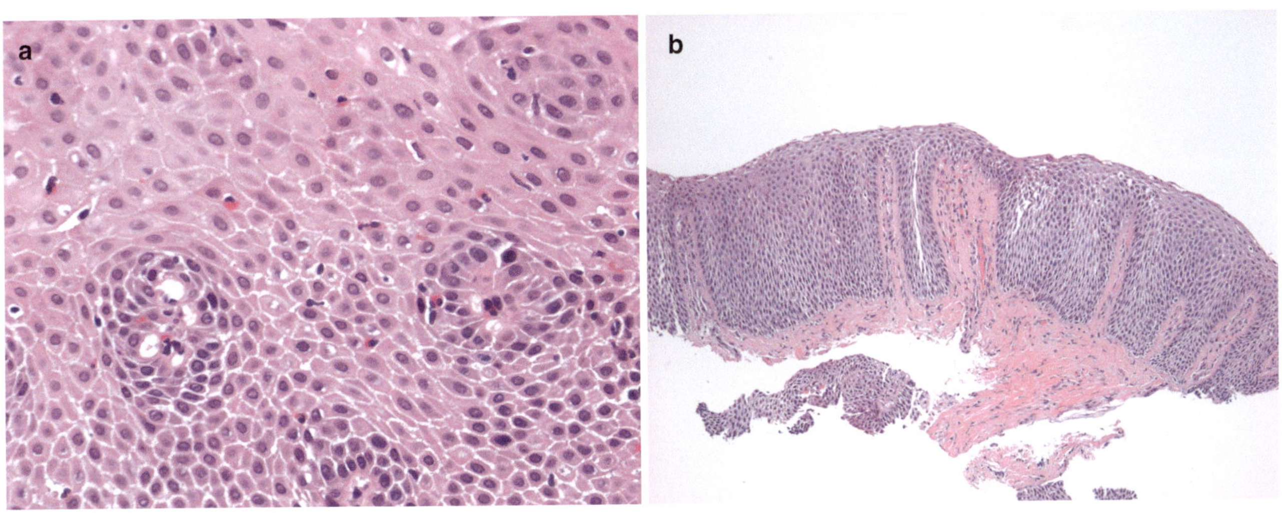

Fig. 3.8 (**a**) Because EE is often a patchy disease, in many cases with obvious changes other biopsies, even fields in single biopsies, are likely not to have the diagnostic changes. In this field from a case of EE with a maximum eosinophil count elsewhere of 50 per high-power field, there are only 5 eosinophils. (**b**) In long-standing EE, lamina propria fibrosis sometimes develops. In this image, the fibrosis extends high into the papillae. This fibrosis may explain some of the structural abnormalities of EE, such as strictures and even the endoscopic rings that are so characteristic

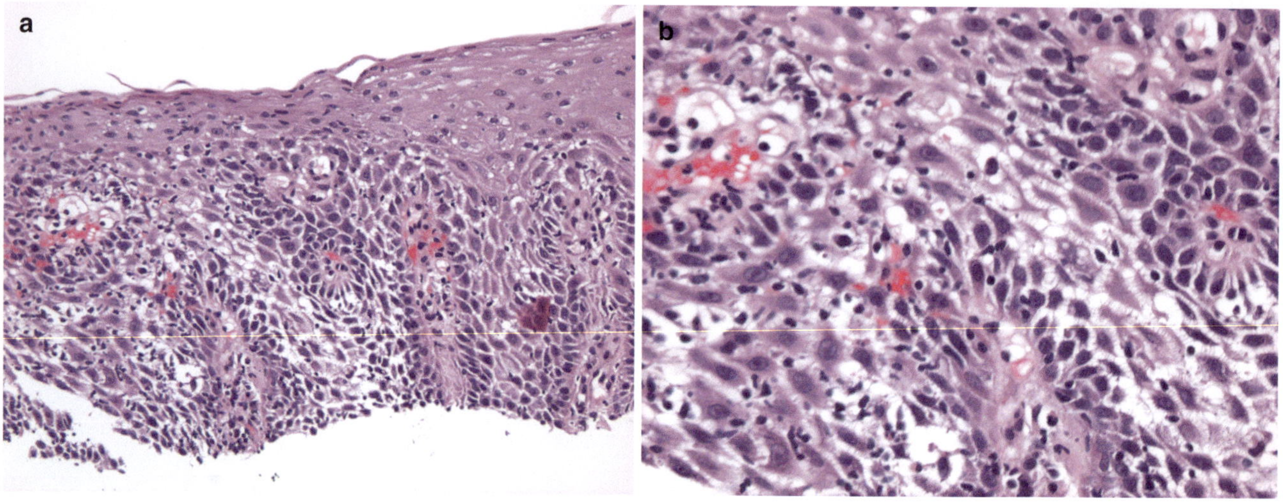

Fig. 3.9 Lymphocytic esophagitis. (**a**) This disease is characterized by lymphocytes within the squamous epithelium accompanied by various degrees of intercellular edema or spongiosis, basal cell hyperplasia and papillomatosis. In this view, all of these changes are present and intense. (**b**) In the high-power view, the intraepithelial lymphocytes both surround the papillae and are present between papillae. Many of them have elongated or wavy nuclei. As a result, they have also been called "squiggle cells" and "cells with irregular nuclear contours"

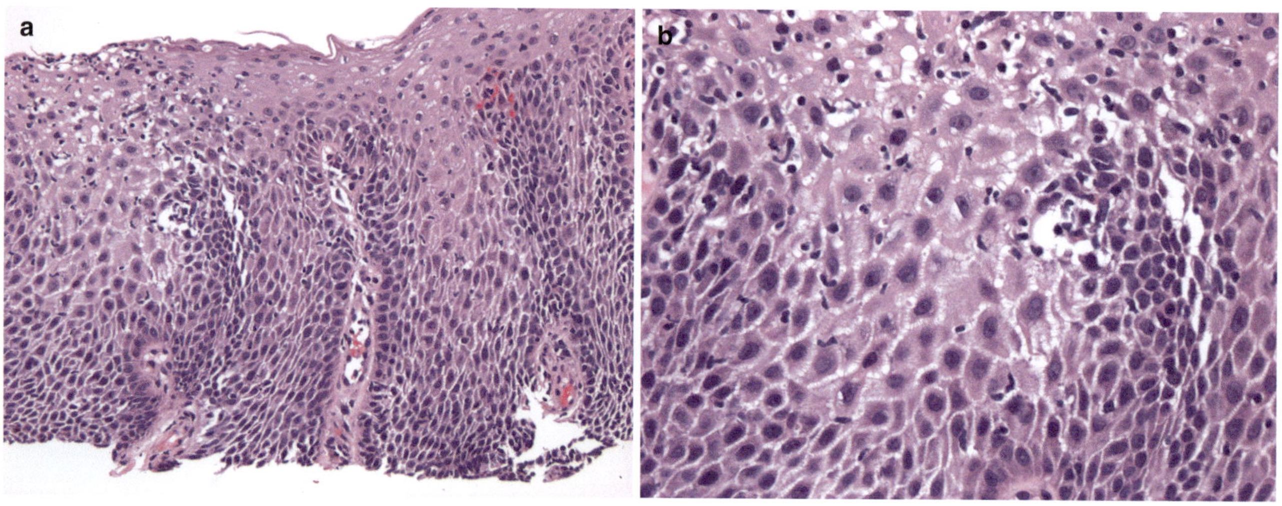

Fig. 3.10 (**a**) A much less severe form, the more intense diagnostic changes are found on the left, whereas on the right, basal cell hyperplasia and papillomatosis are mainly seen. (**b**) A higher magnification of *A* elucidates the irregular shapes of the lymphocyte nuclei. Lymphocytic esophagus is a fascinating condition. First, it is histologically spectacular. The complex of changes is identical to what is seen in contact allergic reactions in the skin, such as those due to poison ivy. Second, the few studies that have analyzed it have found that, in children, it has a significant association with Crohn's disease elsewhere in the gut. Therefore, it is basically a Crohn's equivalent in children. However, in adults, no association has been discovered with any other condition, drug, or infectious agent. It is possible that, based on its similarity to cutaneous contact allergy, that it is a localized allergic reaction to things in the diet. However, in adults, it is an esophagitis in search of a clinical disease. Therefore, it should be diagnosed in children with a comment about its Crohn's association, whereas in adults it can safely be ignored based on what we currently know

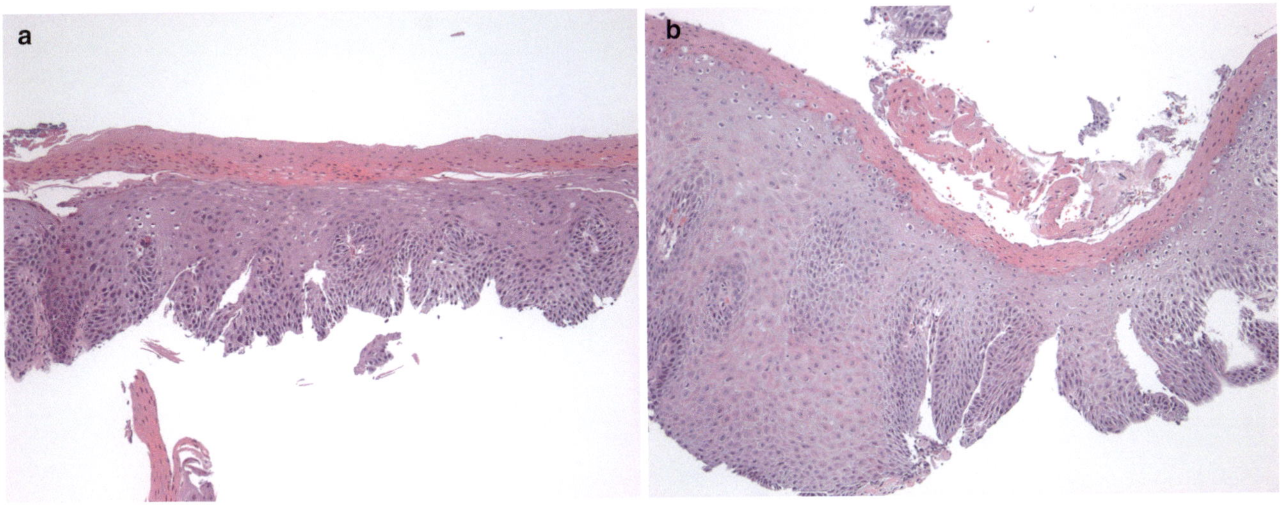

Fig. 3.11 Sloughing esophagitis. Sloughing esophagitis is really not an inflammation but superficial necrosis of squamous epithelium that seems to occur mainly in patients with some form of long-standing debilitation who are taking medications that directly injure the esophagus. (**a** and **b**) At low magnification, the biopsy has a striking two-toned appearance with a superficial layer of dark eosinophilic necrotic squamous cells with pyknotic nuclei. The underlaying squamous epithelium is either normal or slightly reactive

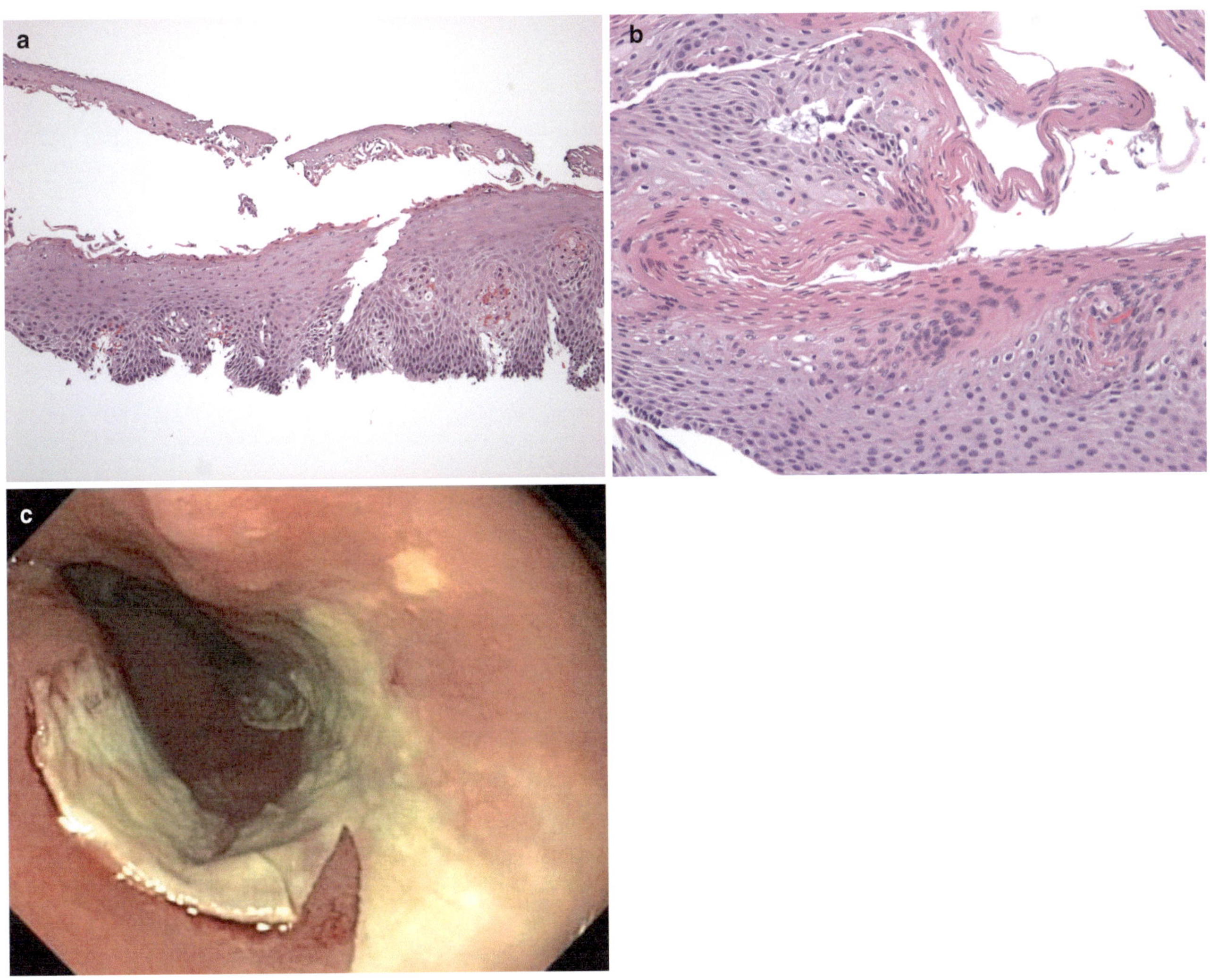

Fig. 3.12 (**a**) In some biopsies, the necrotic layer may be pulled away from the underlying normal epithelium, and in many cases, separate fragments of the necrotic layer may be found in the biopsy. (**b**) In the upper center of this image is the point of separation of the superficial necrotic zone from the underlying, more normal squamous epithelium. (**c**) This separation leads to the typical endoscopic appearance of membranes covering the mucosa that may appear to be separating

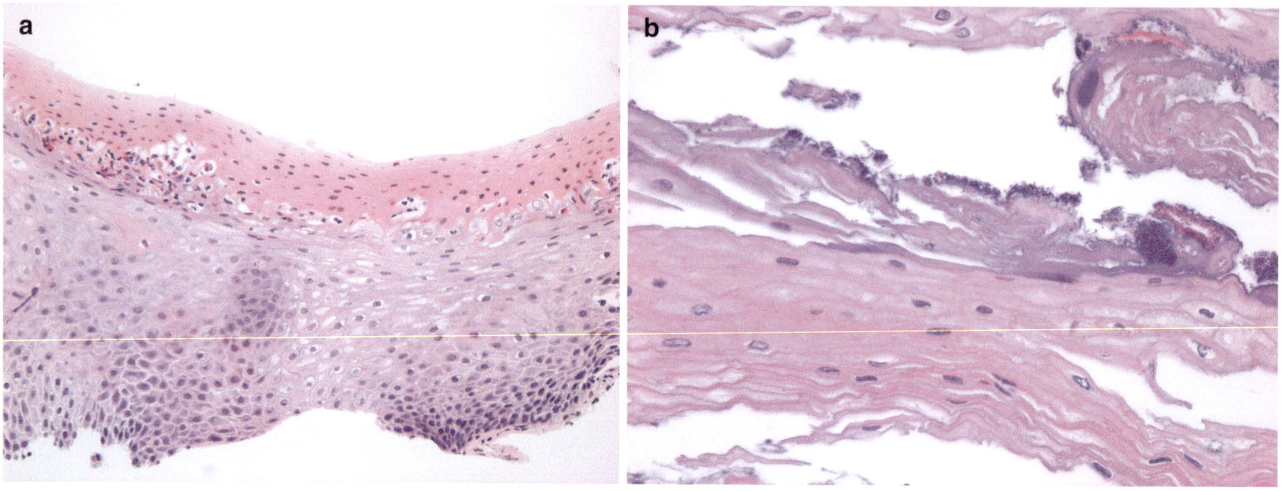

Fig. 3.13 (**a**) In some cases, there may be a layer of neutrophils at the interface, even accompanied by a few eosinophils. (**b**) Sometimes bacteria may colonize the necrotic superficial layer

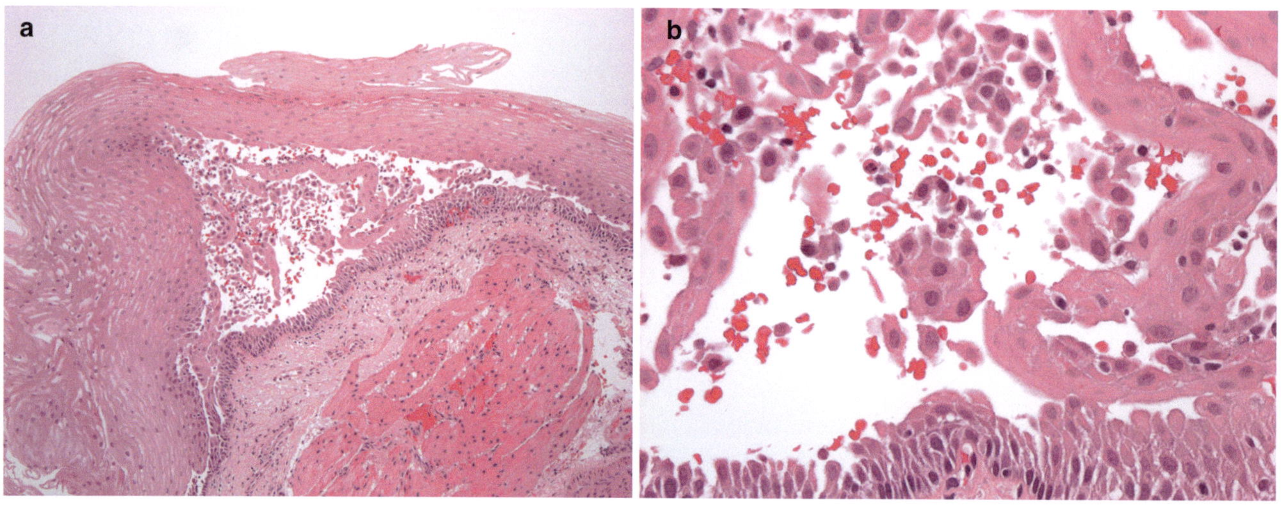

Fig. 3.14 Pemphigus. Just as in the skin, pemphigus in the esophagus has a suprabasal blister with acantholytic cells floating in the blister fluid. The location of the bulla is best seen at low power (**a**), with the acantholytic cells more obvious at high power (**b**). This is one example of a skin disease that on rare occasions affects the esophagus. Other cutaneous diseases with esophageal involvement include lichen planus, Darier's disease, bullous pemphigoid, and acanthosis nigricans

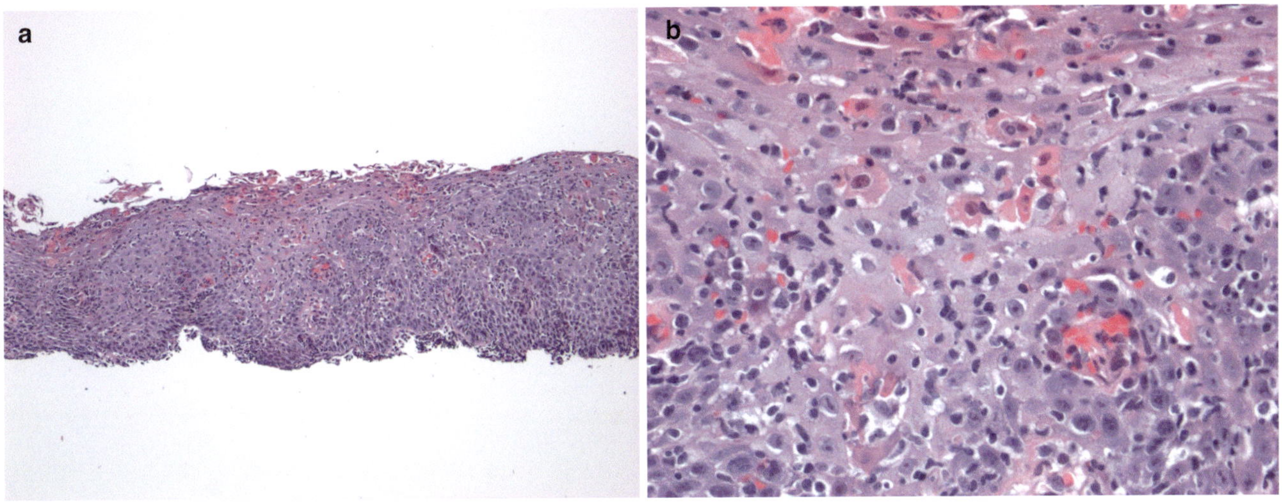

Fig. 3.15 Intense destructive esophagitis of unknown cause. This is a biopsy of a patchy endoscopic inflammation mainly in the distal esophagus. (**a**) At low power, the squamous epithelium is dark and hypercellular, and it has hardly any maturation toward the surface. There are red structures mostly superficial within the epithelium. (**b**) At high power, these same changes become more obvious. The whole epithelium seems to consist of dark basal cells and there is a diffuse intense lymphocytic infiltrate, much more intense than in the usual forms of lymphocytic esophagitis. The red structures are individually necrotic squamous cells. This type of esophagitis has no literature and no name. It was seen by our colleagues in dermatopathology who did not know of any skin disease that looked quite like this, except possibly for a strange, intense variant of erythema multiforme. They raised the possibility of a drug reaction but we never identified a drug. Strange, unclassified inflammations occur in the esophagus and the rest of the gut that tend to remain strange and unclassified. We never see follow-up biopsies, so we have no idea that happens to them with time. It is important to recognize these bizarre inflammations and not classify them as something else. Perhaps some of them will need special treatment or eventually a cause or causes may be discovered

Suggested Reading

Liacouras CA, Furuta GT, Hirano I, et al. Eosinophilic esophagitis: updated consensus recommendations for children and adults. J Allergy Clin Immunol. 2011;128:3–20.

Purdy JK, Appelman HD, McKenna BJ. Lymphocytic esophagitis. Am J Clin Pathol. 2008;130:508–13.

Purdy JK, Appelman HD, McKenna BJ. Sloughing esophagitis is associated with chronic debilitation and medications that injure the esophageal mucosa. Mod Pathol. 2012;25:767–75.

4 Infectious Esophagitis and Organisms

The esophagus is not susceptible to a significant number of infections. There is no esophageal equivalent to *Helicobacter pylori* or *Clostridium difficile* and no epidemic infection to compare with cholera. Instead, a few esophageal infections (*eg*, *Candida* and herpesvirus) that are more likely to occur in immunocompromised individuals infect the surface epithelium and are illustrated in this chapter. Cytomegalovirus (CMV) also involves the esophagus in its usual location (endothelial cells beneath the epithelium), but we omitted this because it looks exactly like CMV-infected endothelium everywhere else in the body. Bacteria are sometimes encountered in esophageal biopsies, and there are a few illustrations of them and their significance. We also included something that looks like a condyloma because human papillomavirus is everywhere these days, and the esophagus is not immune. Finally, we have inserted a surprise organism.

S.R. Owens, H.D. Appelman, *Atlas of Esophagus and Stomach Pathology*, Atlas of Anatomic Pathology,
DOI 10.1007/978-1-4614-8084-6_4,

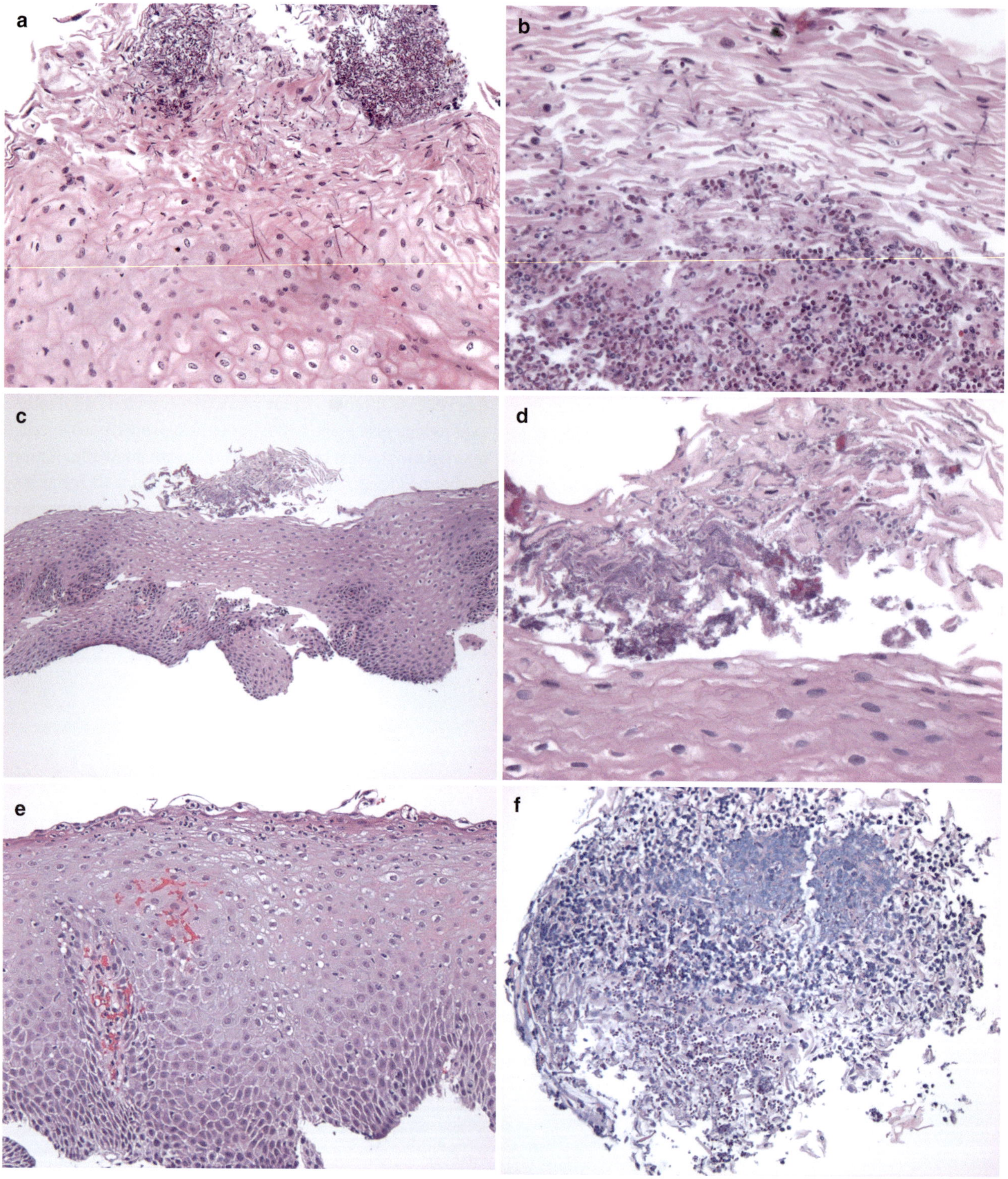

Fig. 4.1 *Candida* esophagitis. *Candida* infection is undoubtedly the most common esophageal infection in our practice. It can have a number of different but related histologic manifestations. (**a**) Sometimes the infection is obvious, as in this view, in which there are pseudohyphae invading the superficial squames and some debris with yeasts on the surface. (**b**) Large chunks of debris and exudate on the surface contain huge masses of yeasts and less common pseudohyphae. (**c**) In some biopsies, the only hint of infection is a small clump of superficial squames barely attached to or even completely detached from the surface. (**d**) This is a closer view of **c**. The clump contains superficial squamous cells that look necrotic with dense pink cytoplasm mixed with both yeasts and pseudohyphae. (**e**) There are even cases where the only hint of infection is a few microabscesses in the superficial-most squamous epithelium. (**f**) This should prompt a search of the entire slide for detached clumps of debris, squames and yeasts, or pseudohyphae as in the large clump in this image

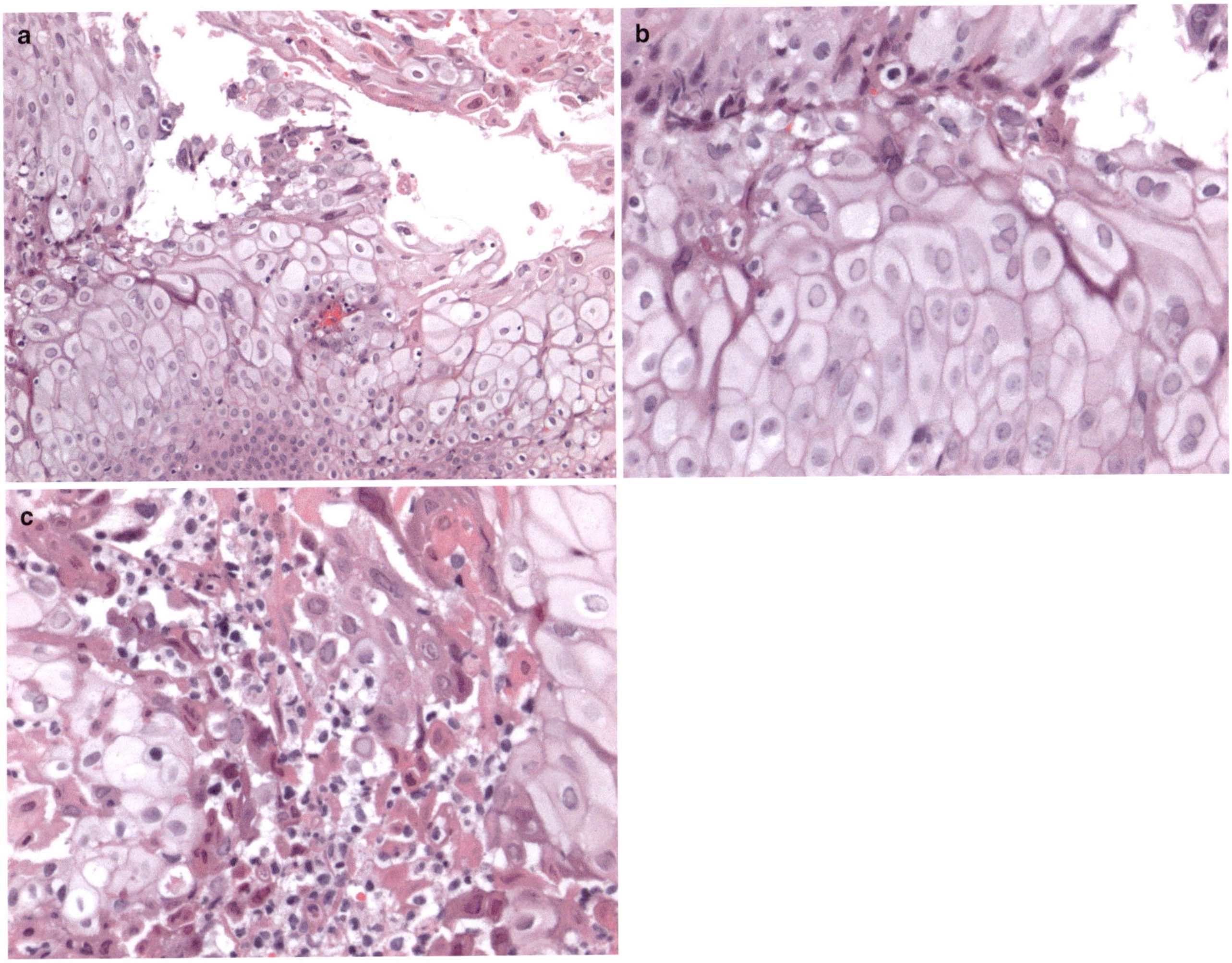

Fig. 4.2 Herpesvirus infection. (**a**) At the bottom, the basal cell layer is thicker than normal, indicating a proliferative response to injury. Above that, the squamous cells are enlarged with smooth or glassy-appearing cytoplasm, and the nuclei have pale centers. In addition, there are scattered squamous cells with more than one nucleus. At the top right, there are detached degenerated or even necrotic squames, most of which have retained large nuclei. (**b**) At this high magnification, the pale nuclear inclusions are more obvious as are the multinucleated cells, each nucleus also containing an inclusion. (**c**) Occasionally, peculiar macrophages with indented or folded nuclei are found toward the base, especially when there is an ulcer. Such cells are also found in CMV esophageal infections. This is a typical example of herpesvirus esophagitis. Most of these infections occur in immunocompromised individuals, so this is a common biopsy in major medical centers with large hematology–oncology and transplant practices. Much less common are the infections in immunocompetent individuals, but there is a literature documenting a small series of such cases [1]

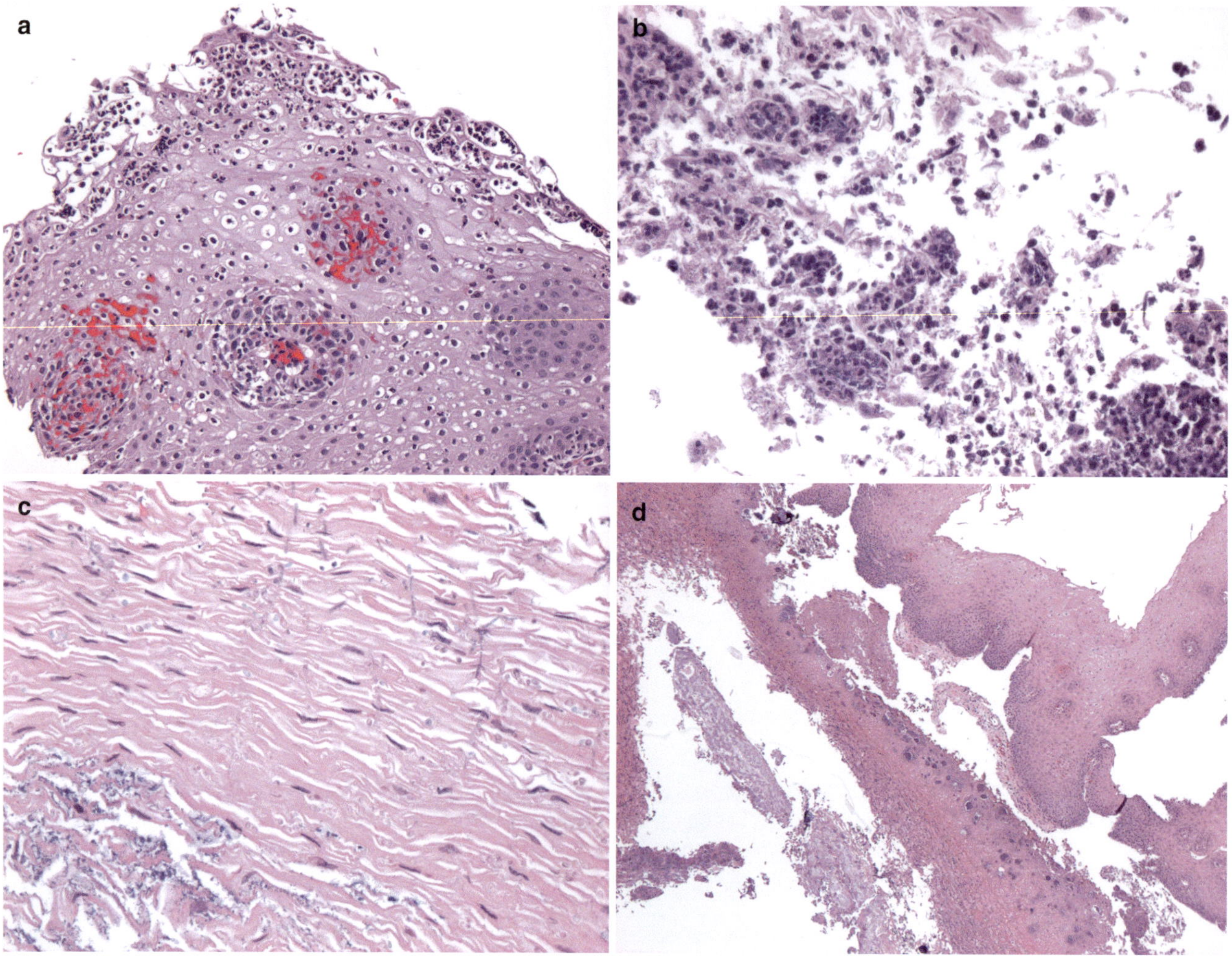

Fig. 4.3 Bacteria in various biopsies. Bacteria appear in biopsies in several settings, most of which have associated epithelial necrosis with sloughing. (**a**) Within the superficial squames, there is an infiltrate of polymorphonuclear leukocytes (PMNs) that forms several intraepithelial abscesses. (**b**) Occasionally small collections of pus and debris with bacteria are also included. Perhaps these bacteria caused the acute inflammation or maybe they are just secondary colonizers of sloughed necrotic superficial squames. Dealing with cases of acute esophagitis such as these is frustrating. Such debris with bacteria might have even come from the mouth and may have absolutely nothing to do with the esophagitis. (**c**) *Candida* pseudohyphae are in the superficial squames and at the base (*lower left*) there are bacteria in the damaged epithelial cells. In such cases we suspect that the *Candida* causes the disease and the bacterial colonization is secondary, although we are not certain. (**d**) In this case of sloughing esophagitis (*see* Chap. 3), there are large bacterial colonies at the interface between the superficial necrotic and deep viable layers of the squamous epithelium. Such colonization of the sloughed layers is not uncommon in sloughing esophagitis. As far as we know, bacterial infection is not the cause of this condition

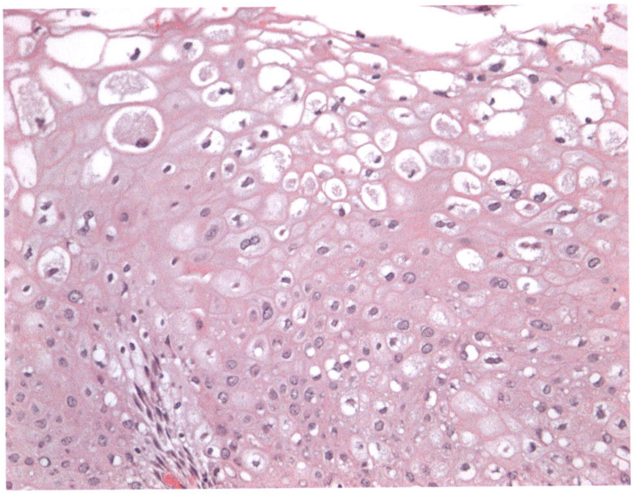

Fig. 4.4 Human papillomavirus (HPV)-like changes. This biopsy came from a patient on long-term immunosuppression for a heart transplant performed 15 years earlier. Recently he developed high-grade squamous intraepithelial neoplasia of the midesophagus. In this non-neoplastic squamous epithelium, there are superficial changes resembling those in HPV infection, including binucleation and enlargement and cytoplasmic pallor of squamous cells with crinkled or raison-shaped nuclei (*ie*, koilocytosis). HPV was not proven by molecular testing in this case because the patient had already developed neoplasia. HPV has been implicated as a cause of both squamous papillomas and squamous carcinomas of the esophagus, even in seemingly immunocompetent individuals

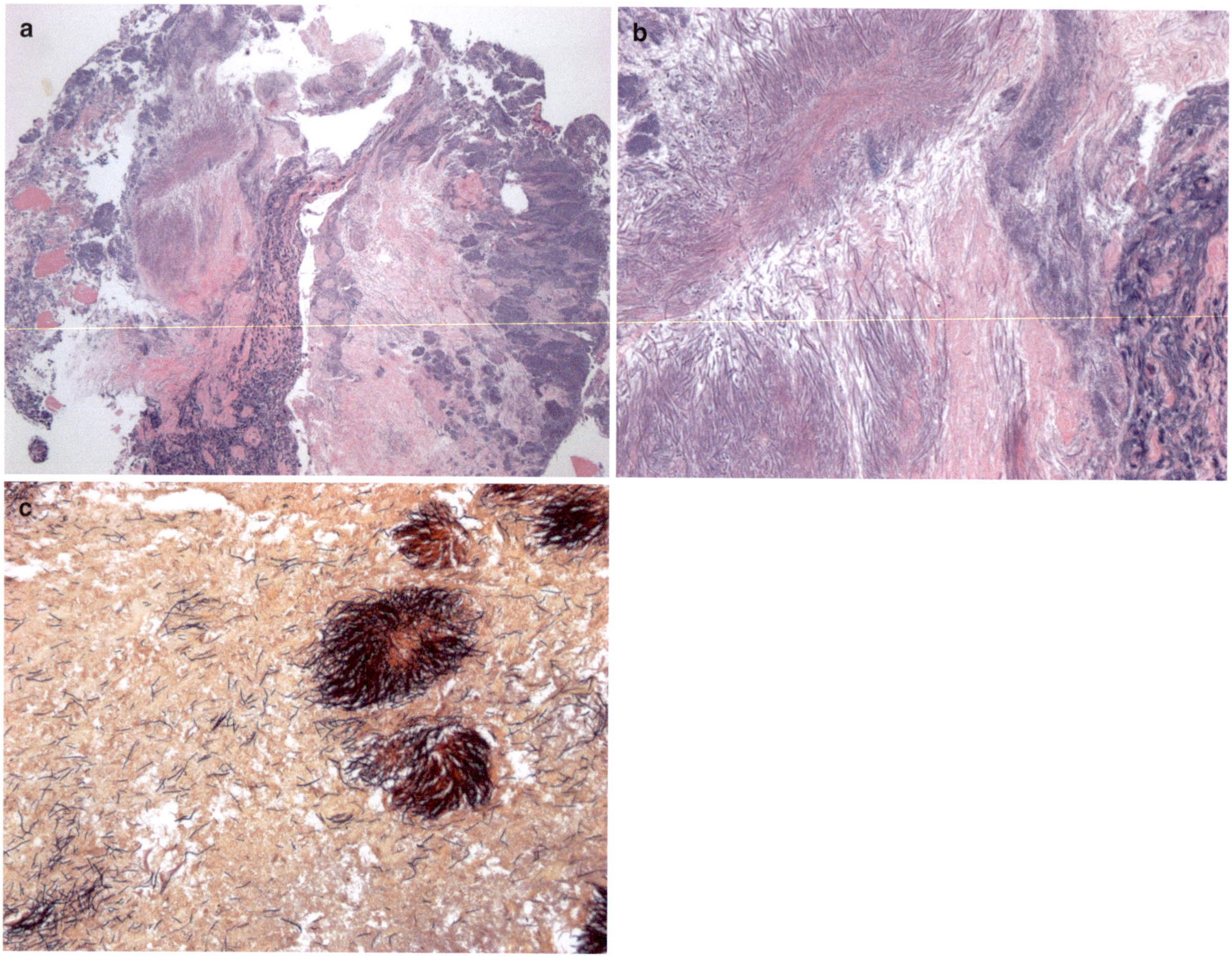

Fig. 4.5 Filamentous organisms and ulcers. (**a**) Occasionally, a gastric biopsy contains clumps or even masses of long, slender, filamentous organisms that tend to mix with debris or food particles, as in this low-power magnification view. (**b**) At high-power magnification, they really do not look like typical bacteria or fungi. They are too thick for *Actinomyces* and too thin for fungi like *Candida*. So far, as best as we can tell, they have no name. However, they occur in a specific clinical setting, namely an ulcer, regardless of the cause. In our experience they are almost always associated with some type of ulcerating esophageal or gastric cancer. In some of the older literature, they were described as occurring over benign as well as malignant gastric ulcers, but we see so few biopsies of benign gastric ulcers that we have no experience with this setting. They do not occur in ulcerating conditions of the intestines. (**c**) These organisms are gram positive

Reference

1. Kato S, Yamamoto R, Yoshimitsu S, et al. Herpes simplex esophagitis in the immunocompetent host. Dis Esophagus. 2005;18:340–4.

5 Benign Squamous Proliferations

There are few esophageal squamous proliferations that are not malignant. In fact, it was challenging to find enough examples for a separate chapter. The two most common are the glycogen acanthosis, a difficult lesion to classify, and the squamous papilloma, which is more likely a benign neoplasm. A few proliferations are sometimes confused with squamous carcinoma, mostly the long prong squamous proliferation at the edge and base of ulcers and squamous hyperplasia with pleomorphic nuclei (*see* Chap. 2). This chapter includes a spectacular, mass-forming, benign-appearing squamous proliferation that we had trouble placing in the squamous chapters. We were not exactly sure what it was, but it did not seem malignant cytologically.

S.R. Owens, H.D. Appelman, *Atlas of Esophagus and Stomach Pathology*, Atlas of Anatomic Pathology,
DOI 10.1007/978-1-4614-8084-6_5,

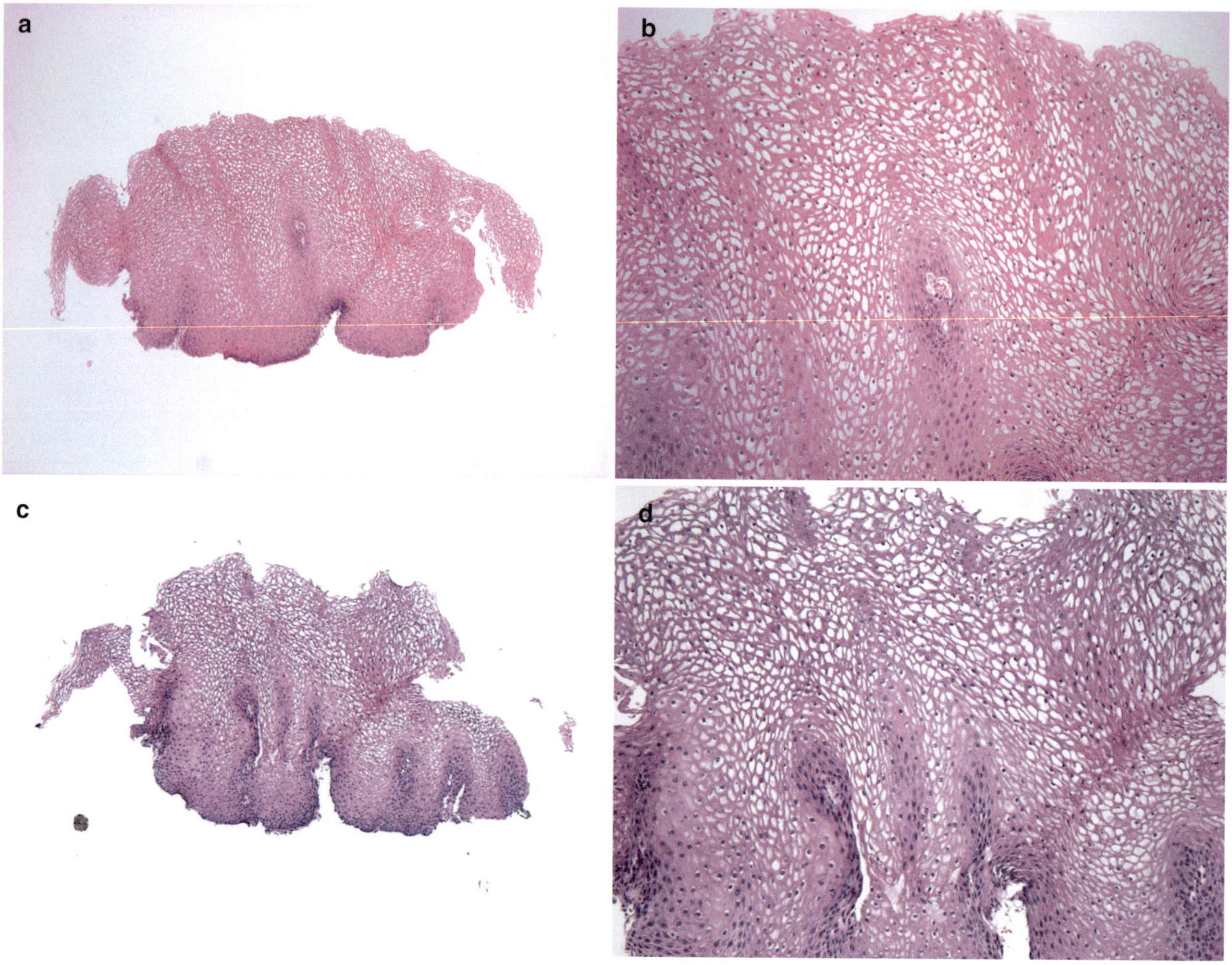

Fig. 5.1 Glycogenic acanthosis. One benign squamous proliferation unique to the esophagus is the glycogenic acanthosis, which is characterized by thick, highly differentiated squamous epithelium with heavily glycogenated cells, appearing as large cells with clear cytoplasm, comprising half or more of the total squamous thickness. These lesions commonly are seen grossly and endoscopically as small plaques oriented longitudinally. They have no relation to specific irritants, inflammations, and neoplasms. It is unknown why and how they develop, but one situation in which they are found frequently is Cowden's Syndrome, the multi-hamartoma syndrome associated with a *PTEN* gene mutation. So, perhaps they are malformations; however, it is common enough that some esophageal experts regard it as a normal variant. (**a** and **b**) Low- and high-power magnification of an almost perfectly oriented lesion captured in its entirety. There is acanthosis, papillomatosis with lamina propria papillae extending close to the surface, and a thick multilayer of cells with clear cells stuffed with glycogen. (**c** and **d**) Low- and high-power magnification of what we more commonly see in a biopsy, a bias cut with part of the top missing. Otherwise, it has exactly the same features as **a** and **b**

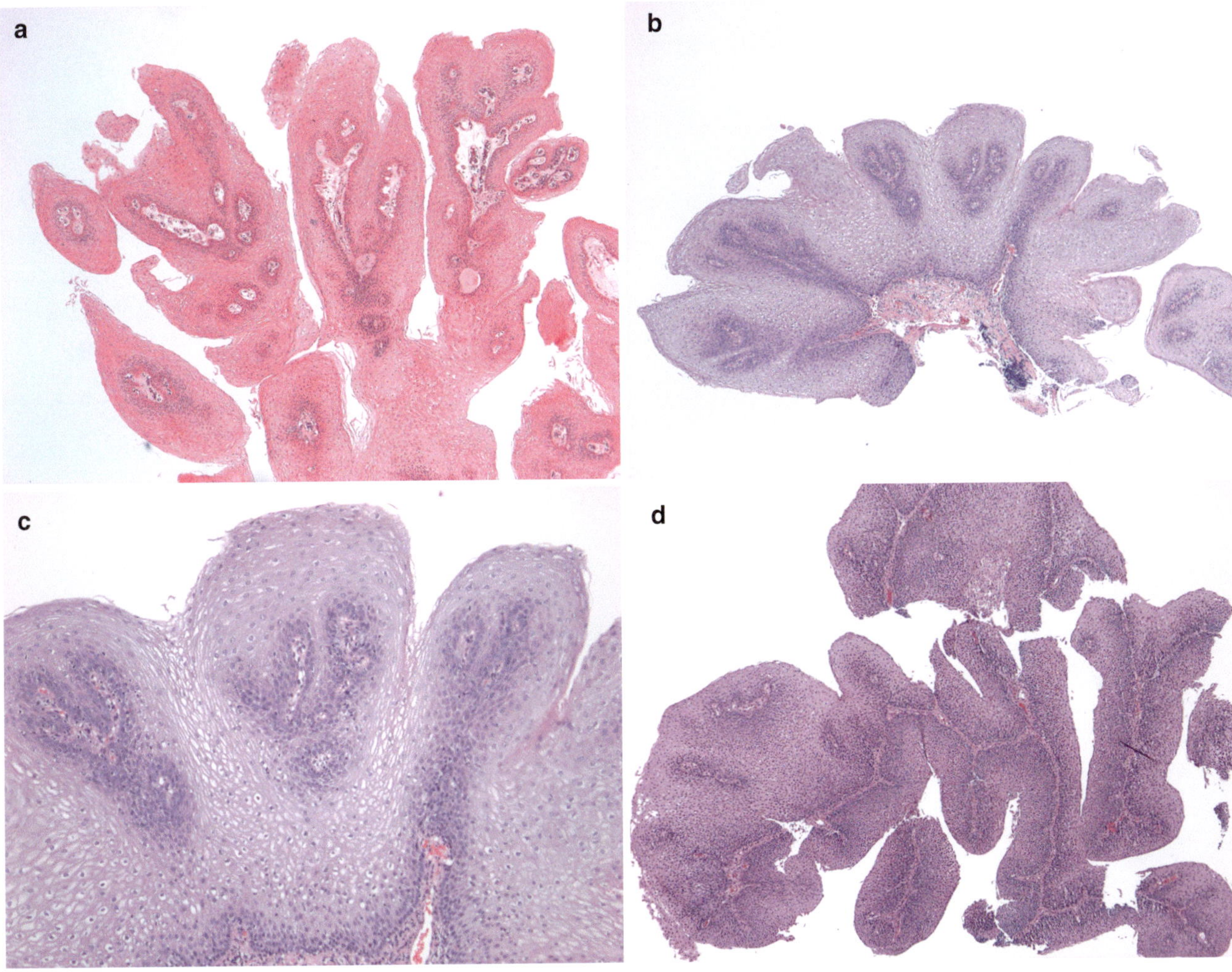

Fig. 5.2 Squamous papillomas. Basically the only benign squamous neoplasm in the esophagus, squamous papillomas appear endoscopically as small polyps at any level. Most are characterized by a core of extended, occasionally branched lamina propria containing small vessels and covered by mature squamous epithelium. This squamous epithelium varies in thickness from one papilloma to another. When the lamina propria expansion and branching is complex, the epithelium may be thinner than normal. Sometimes the superficial layers of squamous cells have koilocytotic changes, suggesting human papillomavirus (HPV) induction, and that may actually be the case. Different reported studies have found remarkably different frequencies of HPV in these papillomas, but these differences may be technic dependent. Occasional papillomas have intraepithelial neoplasia, usually low grade, but they are not cancer associated. (**a**) This papilloma has complex branching papilla of lamina propria and generally thin overlying squamous epithelium. (**b**) A flatter papilloma with shorter papillae that have less branching. (**c**) A close view of the normal-appearing squamous epithelium. (**d**) This papilloma is covered by squamous epithelium that has basal cell hyperplasia comparable to that seen in various injuries, suggesting that this papilloma also suffered from surface damage

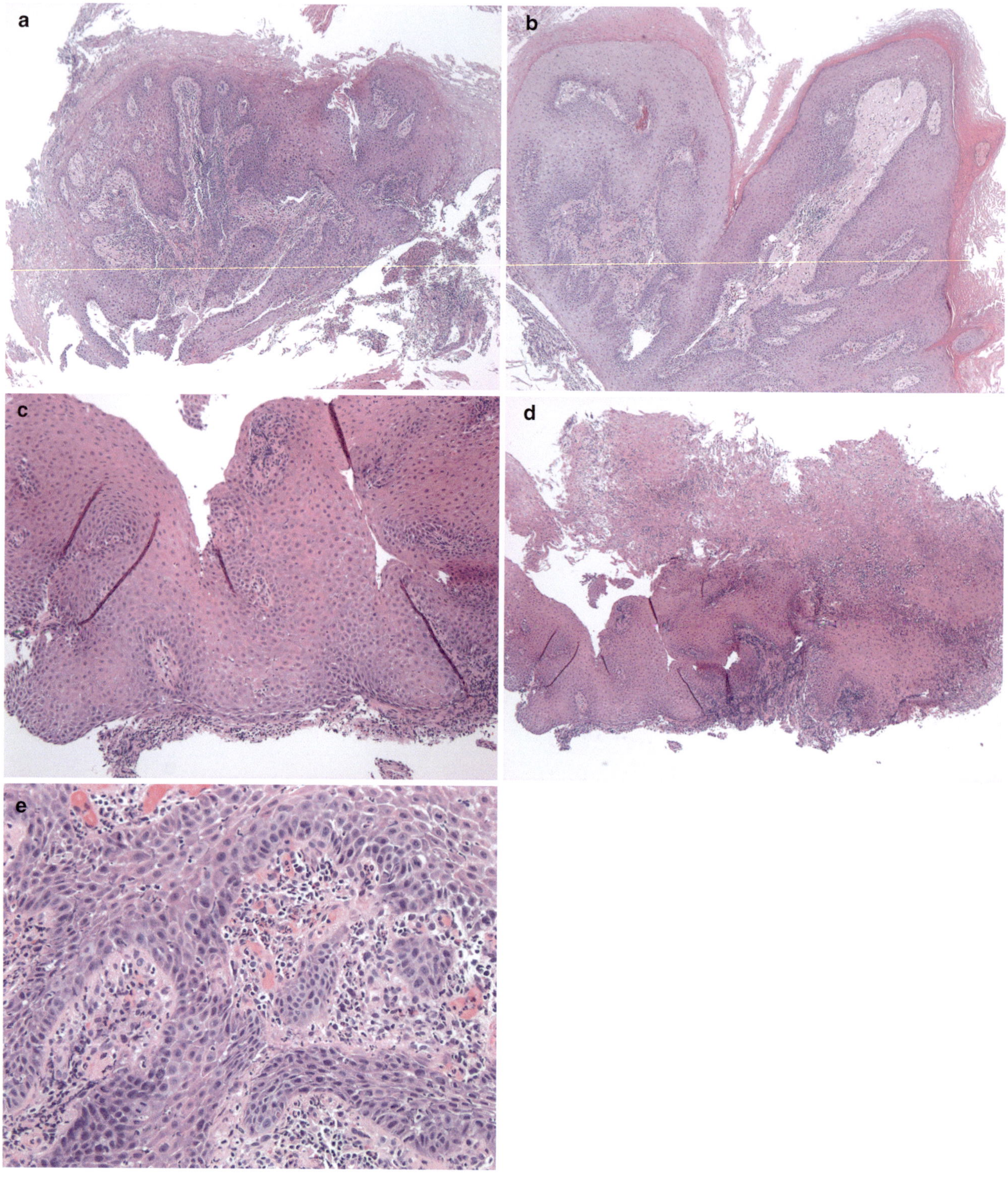

Fig. 5.3 Mass-forming, histologically benign squamous proliferation. We have seen several cases of huge, often obstructing esophageal masses, usually distal, that clinically appear to be malignant but when seen on biopsies and sometimes on resections are histologically benign, usually chronically inflamed, and sometimes eroded. These masses do not seem like variants of verrucous squamous carcinoma, the most benign-appearing squamous carcinoma. They seem to be exuberant forms of pseudoepitheliomatous hyperplasia. The following are different areas from a single lesion that are characteristic of this florid benign squamous proliferation. (**a**) Part of one lesion has irregular interconnecting squamous prongs and a variably thick surface squamous layer with abundant keratin, parakeratin, and debris covering the surface. The lamina propria is intensely, chronically inflamed. (**b**) In some areas, the lamina propria forms elongated papillae, resembling those in a squamous papilloma. (**c**) In some areas, the base is flat, similar to that in normal esophagus. (**d**) The surface is often covered by a thick layer of keratin, debris, and inflammatory cells, and this layer is often colonized by bacteria and *Candida*. (**e**) Some places have long basal prongs of squamous cells that extend into the inflamed lamina propria, similar to the long prongs at the edges and bases of healing ulcers

6 Squamous Intraepithelial Neoplasia

In our part of the world (the upper midwestern United States), squamous epithelial neoplasms of the esophagus have become rare, and the common esophageal carcinoma is the Barrett's adenocarcinoma. As a result, we have had very little recent experience with squamous neoplasms. Therefore, the chapters devoted to these neoplasms may be less informative than comparable chapters written in places where they are still common, such as Japan.

According to the 2010 World Health Organization book on tumours of the digestive system [1], all things previously known as squamous dysplasias and in situ carcinomas are now designated as intraepithelial neoplasias (IEN). Furthermore, IENs are now divided only into two groups: low-grade (LGIEN) and high-grade (HGIEN). The same terminology is used for the squamous anus. However, in the columnar gut, including the metaplastic columnar gut known as Barrett's mucosa, the term *dysplasia* is still preferred. IENs have a mixture of architectural and cytologic changes. The architectural changes generally are the orientation and polarity of the squamous cells, whereas the cytologic changes include decreased cytoplasmic maturation, nuclear hyperchromatism, and pleomorphism, as well as an increase in mitoses that are often higher in the abnormal epithelium compared to normal and that may have atypical features, such as tripolarity. LGIEN has fewer of these features than HGIEN, and they are confined to the lower half or so of the epithelium. HGIEN, therefore, has more of these features than does LGIEN, and they extend higher. However, it becomes obvious that there are epithelia that have low-grade features but with some high-grade features, but not enough of them for a confident high-grade diagnosis. The illustrations in this chapter include a number of variants of IENs, including some that are difficult to classify.

One extraordinarily annoying problem that surfaces when HGIEN is found is how to determine the most incipient invasion. This determination, it seems to us, is often not reproducible from one experienced pathologist to another. Several examples of real or suspected incipient invasion into the lamina propria are included. We offer our interpretations of these foci, but we expect that some readers may disagree.

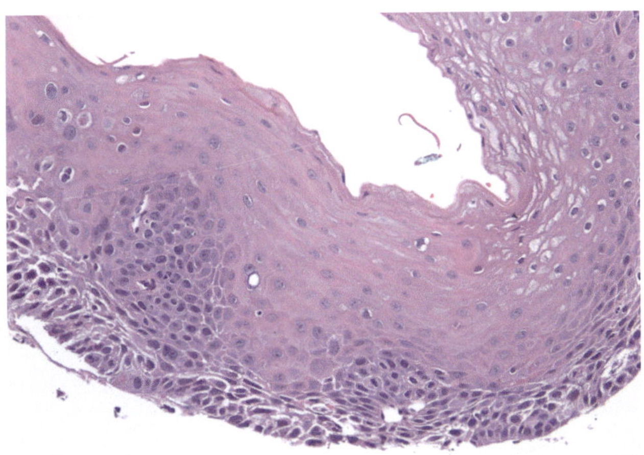

Fig. 6.1 The lowest end of LGIEN has several layers of cells at the base of the epithelium with enlarged, hyperchromatic, and pleomorphic nuclei whereas the superficial layers appear relatively normal, except for a few dysplastic cells higher than the base

S.R. Owens, H.D. Appelman, *Atlas of Esophagus and Stomach Pathology*, Atlas of Anatomic Pathology,
DOI 10.1007/978-1-4614-8084-6_6, © Springer Science+Business Media New York 2014

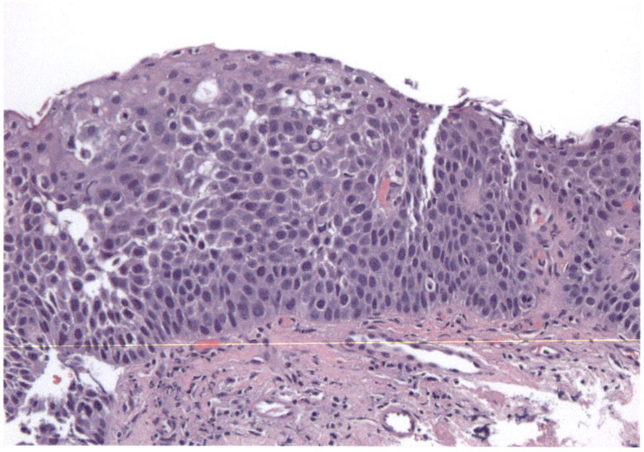

Fig. 6.2 LGIEN in which the cells at the base resemble those in Fig. 6.1, but similar nuclear changes extend higher and, at the same time, there is gradual maturation toward the surface

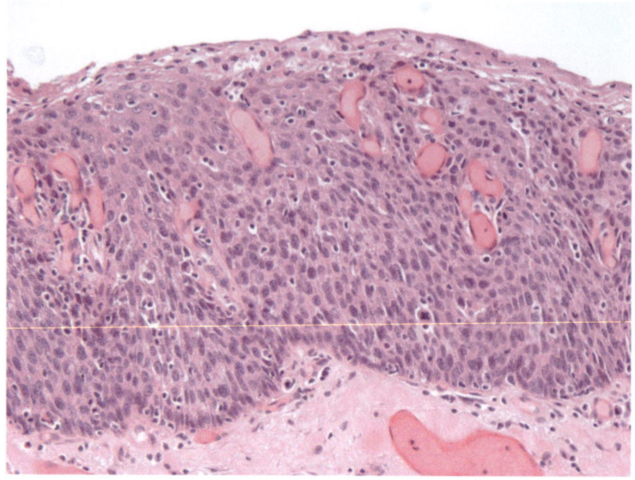

Fig. 6.3 HGIEN. The squamous epithelium is of normal thickness but there is almost full thickness crowding of smaller than normal cells with loss of nuclear polarity. There are only a few thin superficial layers of more mature-appearing squamous cells

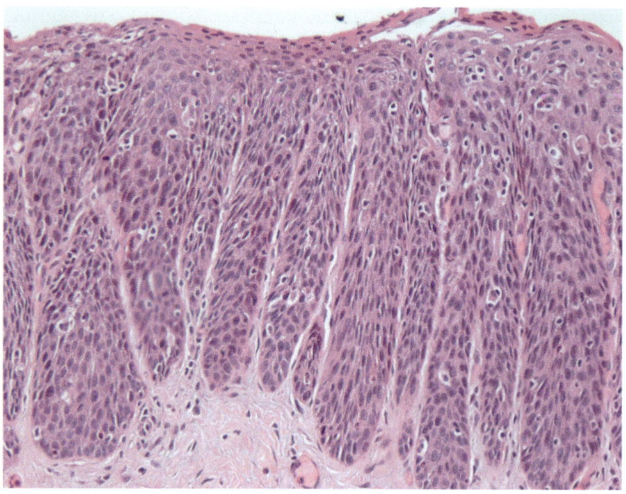

Fig. 6.4 HGIEN with acanthosis. The squamous epithelium is much thicker than normal (acanthotic) with thin basal projections into the lamina propria. The cells are small, elongated, and crowded, thus resembling basal cells. As in Fig. 6.4, there are a few superficial layers of maturing epithelium

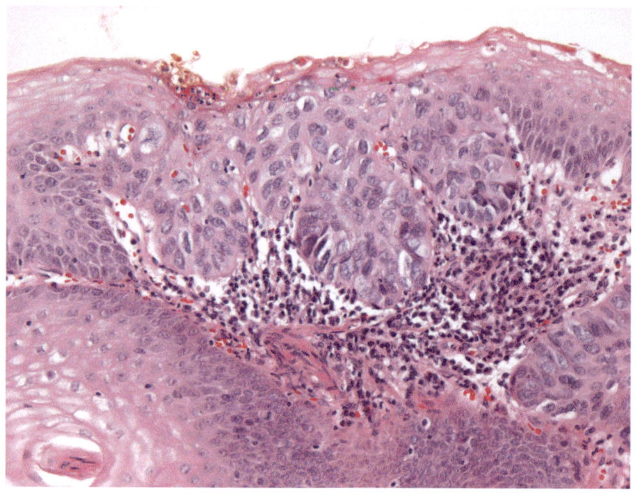

Fig. 6.5 HGIEN with atrophy. The epithelium is much thinner than normal (atrophic). All the cells are large and polygonal with enlarged, strangely shaped, folded and angulated nuclei, which are totally disorganized. This change is almost full thickness with only a thin layer of flattened cells on the surface

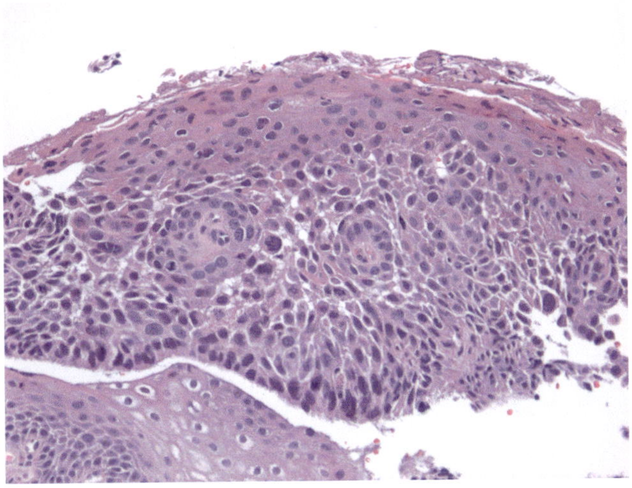

Fig. 6.6 IEN, somewhere in the area of the highest end of LGIEN and the lowest end of HGIEN. The basal half of the epithelium is disorganized whereas the upper half appears to be maturing, although it contains cells that have enlarged and hyperchromatic nuclei

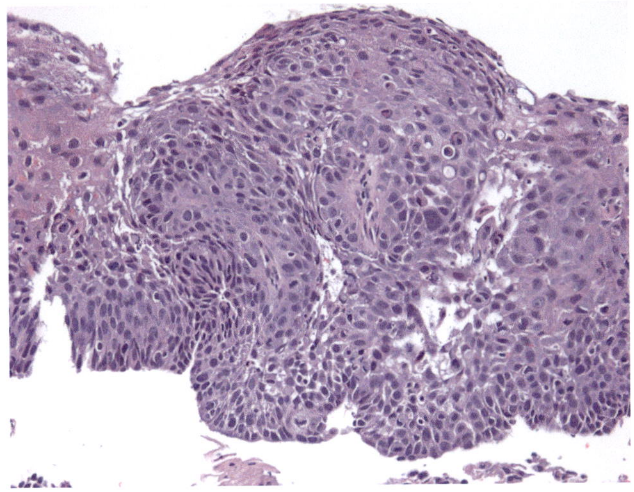

Fig. 6.7 Another example of an IEN somewhere between low and high grade. The epithelium seems to mature toward the surface, although there are nuclei that extend quite high. In addition, there is cellular disorganization with clusters of cells forming discrete small nodules close to the surface. Thus, this has both cytologic and architectural abnormalities, although there is still the sense of maturation

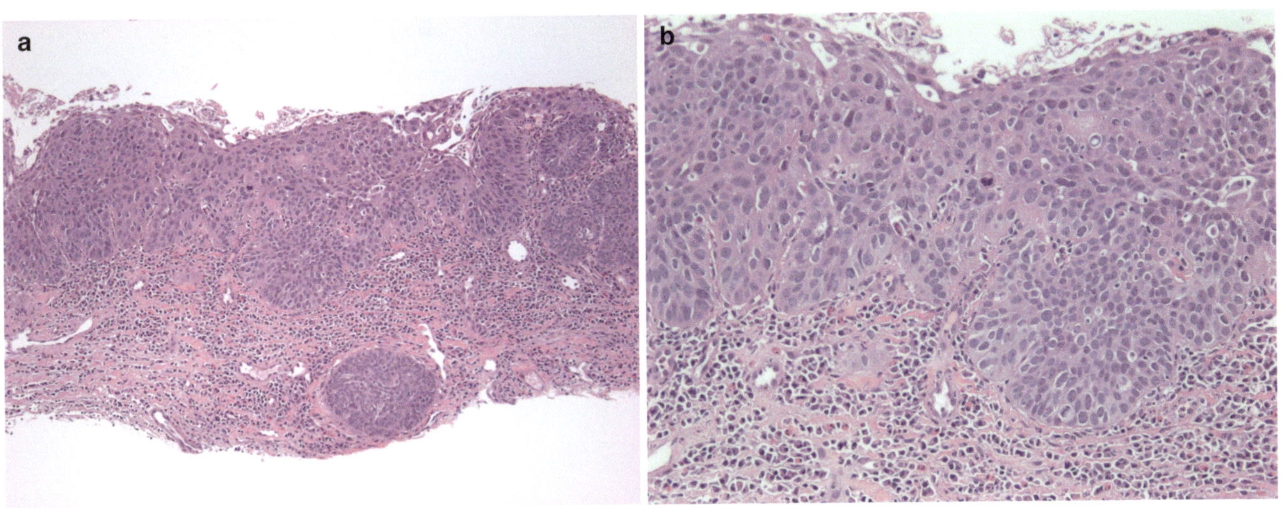

Fig. 6.8 IEN involving the surface and extending into a duct of a submucosal gland. The surface epithelium has the changes of high-grade dysplasia with full thickness involvement and loss of maturation. At the base, there is a round nodule of the same epithelium deep in the inflamed lamina propria. This is a duct of a submucosal gland in which the neoplastic epithelium has replaced the usual cuboidal epithelium. (**a**) Low-power magnification view of the entire focus including the duct. (**b**) High-power magnification view of the neoplastic surface epithelium

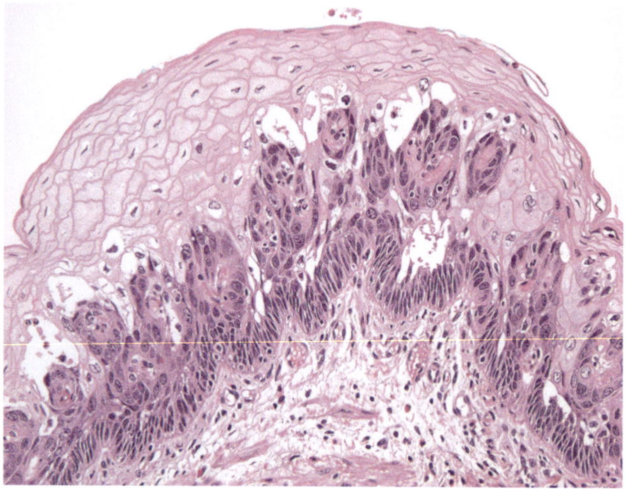

Fig. 6.9 High-grade basal EIN. Several layers of cells at the base, clearly too large to be basal cells, have enlarged and pleomorphic nuclei. These cells extend into the heavily glycogenated superficial cells, probably around papillae of lamina propria. This is an unusual variant of EIN. Cytologically, it looks high grade, yet it only involves the basal third to a half of the total epithelial squamous thickness

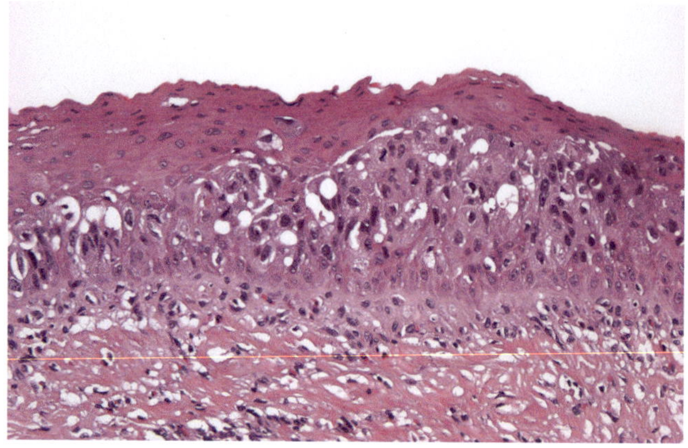

Fig. 6.10 Another variant of HGEIN. In this case, the basal half to two thirds of the epithelium is disorganized and the nuclei are large, hyperchromatic, and pleomorphic. There is sharp separation between the neoplastic and non-neoplastic epithelium, a vaguely pagetoid look

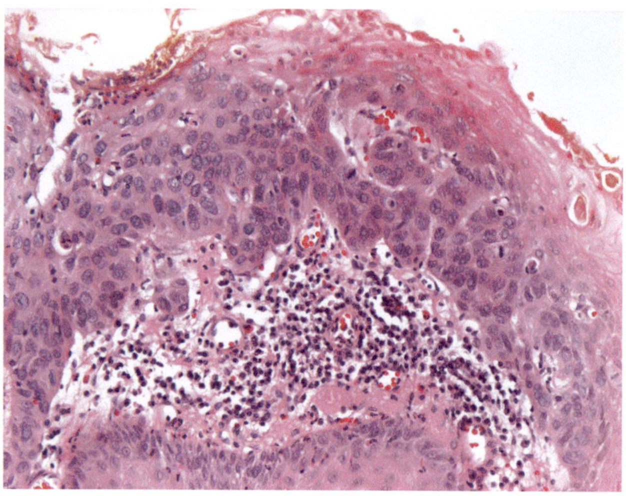

Fig. 6.11 Incipient invasion from HGIEN. This is an atrophic form of HGIEN. At the base toward the left side, there is a cluster of about five cells that may have separated from the base of the IEN. Tiny foci such as this may be the smallest evidence of lamina propria invasion

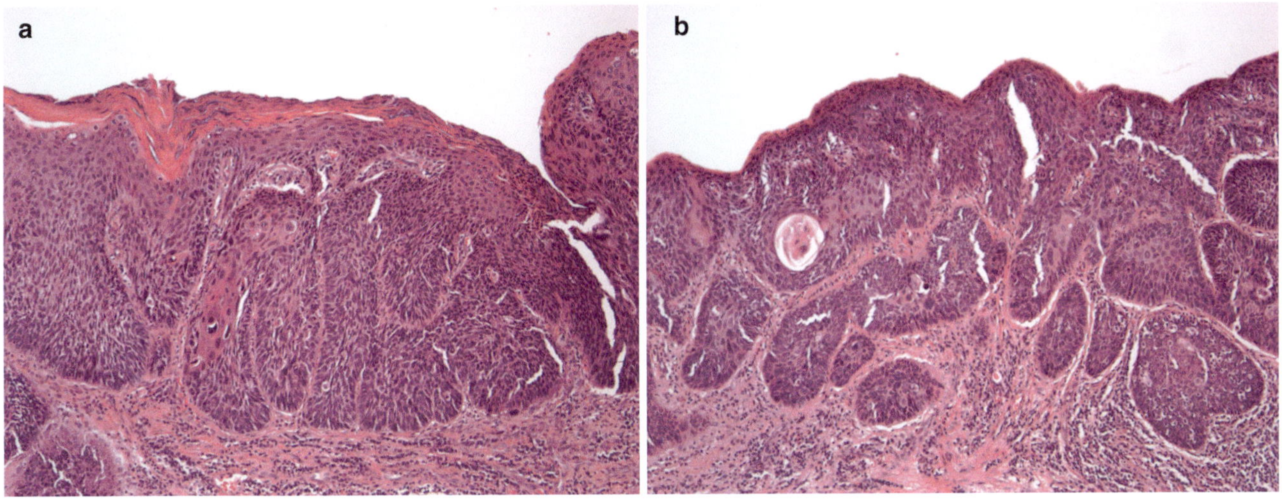

Fig. 6.12 Irregular prongs of IEN extending into the lamina propria. We regard these as noninvasive because of their smooth borders. (**a**) A perfectly perpendicular section that we often do not see. (**b**) A bias cut across the prongs in which they are separate from each other. A bias cut is a common view in a biopsy. We have to extrapolate it to the perpendicular view

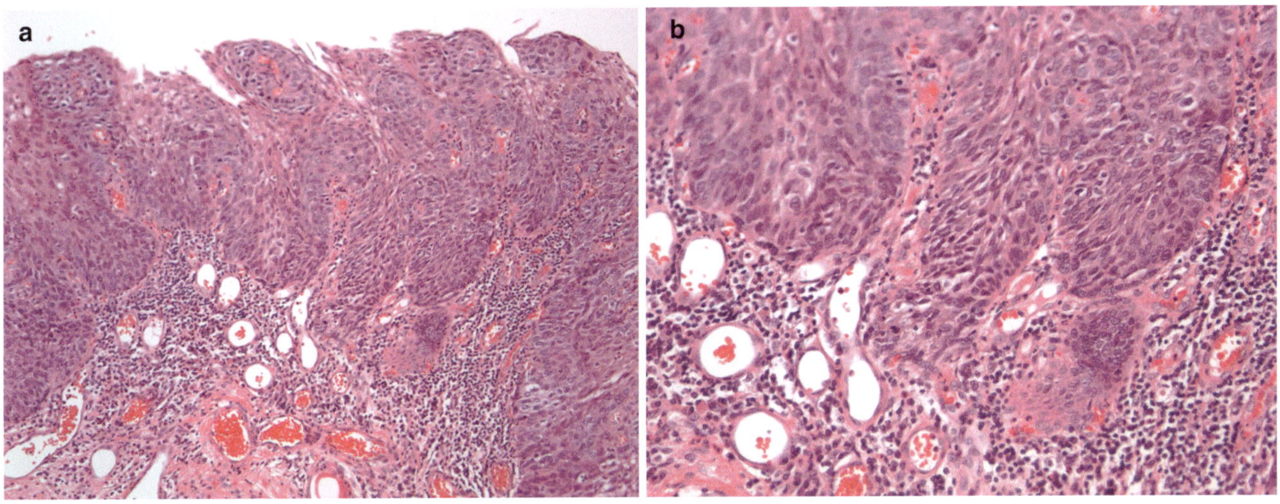

Fig. 6.13 A perpendicular but high-grade IEN with an irregular lower border. We are highly suspicious that this is the most incipient of incipient lamina propria invasion, but this is open to debate. Besides, a diagnosis of suspicious for invasion is not clinically helpful. (**a**) The lower-power view of the full thickness of the IEN. (**b**) A higher-power view concentrating on the irregular lower border of two adjacent prongs

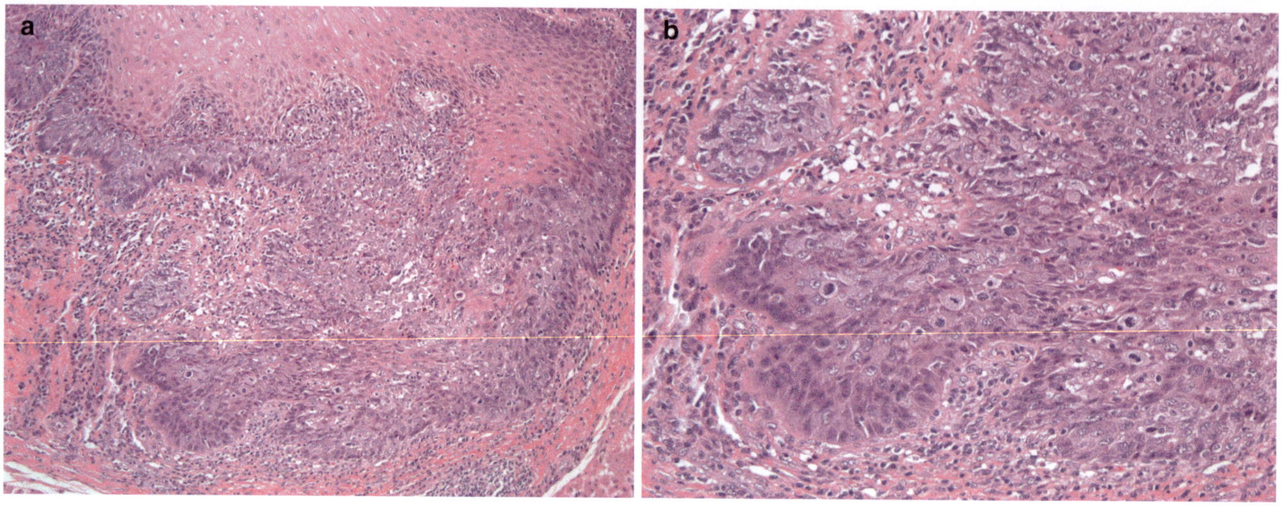

Fig. 6.14 True invasions into the superficial lamina propria. Irregular lower borders to some adjacent prongs of squamous IEN, as well as a separate island of neoplastic cells in the lamina propria. (**a**) Lower-power magnification view. (**b**) Concentrates on the irregular contours and separate island slightly above them

Reference

1. Montgomery E, Field JK, Boffetta P. Squamous cell carcinoma of the oesophagus. In: Bosman FT, Carneiro T, Hruban RH, Theise ND, editors. WHO classification of tumours, 4th ed. Lyon: IARC; 2010.

7 Invasive Squamous Cell Carcinoma

We see so few invasive squamous cell carcinomas these days that we have a paucity of cases to use as illustrations. As such, we have included the few cases we have seen recently. Some invasive squamous carcinomas keratinize whereas other do not, and the amount of keratin formation varies from a tiny focus to a lot. The cancers also vary in differentiation from very well (a good caricature of normal) to very poorly, which looks nothing like normal. In the 2010 World Health Organization book [1], invasive squamous cancers are divided into well, moderate, and poor differentiation, with mention that the most common type is moderately differentiated, but there are no definite histologic criteria for making this determination. What is apparent is that a squamous esophageal carcinoma is likely to be heterogeneous with different areas looking quite different histologically. We have chosen to illustrate different squamous cancers and we will leave it to the reader to determine the degree of differentiation of each tumor. The issue of incipient invasion into the lamina propria is covered in depth at the end of Chap. 6.

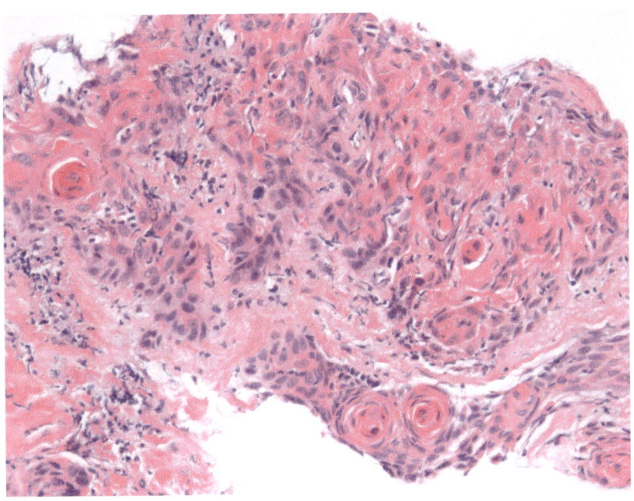

Fig. 7.1 This is a biopsy of a differentiated keratinizing carcinoma. The tumor forms small nests and with central keratinizing pearls, all embedded in a collagen-rich desmoplastic stroma. We leave it to the reader to decide if this is well or moderately differentiated

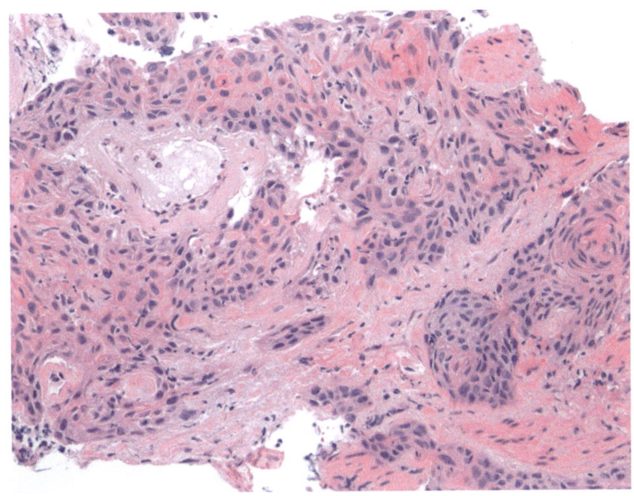

Fig. 7.2 A biopsy of a differentiated nonkeratinizing carcinoma. The nests contain squamous cell pearls, but no or little keratin. Again, readers have their choice in differentiation

S.R. Owens, H.D. Appelman, *Atlas of Esophagus and Stomach Pathology*, Atlas of Anatomic Pathology,
DOI 10.1007/978-1-4614-8084-6_7, © Springer Science+Business Media New York 2014

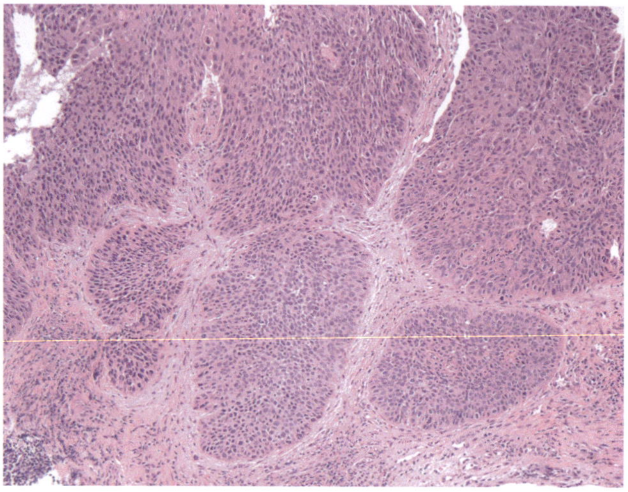

Fig. 7.3 A biopsy of a poorly differentiated nonkeratinizing carcinoma. The tumor forms solid nests and thick cords. There is only a hint of squamous differentiation with some larger cells in the center of the nests

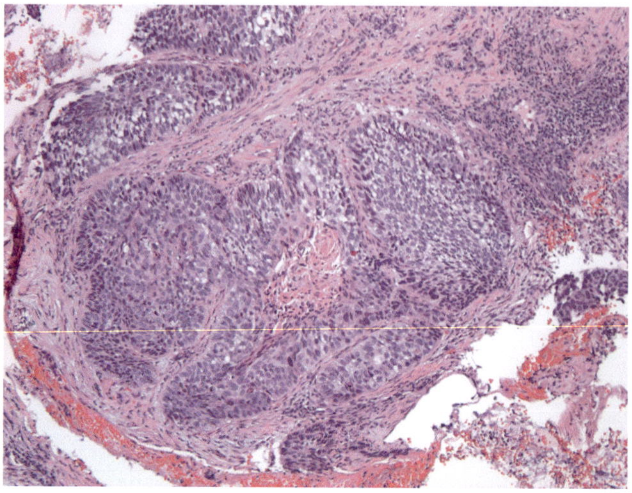

Fig. 7.4 A squamous carcinoma that is virtually undifferentiated except for clear-cut, central keratinization. Presumably, since this has both poor and definite differentiation, this fits into the moderately differentiated category

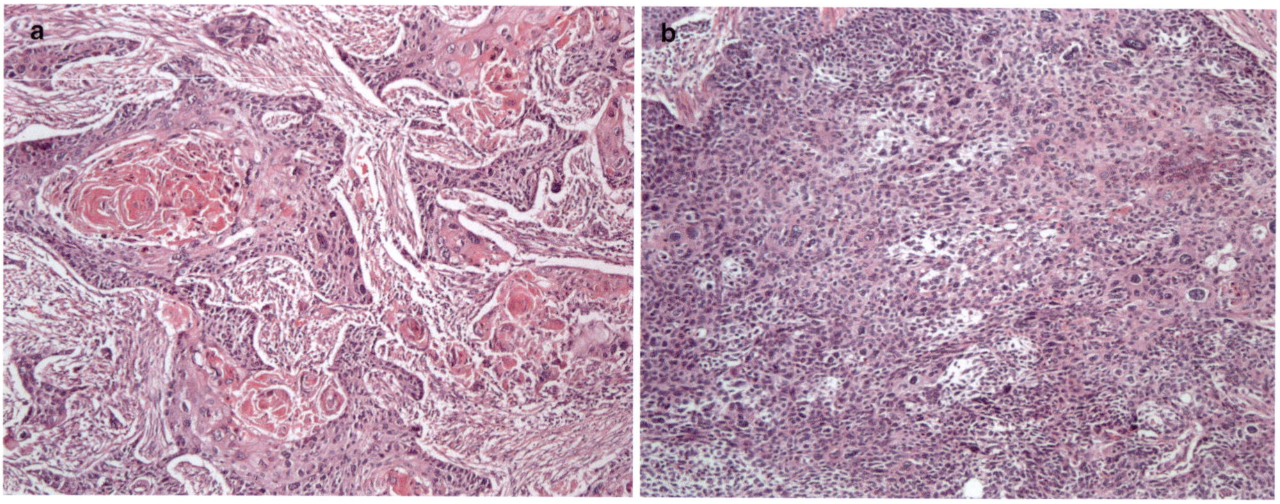

Fig. 7.5 Two fields from the same invasive carcinoma. (**a**) Differentiated and keratinizing. (**b**) Very poorly differentiated and barely recognizable as squamous

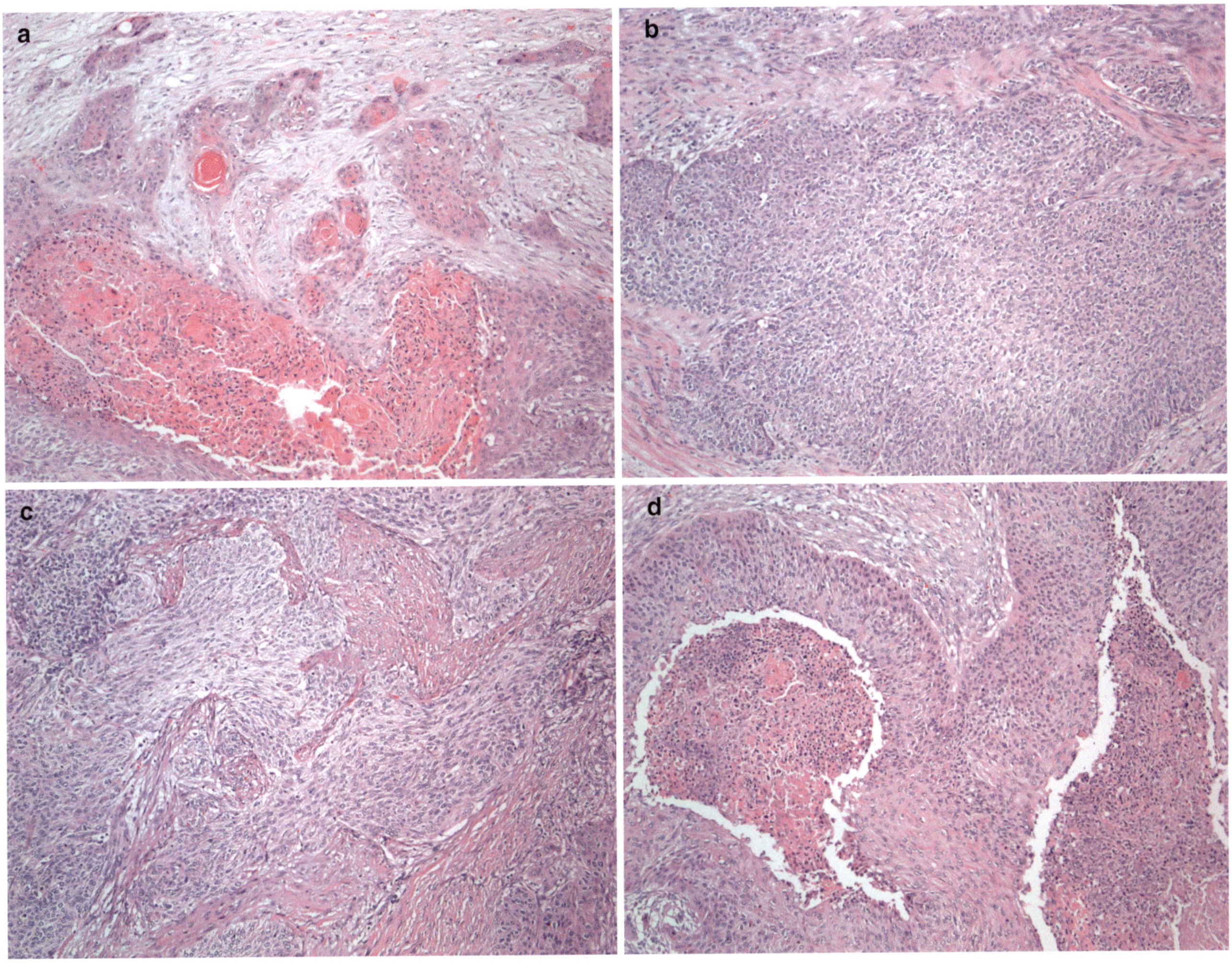

Fig. 7.6 Four totally different fields from a single invasive carcinoma. (**a**) A focus of differentiated and keratinizing carcinoma. (**b**) A focus that is solid and minimally differentiated at best. (**c**) A solid area with no squamous differentiation but with spindle cells that form fascicles. (**d**) A solid area with minimal squamous differentiation and central necrosis

Reference

1. Montgomery E, Field JK, Boffetta P. Squamous cell carcinoma of the oesophagus. In: Bosman FT, Carneiro T, Hruban RH, Theise ND, editors. WHO classification of tumours, 4th ed. Lyon: IARC; 2010.

8 Unusual Carcinomas, Including Squamous Variants

This chapter includes nontraditional carcinomas including unusual but interesting squamous carcinoma variants and endocrine tumors. They do occur, although infrequently, so we must be aware of their presence and their appearances, especially in biopsies. The purpose of this chapter is to illustrate these rare cancers to give the reader some pictures with which to compare biopsies of carcinomas that do not look like either typical squamous cell carcinomas or typical adenocarcinomas.

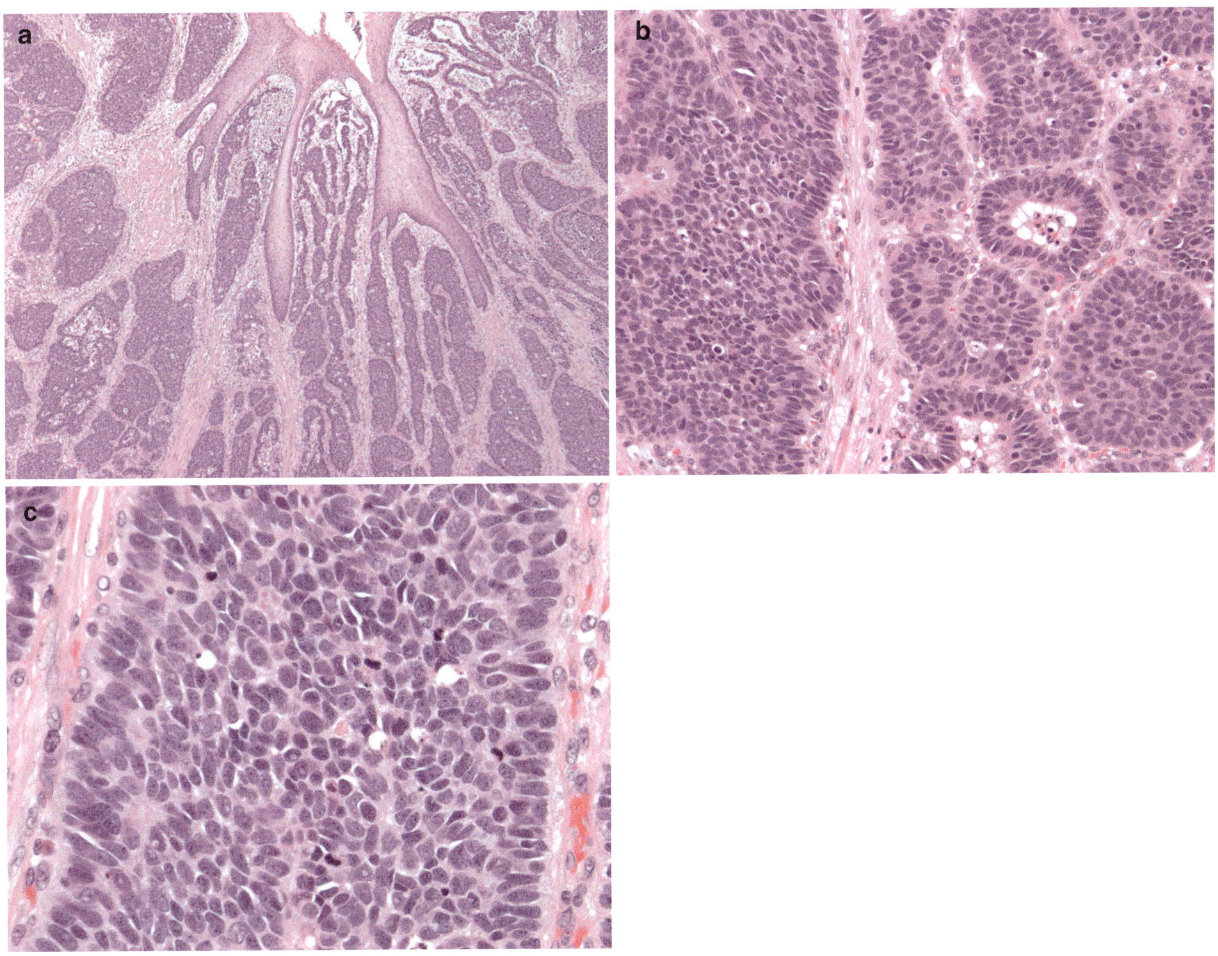

Fig. 8.1 Basaloid squamous carcinoma. One very peculiar esophageal carcinoma is the basaloid squamous cell variant. This carcinoma is much more common in the head and neck than in the esophagus. (**a**) It is characterized by discrete nests of cells with a high N:C ratio. These tumors are situated beneath a squamous surface that may be nonneoplastic. The nests of carcinoma often grow superficially to touch the base of this overlying epithelium. (**b**) There is a vague hint that the peripheral cells in the nests are palisaded. (**c**) The carcinoma cells have high-grade nuclei and frequent mitoses

S.R. Owens, H.D. Appelman, *Atlas of Esophagus and Stomach Pathology*, Atlas of Anatomic Pathology,
DOI 10.1007/978-1-4614-8084-6_8,

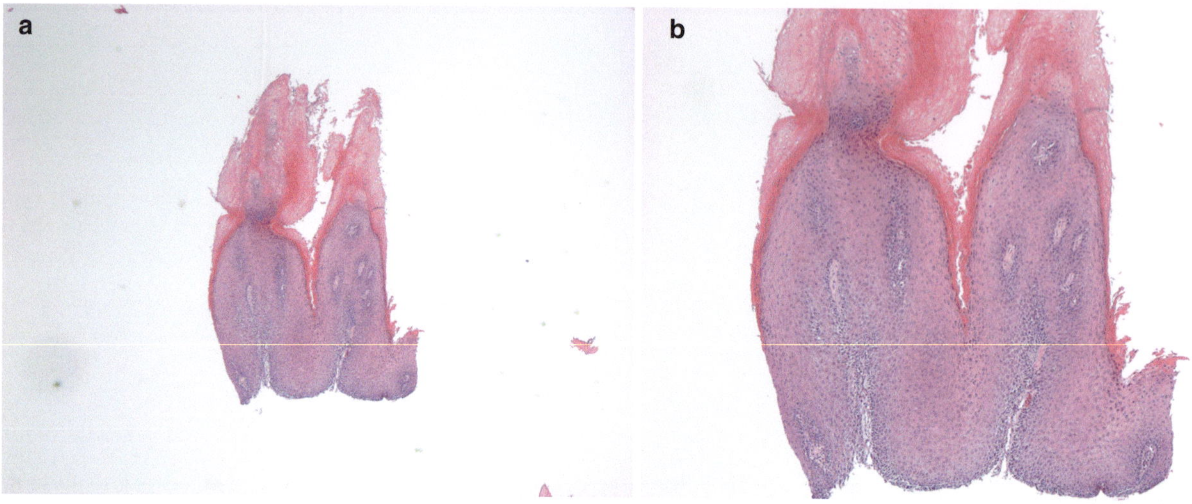

Fig. 8.2 Verrucous squamous cell carcinoma. (**a**) This is a biopsy of a squamous proliferation characterized by acanthosis with bulbous basal prongs. (**b**) In a higher-power view, it is clear that this is a highly differentiated proliferation. In addition, there is papillomatosis with papillae of lamina propria extending close to the surface. These are all the classic findings of verrucous squamous carcinoma, an extraordinarily rare carcinoma in the esophagus. Many cases reported as verrucous esophageal carcinomas really are other things, because they do not satisfy the diagnostic criteria

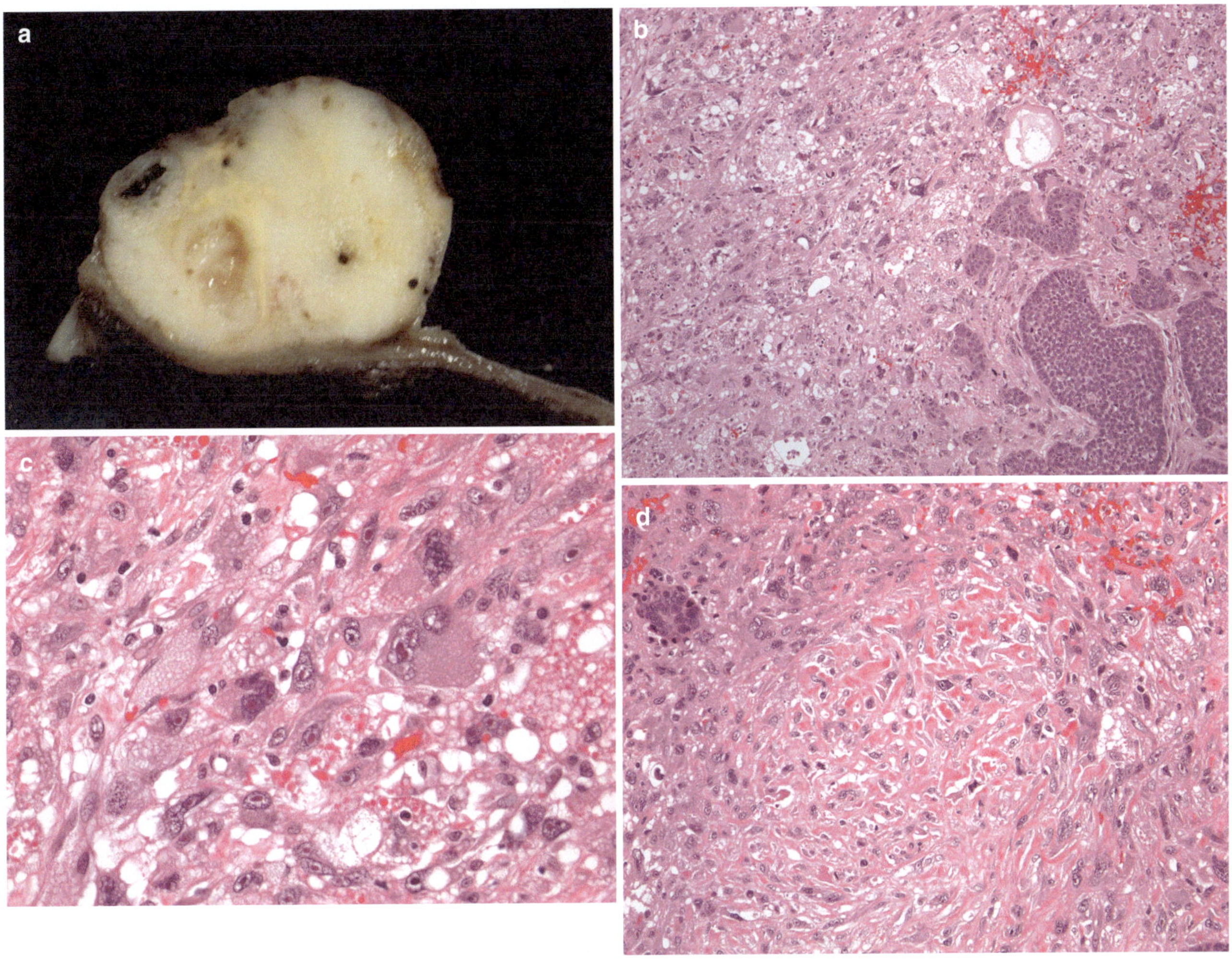

Fig. 8.3 Spindle cell squamous carcinoma (sarcomatoid carcinoma, carcinosarcoma, pseudosarcomatous squamous cell carcinoma). (**a**) These tumors usually produce exophytic masses that can grow to enormous sizes, yet are only superficially invasive. In this cross-section, such an exophytic mass extends above the esophageal wall. It invades into the submucosa and has an expansile lower border that abuts the muscularis propria. (**b**) In this low-power view, there is a mixture of carcinomatous nests (*right*) and stroma with pleomorphic spindle and stellate cells (*left*). (**c**) A high-power view of the pleomorphic cells in the stromal component. (**d**) There is pink matrix that resembles osteoid with a carcinoma nest (*upper left*). These tumors are comparable to similar mixed tumors in other sites such as the mixed Müllerian tumors of the female genital tract. They are thought to be squamous carcinomas in which some carcinoma cells undergo transformation or metaplasia to stromal cells, which on occasion can produce matrix-like osteoid or chondroid or even develop skeletal muscle characteristics. Because of their limited invasion, they tend to have a much better prognosis than usual squamous cell carcinomas of similar size that are deeply invasive

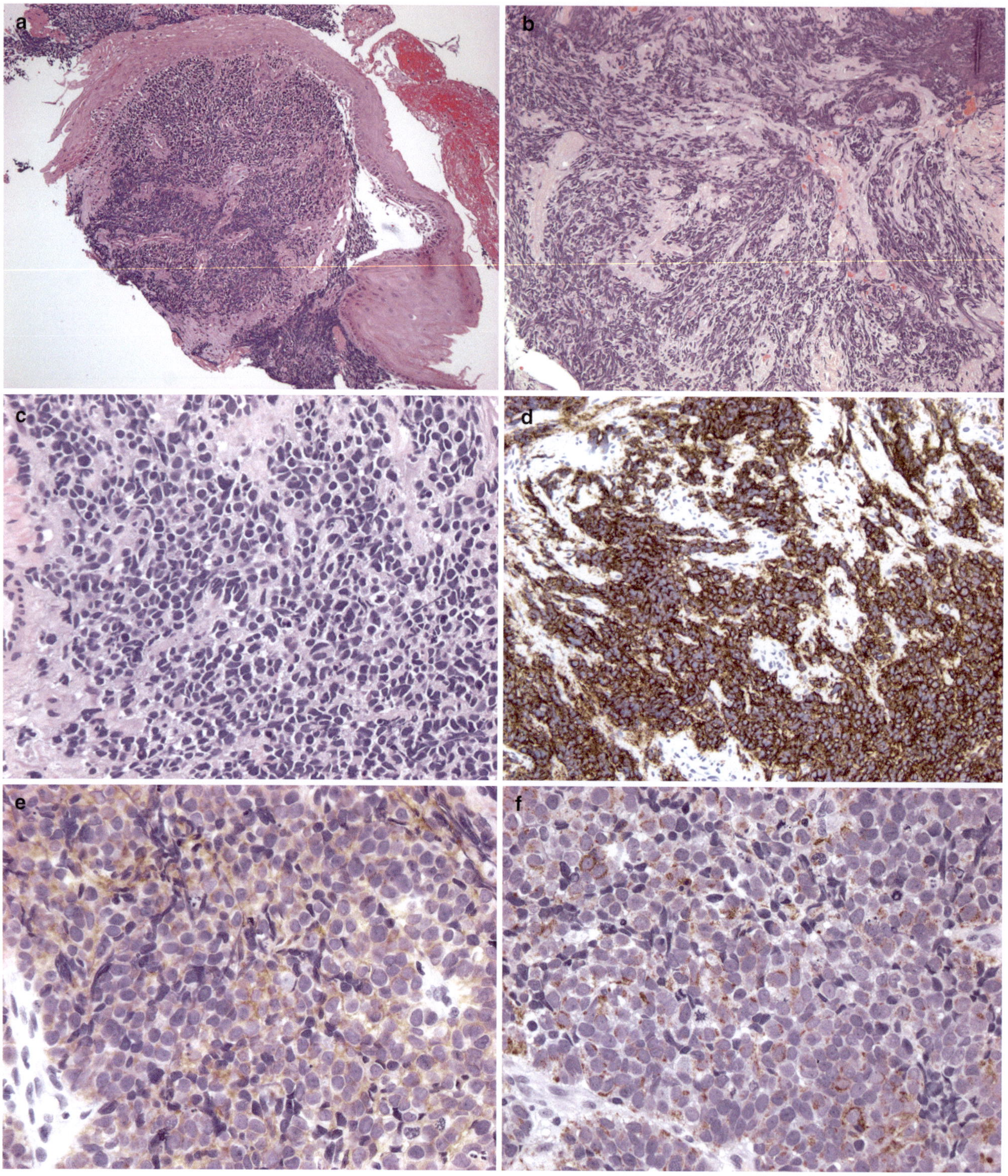

Fig. 8.4 Small cell carcinoma. Small cell carcinomas, which are identical to those in the lung, occur as esophageal primaries. Considering that they are so much more common in the lung, a biopsy of an esophageal mass that contains small cell carcinoma is immediately suspicious for either a metastasis or extension from a lung primary. There is no way that pathologists can determine whether the primary is lung or esophagus based on a biopsy. Clinicians must make that determination. (**a**) At low power, a blue mass abuts the squamous epithelium. (**b**) At higher power, much or even most of the neoplasm is likely to be crushed, but this crushing should immediately raise the suspicion of a small cell carcinoma or perhaps a lymphoma. Here, the crushed cells interdigitate with stromal areas containing small vessels, a common pattern in small cells carcinomas. (**c**) Some areas, hopefully, will not be crushed and look like this with small cells containing round to oval, primitive nuclei and little cytoplasm. There are mitoses and considerable fine granular necrotic debris in the background. (**d**) Immunostains for endocrine markers are likely to be positive. The CD56 is usually positive, sometimes very strongly and diffusely as in this field. (**e**) Some CD56 staining is much weaker and more focal as in this field. (**f**) Other endocrine markers such as chromogranin are sometimes positive as in this field where the staining is punctate and cytoplasmic. Sometimes synaptophysin is positive

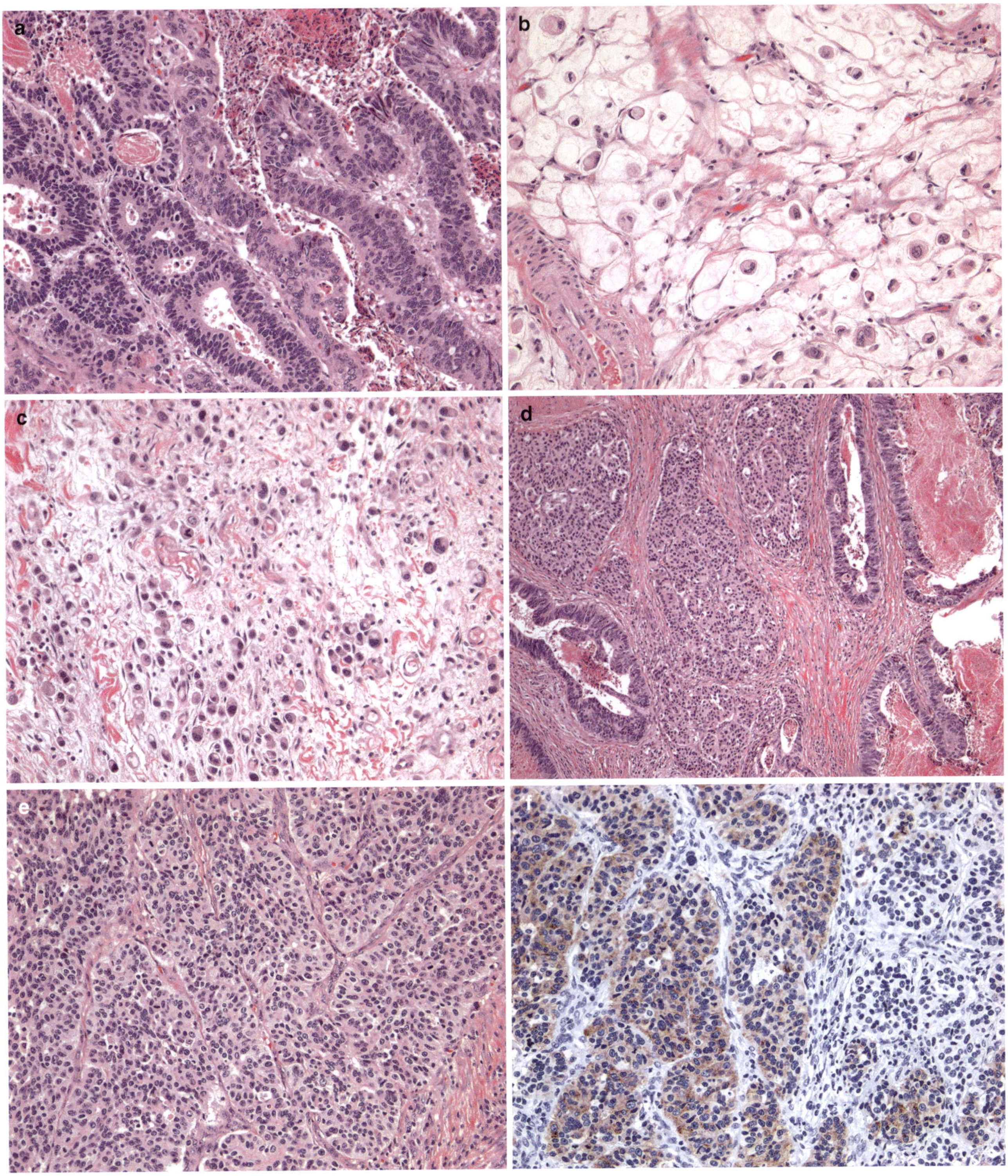

Fig. 8.5 Mixed carcinoma with adenocarcinoma and endocrine tumor components. Endocrine tumors of all types are really very rare in the esophagus. The small cell carcinoma is by far the most common. Typical carcinoid tumors are so rare that we do not even have a case to use as an illustration. However, every so often, an adenocarcinoma, arising in Barrett's mucosa, has an endocrine component, a composite tumor. Such tumors arise throughout the gastrointestinal tract. (**a**) Part of this carcinoma is differentiated, tubule forming. (**b**) Another area had mucinous differentiation with pools of mucin containing detached cancer cells or small collections of cells. (**c**) Still another area had signet ring cells growing in a diffuse, spreading pattern. (**d**) This is the interface in which both the differentiated adenocarcinoma on the sides and the differentiated endocrine neoplasm in the middle are present. (**e**) The endocrine component really resembles a carcinoid tumor—*ie*, what we now call a neuroendocrine tumor (NET)—but there is much more pleomorphism, more mitoses, and more disorganized nests. However, the typical thin fibrovascular septa are present; they produce the typical organoid pattern of endocrine tumors. (**f**) Some endocrine cell nests stain strongly with the antibody to synaptophysin

9 Nonneoplastic Barrett's Mucosa

In the United States and in many other countries, Barrett's mucosa is defined in a 2008 position paper from a group sponsored by the American College of Gastroenterology [1] as "a change in the distal esophageal epithelium of any length that can be recognized as columnar type mucosa at endoscopy and is confirmed to have intestinal metaplasia by biopsy of the tubular esophagus." In 2011, in another position paper by a group sponsored by the American Gastroenterological Association [2], this definition was modified as "the condition in which any extent of metaplastic columnar epithelium that predisposes to cancer development replaces the stratified squamous epithelium," with a further statement that "Presently, intestinal metaplasia is required for the diagnosis … because intestinal metaplasia is the only type of esophageal columnar epithelium that clearly predisposes to malignancy."

These two definitions are actually similar in that they require intestinal metaplasia with goblet cells being the sole marker of that condition. In contrast, in a 2006 position statement from the British Society of Gastroenterology [3], Barrett's mucosa was defined as "an endoscopically apparent area above the oesophagogastric junction that is suggestive of Barrett's which is supported by the finding of columnar lined oesophagus on histology." In this definition, intestinal metaplasia is not a requirement for diagnosis; however, both the British and the American definitions require that there be endoscopic changes that look like Barrett's. In this chapter, we have included variations that meet the requirements of diagnosis depending on which definition of Barrett's the reader prefers.

Although goblet cells are required for diagnosis in our practice, Barrett's is actually a metaplasia with a variety of cell types and architectural patterns. Barrett's is not generally a uniform mucosa, but it varies greatly in its composition from one area to another, even within a single microscopic field. So, all Barrett's does not look alike.

Furthermore, it is not simply an epithelial abnormality, but it also has a stromal component that makes it a remarkably complex mucosa.

This chapter will include variations commonly seen in Barrett's biopsies, all the different epithelial types, the stromal components, and other variations that do not conform to our definition of Barrett's but may satisfy the diagnostic criteria in other countries.

S.R. Owens, H.D. Appelman, *Atlas of Esophagus and Stomach Pathology*, Atlas of Anatomic Pathology,
DOI 10.1007/978-1-4614-8084-6_9,

9.1 Typical Barrett's Mucosa

Barrett's mucosa is a metaplastic columnar mucosa that replaces variable lengths of esophagus from the esophagogastric junction proximally. As in the rest of the tubular gut, this mucosa has epithelial structures and lamina propria mixed together in contrast to the normal squamous esophagus in which the epithelium and the lamina propria form separate layers with little mixing. The surface can be flat, undulating, and villiform with surface projections and any mixture. Barrett's mucosa usually has two components, sort of like gastric mucosa: (1) tubular structures extending downward from the surface and (2) mucus glands that tend to be sparse and often clustered. The tubules roughly correspond to pits in the stomach and crypts in the intestines, but they actually do not have a standard name, so they are often referred to as pits or crypts or even glands. We just call them "tubules."

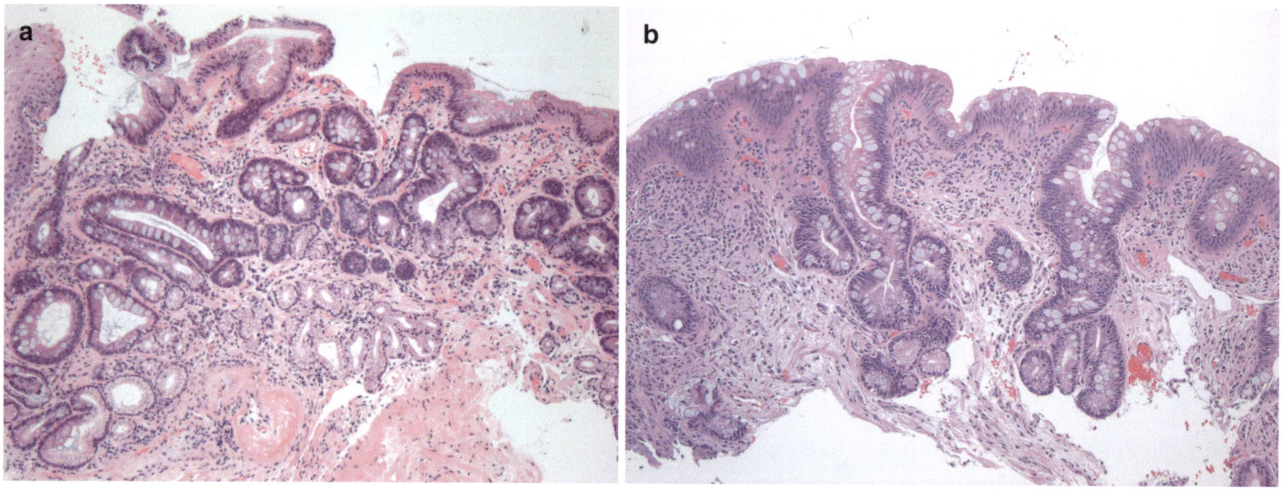

Fig. 9.1 Typical Barrett's mucosa. (**a**) In this example, the surface is undulating. The tubules are close together separated by small amounts of lamina propria, and the basal gland cluster is large, at least in Barrett's terms. The surface epithelium and some of these tubules are lined by epithelium that is a mixture of gastric type surface columnar cells with apical mucin and discrete goblet cells. This has been designated as the specialized type of mucosa in Barrett's. It is identical to incomplete intestinal metaplasia in the stomach. The deep glands resemble cardiac glands and contain cuboidal to low columnar cells with apical mucin that sometimes looks granular. (**b**) In this Barrett's mucosa from a different individual, the surface is a mixture of flat and undulating. The cells covering the surface and lining the tubules are the typical mixture of columnar cells with apical mucin resembling gastric surface epithelium and plump goblet cells. Compared to the previous view, there are fewer tubules and glands and much more inflamed lamina propria

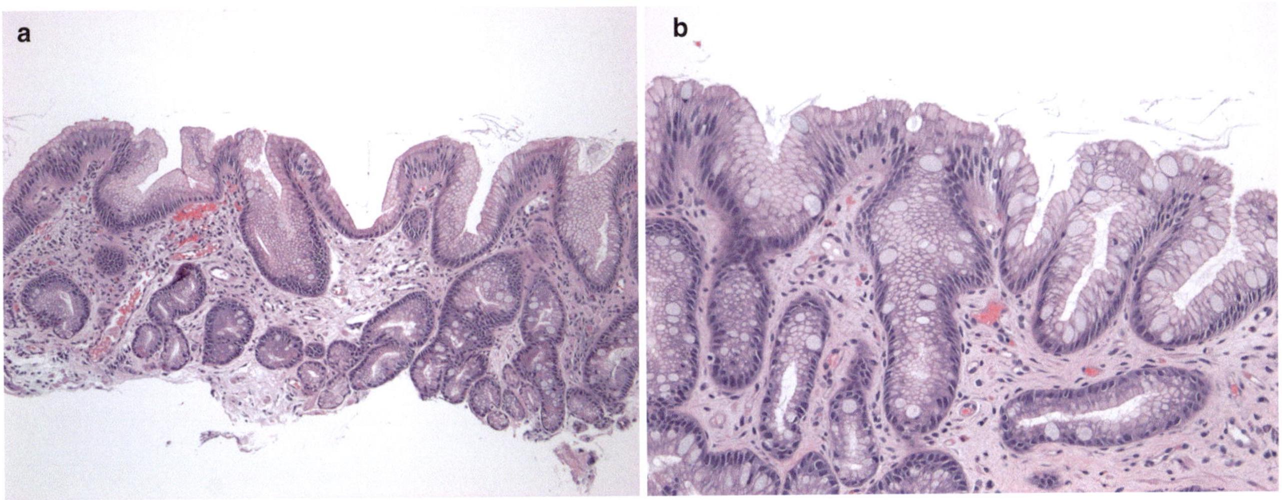

Fig. 9.2 (**a**) In this Barrett's mucosa, the surface has both short projections and undulations. The tubules are more evenly spaced and there is little inflammation in the lamina propria, which is also more vascular than in the previous two examples. There are very few mucus glands at the base. (**b**) The surface columnar cells usually contain pink-staining neutral mucins, much like normal gastric surface and pit cells. In this focus, goblet cells are numerous and easy to find

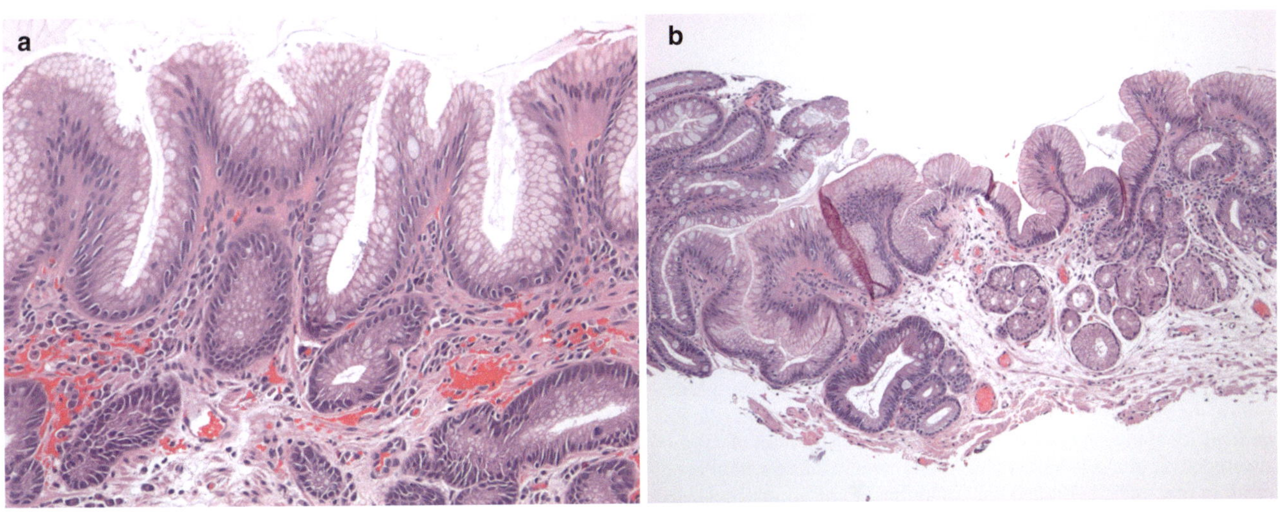

Fig. 9.3 (**a**) In this area, there are few goblet cells and they are mixed with columnar cells that have large rounded apical mucus vacuoles so that they resemble goblet cells, but they have pink-staining neutral mucin, like typical apical gastric surface cell mucin and not like the blue-staining goblet cell acid mucin. Because of the resemblance of these distended surface cell to goblet cells, they are sometimes referred to as "pseudogoblet cells." (**b**) Mosaic mucosa in a Barrett's biopsy. As in this field, it is common for stretches of typical Barrett's mucosa with goblet cells (*left*) to be mixed with nonintestinalized mucosa resembling cardiac mucosa (*right*). Such a biopsy may come from the Barrett's–cardiac junction, but it also may come from within an endoscopic Barrett's segment

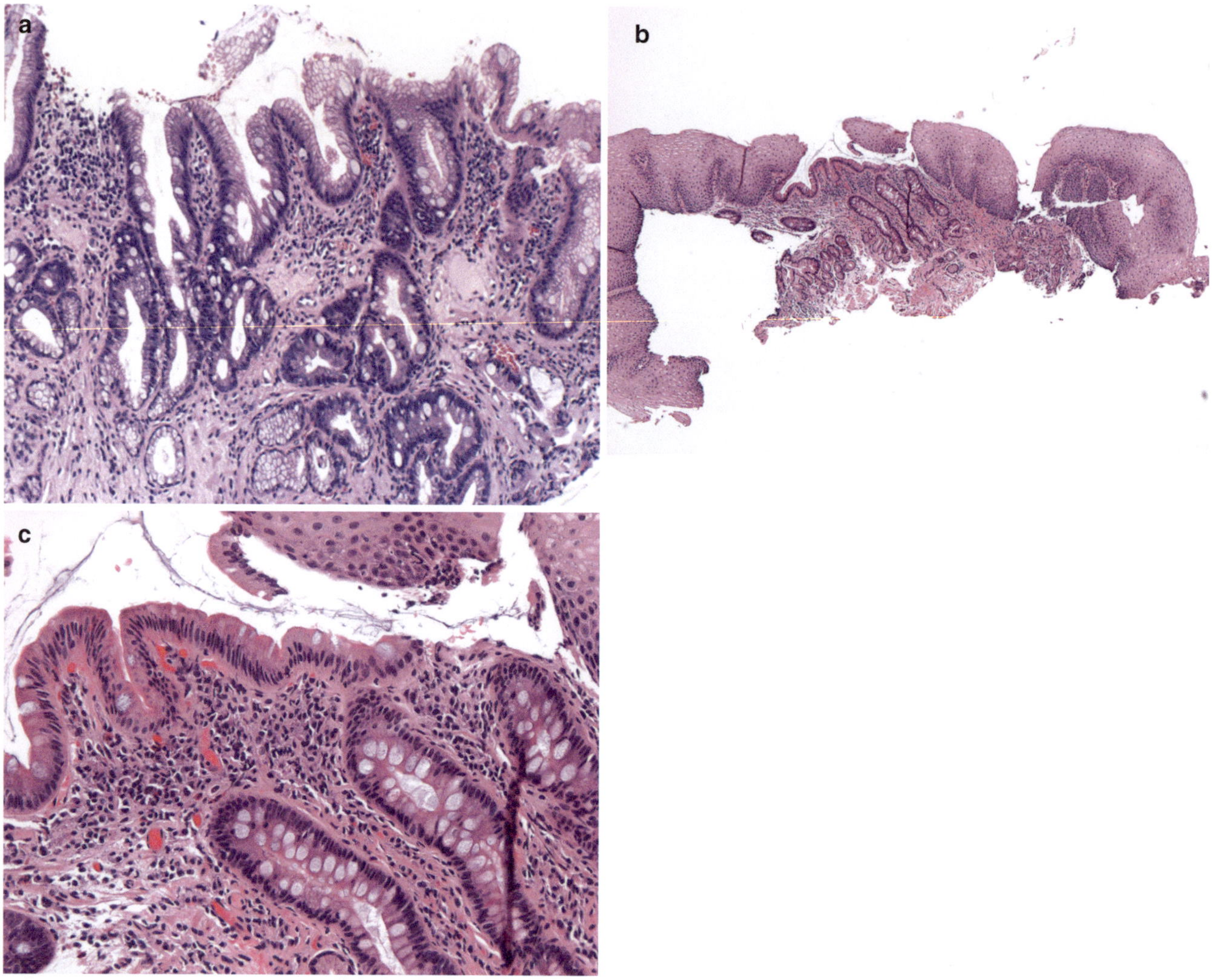

Fig. 9.4 (**a**) Chronic inflammation, characterized mainly by plasma cells in the lamina propria, is common in Barrett's mucosa. In fact, it is unusual for Barrett's mucosae not to have at least a light dusting of superficial plasma cells. The cause of this chronic inflammation is not clear. In one study, published only in abstract form, it was concluded that the inflammation was due to the reflux that was thought to cause Barrett's mucosa in the first place. (**b**) Complete intestinal metaplasia. In this low-power view of a biopsy from what looked endoscopically like a 1 cm segment of Barrett's mucosa, there is a central patch of goblet cell containing mucosa between two areas of squamous surface. (**c**) At high magnification, this epithelium is purely intestinal—*ie*, all the cells are intestinal type with goblet cells interspersed among cells that look exactly like small intestinal absorptive cells. In fact, the surface epithelium seems to have a brush border identical to that in normal small intestinal mucosa. In contrast, Barrett's mucosa typically has epithelium that is mainly gastric type surface cells with scattered goblet cells, often referred to as incomplete intestinal metaplasia. The incomplete form is known to be cancer associated in the stomach, whereas no data link the complete form with carcinoma. Since Barrett's mucosa is only important because of its cancer risk, it seems reasonable to limit the Barrett diagnosis only to incomplete intestinal metaplasia. However, there is no published information about whether the complete form, as in this illustration, is also diagnostic of Barrett's

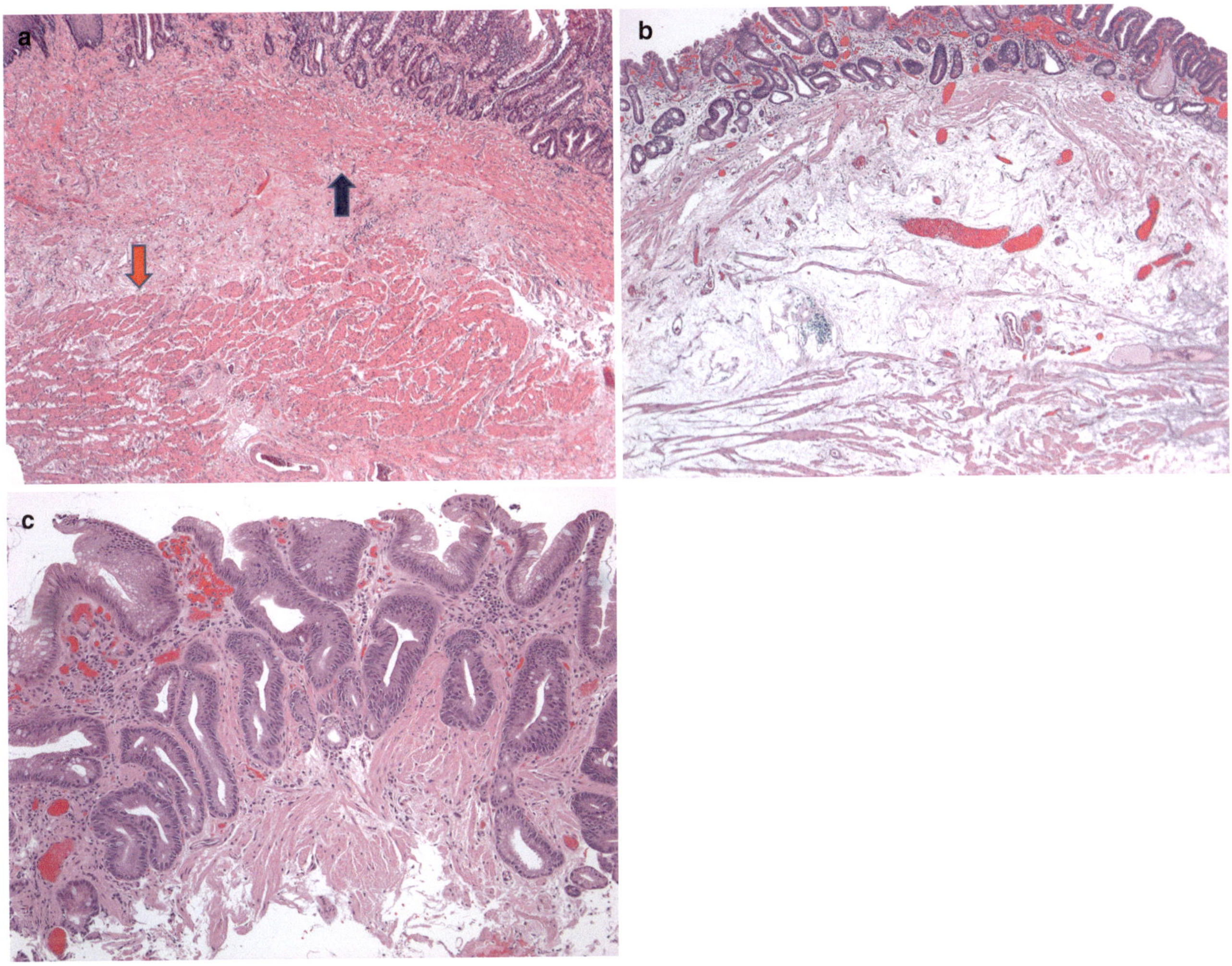

Fig. 9.5 Although the epithelium is almost always the featured component, Barrett's mucosa is really much more complicated. It is actually a complex epithelial–stromal change. The stromal changes involve smooth muscle alterations that tend to be spectacular but totally unexplained. Presumably whatever induces the columnar metaplasia also induces the stromal changes. (**a**) The double muscularis mucosae. In most Barrett's mucosae, there is a new layer of smooth muscle (*blue arrow*) beneath the metaplastic mucosa that parallels the muscularis mucosae; in other words, a duplication of the muscularis mucosae. This layer is often composed of loosely arranged muscle bundles and individual fibers. Beneath this new muscle layer is a loose fibrovascular layer that is actually lamina propria, thus a second or duplicated lamina propria. The deep smooth muscle layer (*red arrow*) is actually the original muscularis mucosae, and beneath this, as expected, is the submucosa. This duplication of the muscularis mucosae was discovered by a Japanese investigator [4, 5], which is remarkable because of the rarity of Barrett's mucosa in Japan. As a result of these muscle changes, Barrett's mucosa becomes a very thick mucosa with four discrete layers: (1) the mucosa containing the epithelium and lamina propria, (2) the duplicated muscularis mucosae, (3) the deep lamina propria between the two muscle layers, and (4) the original muscularis mucosae. A carcinoma that is limited to the mucosa can involve a lot of area in this setting. (**b**) Sometimes strips of smooth muscle fibers extend across the deep layer of lamina propria and connect the duplicated and original muscularis mucosae. (**c**) In some Barrett's mucosa, abundant smooth muscle, both in short bundles and single fibers, extends into the base of the mucosa, separating the glands and tubules. This muscle is an extension of the duplicated inner layer of muscularis mucosae (*see* Fig. 9.2a). Peculiarly, in such areas, the tubules surrounded by the muscle tend to have dark epithelium with enlarged, often stratified nuclei and diminished cytoplasmic mucus, thus mimicking low-grade dysplasia. This muscle-rich basal Barrett's may be the same as the abnormality referred to as the musculofibrous anomaly in Barrett's mucosa. It is unknown why this muscle rich lamina propria occurs. We tend to blame prolapse when we see such muscle in the mucosa in other parts of the gut, but there is no reason to blame prolapse for such changes in flat Barrett's mucosa

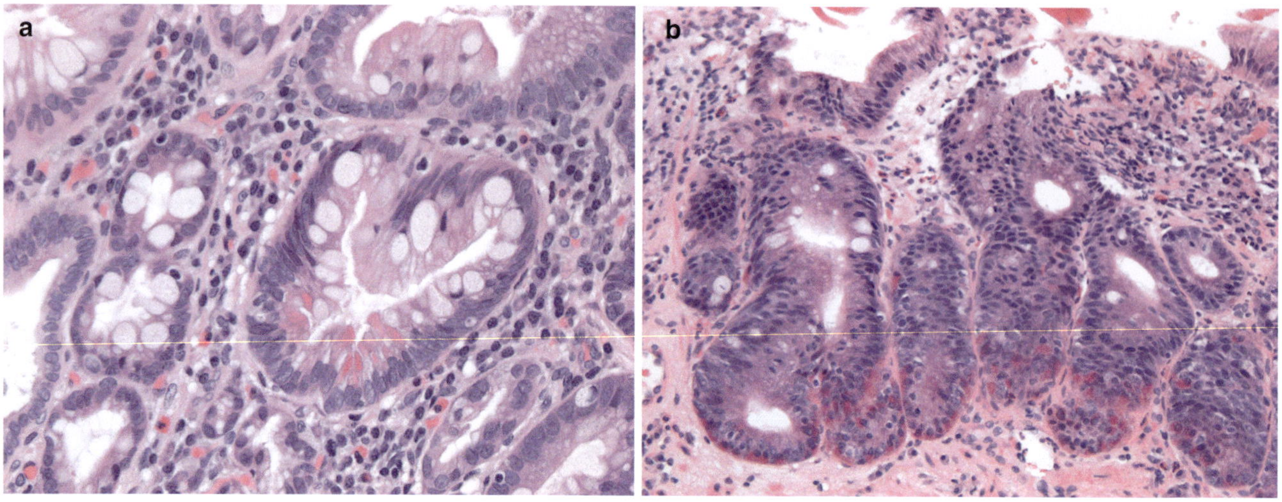

Fig. 9.6 Other epithelium in Barrett's mucosa. Fig. 9.1 includes all the typical epithelium found in every case of Barrett's mucosa, including the goblet cells, the columnar cells that separate the goblet cells, and the deep mucus glands. However, Barrett's mucosa is far more capable of epithelial diversity, so it is not uncommon to find additional epithelial types. (**a**) Some Barrett's mucosae have Paneth cells at the base of the tubules or even in the glands, although this is not well publicized. Theoretically, since Paneth cells are definitely intestinal cells, like goblet cells, they should be given the same stature as goblet cells in diagnosing intestinal metaplasia, but it seems that they have almost been completely ignored. (**b**) Some Barrett's mucosae contain endocrine cells toward the base of the tubules. This is an exaggerated example with multiple endocrine cells containing fine basal granules. These cells have been studied in small series, and they contain a variety of hormones and amines, mostly serotonin and somatostatin, but also pancreatic polypeptide and glucagon

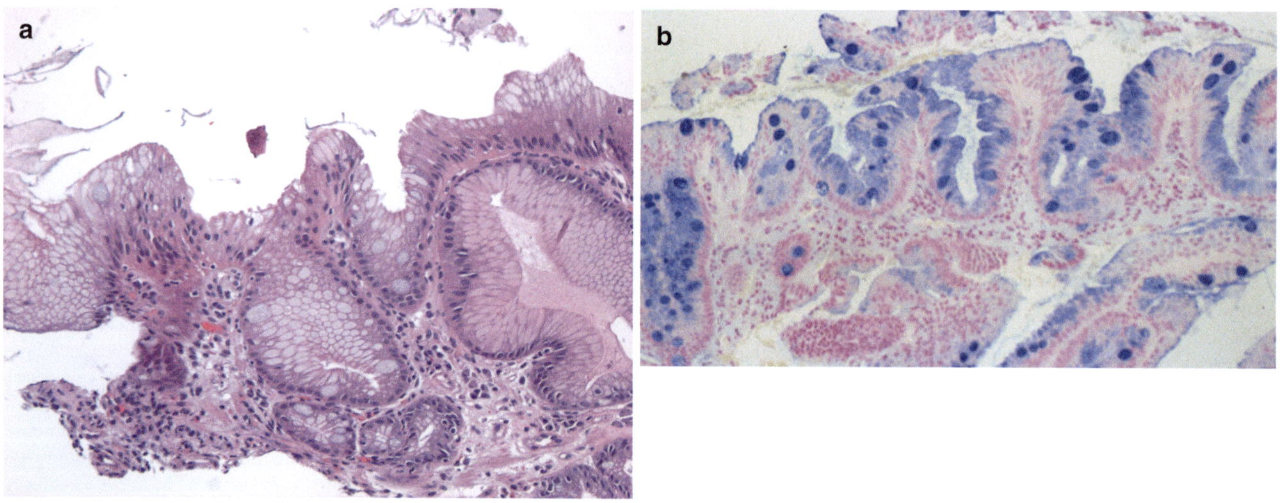

Fig. 9.7 (**a**) There are three types of mucin-containing columnar epithelia in this field. First, there are the goblet cells distended by pale blue-staining acid mucin in the center of the field. Second, mostly in the large tubule on the right, there are columnar cells with light pink-staining neutral mucin. These cells are identical to the cells that are on the surface of gastric mucosa and line the pits. Third, mainly on the left, there are columnar cells with gray or pale blue, rather than pink, mucin. These cells contain acid mucin similar to that in the goblet cells. In the large tubule in the center, these cells are mixed with goblet cells. (**b**) In the Alcian blue stain that stains acid mucins, the goblet cells are dark blue, but most of the cells that stain are the columnar cells that have pale blue mucin on hematoxylin and eosin (H and E). Because of the tinctorial qualities of the mucin, these cells have been named "columnar blues." They are sometimes confused with goblet cells. They definitely are metaplastic cells in terms of their mucin content, but they have not been given the same stature as goblet cells in defining intestinal metaplasia and in diagnosing Barrett's mucosa

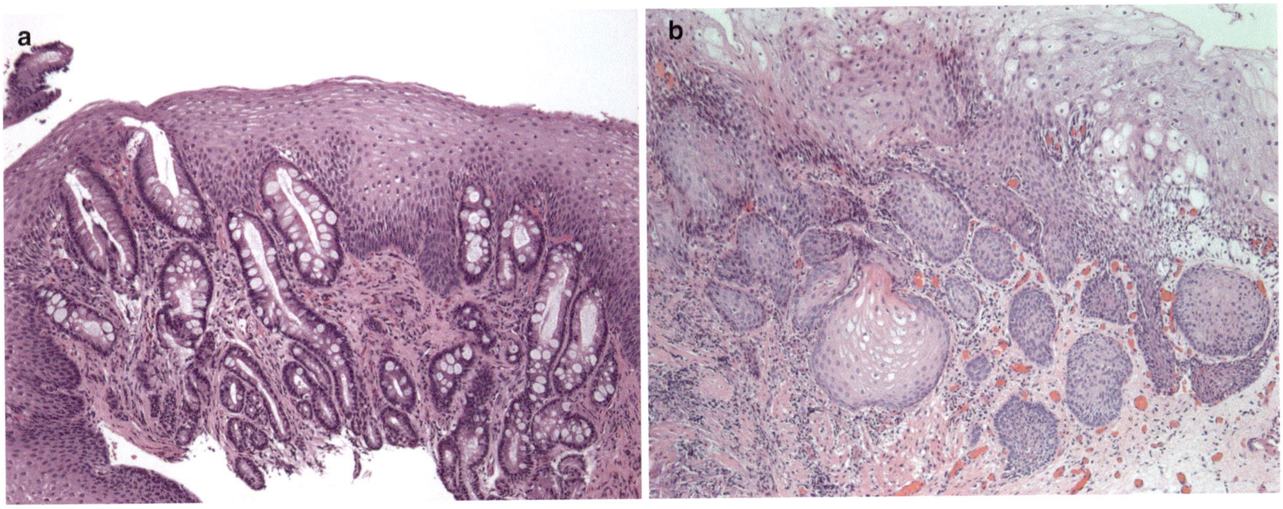

Fig. 9.8 (**a**) Squamous metaplasia. Barrett's esophagus, a columnar metaplasia of a squamous mucosa, can undergo a return to a squamous surface; in other words, squamous metaplasia of the columnar metaplasia. This can occur in two ways. First, squamous epithelium from proximal to the Barrett's segment can grow distally covering the Barrett's tubules and burying them as in this view. These buried tubules may be endoscopically invisible. (**b**) Sometimes, the metaplastic squamous epithelium grows down into the Barrett's tubules eventually replacing them, resulting in club-shaped prongs of mature squamous epithelium extending into the lamina propria where many are cut across producing this peculiar architecture. This looks identical to the common squamous metaplasia in the uterine cervix. It also can be confused with invasive squamous carcinoma

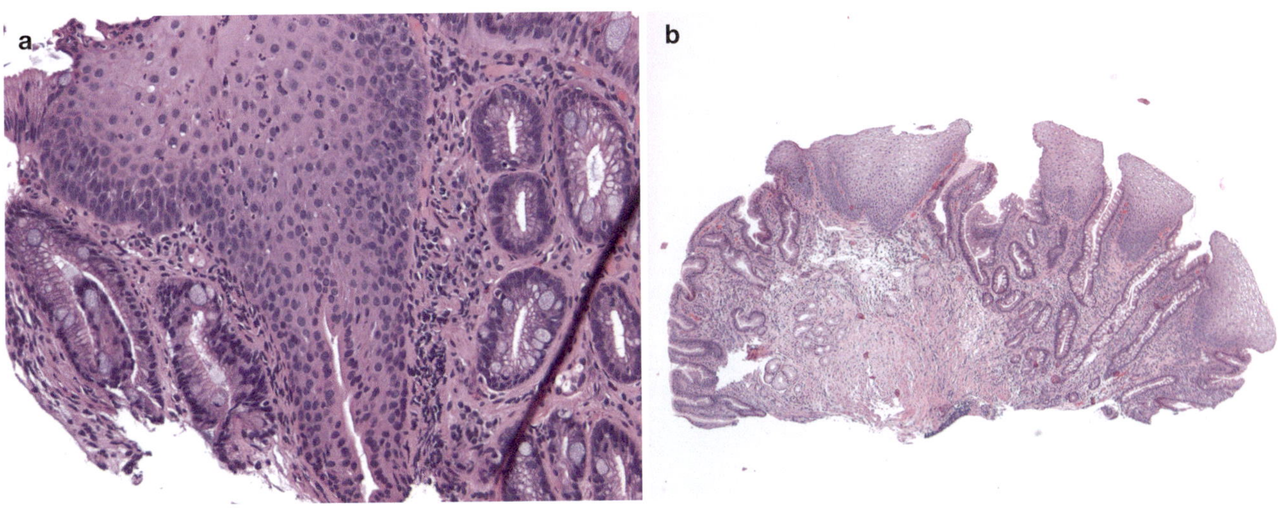

Fig. 9.9 (**a**) The second form of metaplasia is the squamous island, a patch of squamous epithelium in the middle of a stretch of Barrett's mucosa. These islands seem to develop exclusively over the orifices of esophageal submucosal gland ducts, and such a duct can be seen at the base of the squamous island in this image. (**b**) We suspect that squamous islands can spread or even coalesce with adjacent islands. In this image, there are four such islands so close together that it does not take much imagination to merge them. Large squamous islands can be seen endoscopically as pale foci surrounded by the pink Barrett's mucosa. It is thought that the use of proton pump inhibitors may stimulate one or both patterns of squamous metaplasia

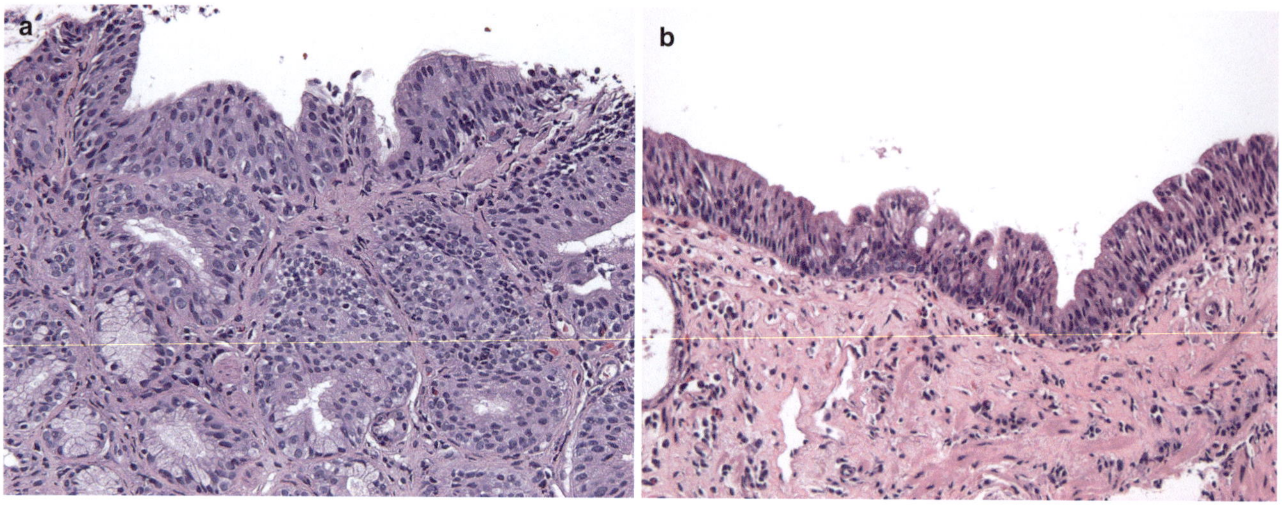

Fig. 9.10 (**a**) Multilayered epithelium: a final type of epithelium is the multilayered epithelium, seen on the surface in this field. It has a squamous look to the base and there are often cells with apical mucus on the surface. This is another type of metaplastic epithelium. It is thought by some Barrett's devotees that this epithelium is the intermediate between normal squamous and Barrett's, but it also resembles immature squamous metaplasia in the uterine cervix, so perhaps it is a precursor of squamous metaplasia. It also occasionally is found in the gastric cardia. (**b**) In some Barrett's mucosae, this multilayered epithelium even resembles the epithelium of the anal transitional zone

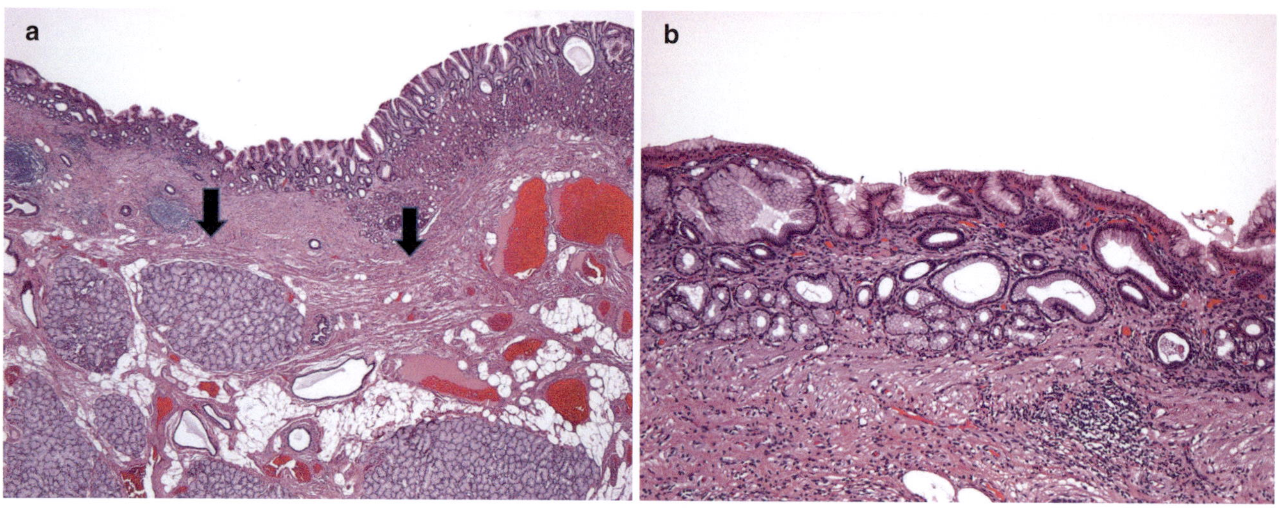

Fig. 9.11 Columnar epithelia in biopsies said to come from the tubular distal esophagus that are not diagnostic of Barrett's mucosa in the United States but may satisfy the Barrett's diagnosis elsewhere. It is not uncommon for biopsies said to come from the distal esophagus to have columnar epithelium but no goblet cells or Paneth cells. According to the diagnostic criteria for Barrett's mucosa currently accepted in the United States and many other countries, goblet cells are required, because their presence is the only proven marker of a metaplastic epithelium at risk for the development of adenocarcinoma. However, the goblet cells must be accompanied by the endoscopic findings of mucosa that resembles Barrett's mucosa and is clearly within the tubular esophagus. However, the current diagnostic criteria for Barrett's in the United Kingdom and in several countries do not require goblet cells, but they do require columnar mucosa that is proven to be in the tubular esophagus by endoscopic examination. The following are a few examples of this non-goblet cell–containing esophageal columnar epithelium. We are not certain how to explain its presence in the esophagus. Perhaps it is truly a metaplasia, but one without cancer risk or perhaps it is a normal variant—that is, distal esophagus lined by proximal gastric mucosa. (**a**) This image was taken from a resected esophagus. The glands toward the bottom are typical normal submucosal esophageal glands, proof that this field is within the tubular esophagus. The covering mucosa is gastric body (oxyntic) mucosa with its typical large glandular compartment and smaller pit compartment on the right. Thinner columnar mucosa extends from there all the way to the left edge of the photo. There was not a single goblet cell in this columnar mucosa, so, therefore, it was not Barrett's in the United States, but it is Barrett's in the United Kingdom. The muscularis mucosae is situated over the glands (*arrows*). (**b**) This is a closer look at the columnar mucosa covering the distal esophagus. It looks like cardiac mucosa with equal thickness of both pits and mucus gland. Notice, however, a layer of smooth muscle under this mucosa, so it appears that this is a duplicated muscularis mucosae, identical to that in Barrett's mucosae. However, as of now, duplicated muscularis mucosae is not part of the diagnostic criteria for Barrett's mucosa

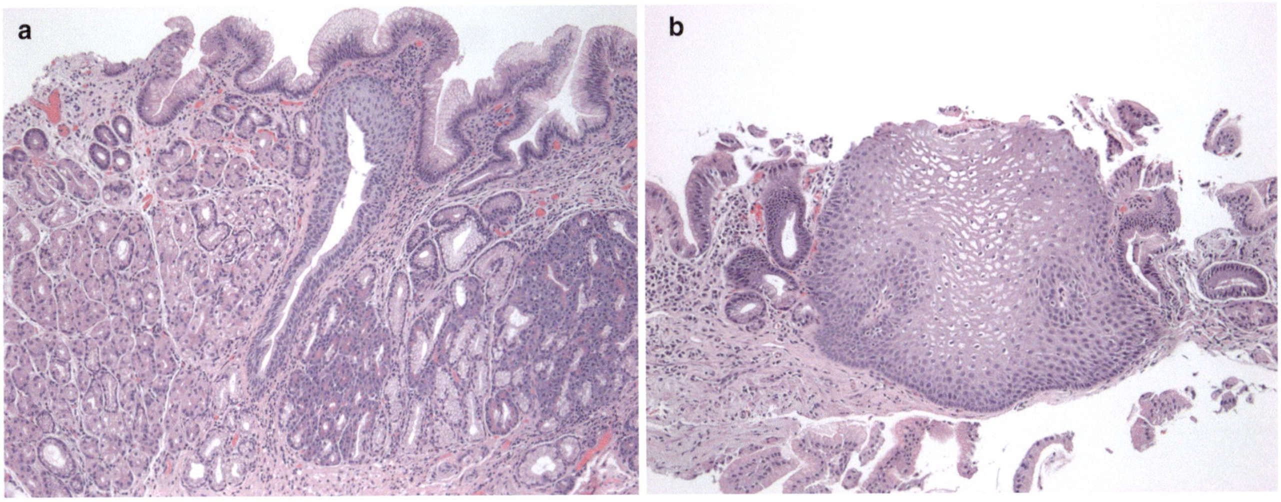

Fig. 9.12 (**a**) In this biopsy, in the center of the mucosa, there is a duct of a submucosal gland, clear evidence of location if the tubular esophagus. On the left of the duct, the mucosa looks like gastric body or oxyntic mucosa with parietal cells in the glands. On the right of the duct, there is a patch of glands with mucus cells mixed with dark cells that are pancreatic acinar cells. This peculiar change is referred to as pancreatic acinar metaplasia, an extraordinarily common finding in gastric cardia mucosa but a very rare finding in Barrett's mucosa, if it even occurs there. There are no goblet cells needed to diagnose Barrett's. (**b**) In this field, in the middle of columnar mucosa resembling cardiac mucosa without goblet cells, there is a squamous island. Since these islands develop over the orifices of submucosal gland ducts, this biopsy must have come from the tubular esophagus. We do not diagnose this as Barrett's because it lacks goblet cells

References

1. Wang KK, Sampliner RE. Updated guidelines 2008 for the diagnosis, surveillance and therapy of Barrett's esophagus. Am J Gastroenterol. 2008;103:788–97.
2. Spechler SJ, Sharma P, Souza RF, et al. American Gastroenterological Association Medical Position Statement on the Management of Barrett's Esophagus. Gastroenterology. 2011;140:1084–91.
3. Playford RJ. New British society of gastroenterology (BSG) guidelines for the diagnosis and management of Barrett's oesophagus. Gut. 2006;55:442–3.
4. Kato H, Iizuka T, Watanabe H, et al. Double adenocarcinoma in Barrett's esophagus. Jpn J Clin Oncol. 1981;11:523–30.
5. Takubo K, Sasajima K, Yamashita K, et al. Double muscularis mucosae in Barrett's esophagus. Hum Pathol. 1991;22:1158–61.

10 Dysplasia and Dysplasia Mimics in Barrett's Mucosa

Dysplasia in the gastrointestinal tract, including that in Barrett's mucosa, is defined as epithelium that is unequivocally neoplastic, a determination that is currently the responsibility of pathologists. Pathologists identify unequivocally neoplastic epithelium based on a set of microscopic features that are both cytologic and architectural. Among the cytologic features is loss of cytoplasmic maturation, which actually means lack of mucin. However, most cytologic features involve the nuclei and include enlargement, hyperchromatism, pleomorphism, and increased number of mitoses, especially atypical mitoses. Among the architectural features are stratification of these atypical nuclei. Additional architectural changes include crowding of tubules lined by these cells in places where tubules in nondysplastic mucosa are not found, such as superficially beneath the surface epithelium. An exaggerated villiform surface with elongated surface projections is another potential dysplastic architectural change. In addition, as the grade of dysplasia increases, there may be additional architectural abnormalities such as budding and branching of tubules. All of these abnormalities vary in intensity or degree. In simple terms, low-grade dysplasia has enough of these features to indicate to the pathologist that the epithelium is more atypical than any reactive or regenerative epithelium, but not as many of these features are present as in high-grade dysplasia. Low-grade dysplasia is not a single histologic entity but a collection of histologic entities that we decide to call by that name. As a result, published studies on low grade dysplasia are not dealing with a single entity but with the many epithelia placed in that category. Furthermore, since agreement on the diagnosis of low-grade dysplasia, even among experienced pathologists, is known to be poor, such published studies may not even be dealing with the same entities.

High-grade dysplasia has more of these features than pathologists allow for low-grade dysplasia. Like low-grade dysplasia, published studies of high-grade dysplasia also do not deal with a single entity but with a collection. However, since there is better agreement among different pathologists on the diagnosis of high-grade than of low-grade dysplasia, studies of high-grade dysplasia are likely to include more similar entities.

Management of patients depends on whether there is dysplasia or not, and if there is, whether it is low- or high-grade. Thus, the two critical distinctions are (1) between nondysplastic and low-grade dysplasia and (2) between low- and high-grade dysplasia. Unfortunately, no specific guidelines separate the highest end of low grade from the lowest end of high grade, and no specific features separate the lowest end of low-grade dysplasia from the most intense regenerative epithelium that shares histologic features with low-grade dysplasia.

The illustrations in this chapter are our attempt to give the viewer some insight as to how we diagnose dysplasia and how we give it a grade. These images are taken from our in-house cases and cases sent to us in consultation by other pathologists. As a result, it becomes obvious that there are differences in preparation from one illustration to the next. We expect that some viewers may not agree with our diagnoses, and this is more likely to occur in cases we label as low-grade dysplasia. It has been proven in numerous studies that most disagreement on diagnosis, even among pathologists with extensive experience in Barrett's epithelial changes, occurs at the low-grade end of the spectrum. Finally, there are epithelial changes that almost appear like dysplasia to some—not necessarily all—pathologists, even the most experienced. These are the epithelia that are thrown into the broad, undefined category known as "indefinite for dysplasia." This chapter, as almost all other chapters dealing with Barrett's mucosa, concentrates on images from biopsies, since these are what pathologists mainly see.

S.R. Owens, H.D. Appelman, *Atlas of Esophagus and Stomach Pathology*, Atlas of Anatomic Pathology,
DOI 10.1007/978-1-4614-8084-6_10,

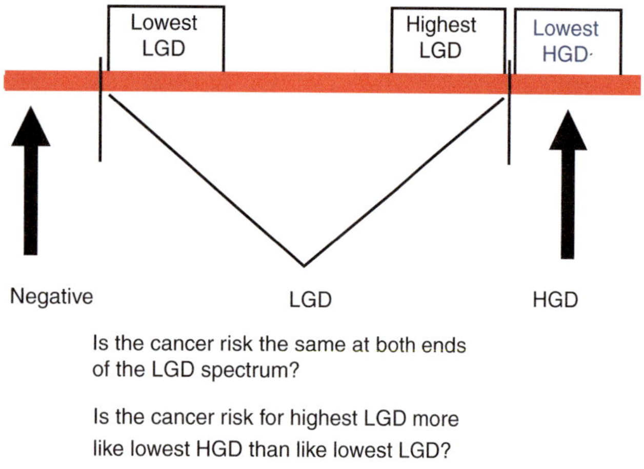

Fig. 10.1 Management of patients depends on existence of dysplasia and whether it is low-grade dysplasia (LGD) or high-grade dysplasia (HGD). Thus, critical distinctions exist between (1) nondysplastic and low-grade dysplasia and (2) low- and high-grade dysplasia. In this cartoon, the LGD area is expanded to emphasize the fact that there are both a lowest end and a highest end of LGD. There are two important distinctions we pathologists are asked to make, the point where nondysplastic or indefinite epithelium ends and the lowest end of LGD begins and the point where the highest end of LGD ends and the lowest end of HGD begins. Management decisions depend on our being able to make these distinctions, which, as is clear from this cartoon, are virtually impossible distinctions

10.1 Low-Grade Dysplasia from the Lowest End to the Highest

What exactly is low-grade dysplasia? The answer is obvious. It is dysplastic epithelium because some pathologist has decided that it is unequivocally neoplastic, and it has the changes listed in the introduction to this chapter, but it does not have those changes in the intensity or degree of high-grade dysplasia. In other words, low-grade dysplasia looks worse than nondysplastic epithelium and better than high-grade dysplasia. This is unassailable truth. In more concrete terms, low-grade dysplasia has nuclear enlargement but little pleomorphism, so nuclear uniformity is the rule. Furthermore, the nuclear stratification is limited mainly to the basal two thirds of the cells. Then there is clear cytoplasmic maturation with mucin and maybe even goblet cells. Thus, this epithelium sort of resembles that in typical colorectal adenomas. The tubules lined by this epithelium may be crowded toward the surface but not so crowded as to obliterate the lamina propria between them. Unfortunately, some of these characteristics are shared with intensely regenerating epithelium, which makes separating these two epithelial types often challenging. Figure 10.2 provides some examples of epithelia that satisfy our concepts of low-grade dysplasia and some that pose problems for us, and likely for readers as well.

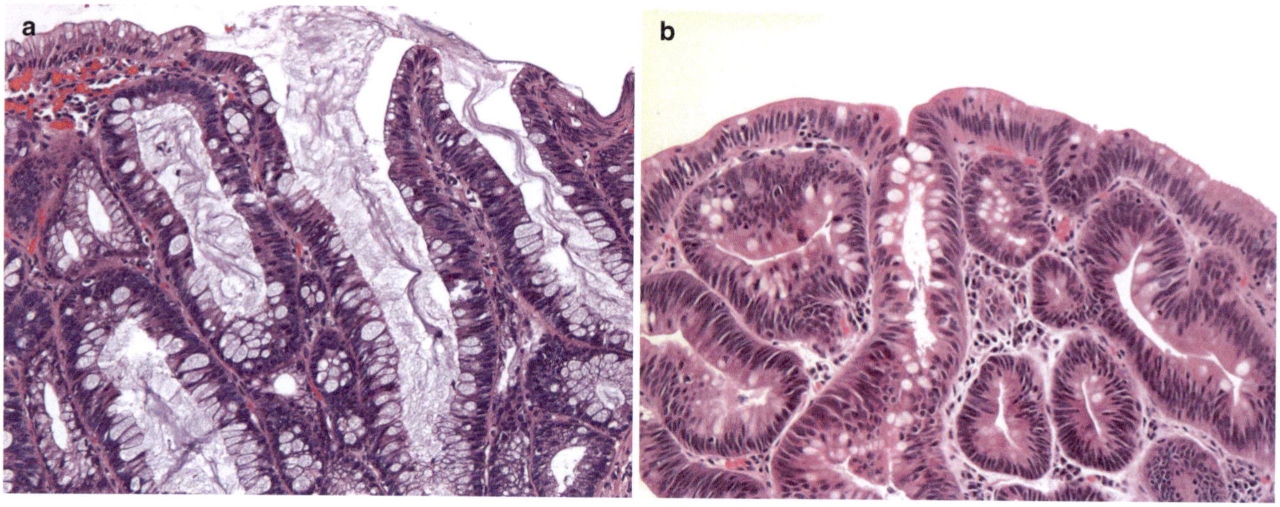

Fig. 10.2 (**a**) This low-grade dysplasia has prominent cytoplasmic maturation with numerous goblet cells and cells with apical mucus. The nuclei are elongated (penicillate) but are remarkably uniform, with stratification limited to the basal half of the cells. The tubules are uniform in size and orientation. (**b**) In this example, crowded superficial tubules vary somewhat in size, shape, and orientation (unlike in **a**) but plenty of lamina propria also separates them. The cells lining the tubules and extending onto the surface have enlarged and hyperchromatic nuclei that stratify about halfway up the cell height, and they are slightly less uniform than in **a**. There is obvious cytoplasmic maturation with goblet cells and cells that have apical pink mucus. In general, there is more cytoplasmic maturation toward the surface than at the base. The nuclei are the most uniform in size, shape, and orientation in the surface epithelium

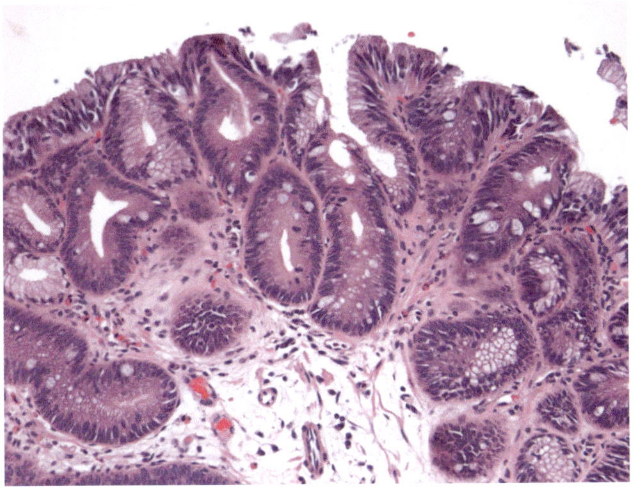

Fig. 10.3 In this example, there are fewer goblet cells but more cells with apical mucus and more cells without apparent cytoplasmic maturation. However, the nuclei are remarkably uniform and basally stratified. There are also more mitoses than in the previous examples. The superficially crowded tubules are all the same size.

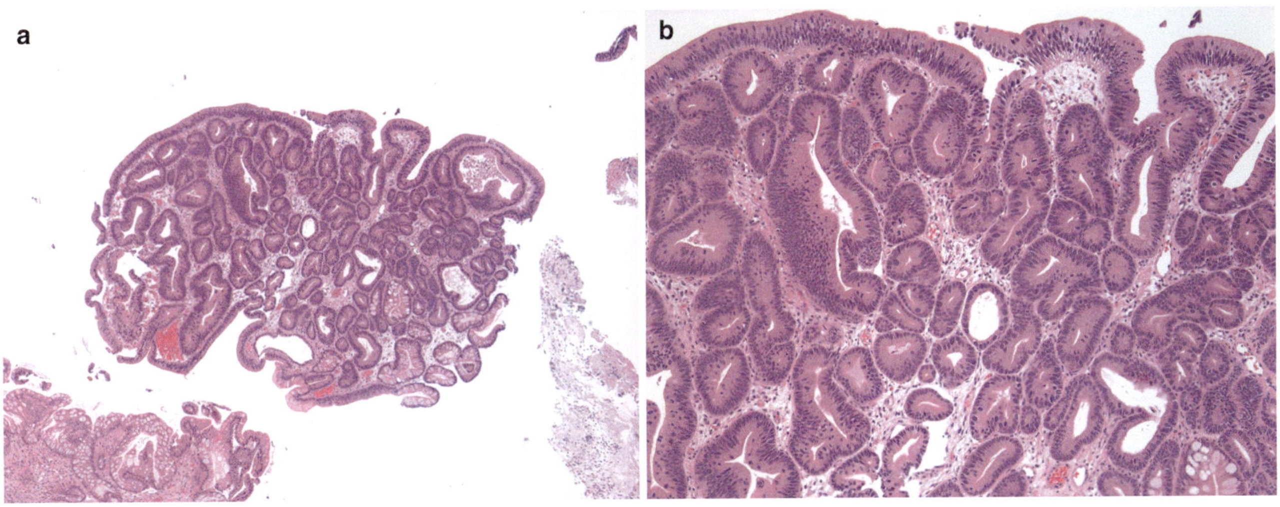

Fig. 10.4 (**a**) This was a small polyp in the middle of a Barrett's segment. At low power, there are clustered tubules, most of which are small and uniform, but there are some larger, irregularly shaped forms. This polyp closely resembles a typical colonic adenoma (**b**) At higher magnification, the dysplastic epithelium has little cytoplasmic mucin or goblet cells. The nuclei are mostly uniform, elongated, and stratified in the lower half of the cells, but there are scattered larger, rounder nuclei, suggesting perhaps the emergence of some subtle high-grade features. Nevertheless, we still grade this as low because of the dominant uniformity

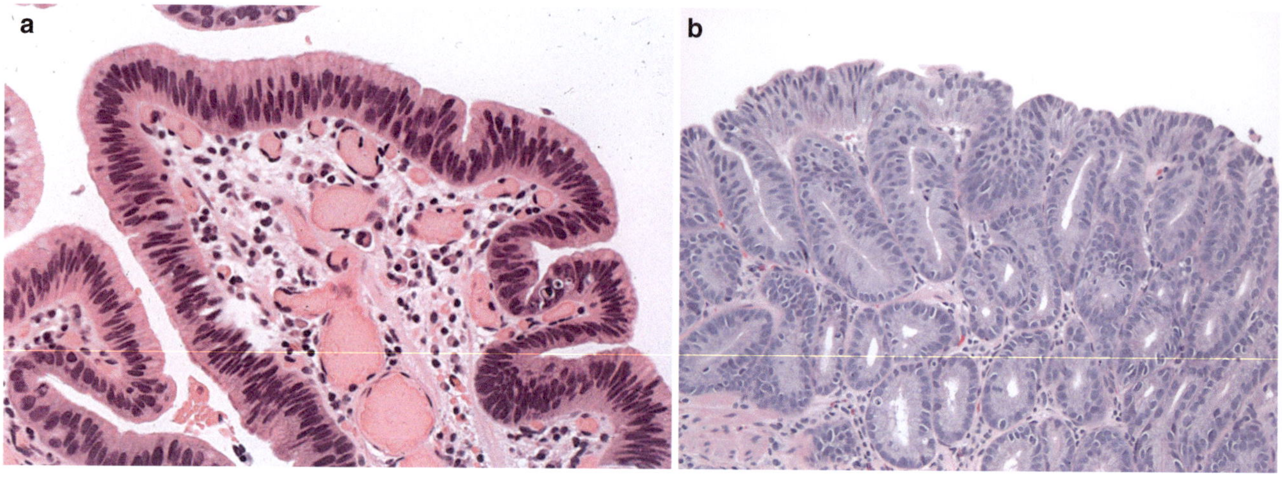

Fig. 10.5 (**a**) The highest end of low-grade dysplasia versus the lowest end of high-grade dysplasia. This is a tough epithelium to grade. The cells have very little apical mucus, so there is hardly any maturation. The nuclei are totally uniform, elongated, and confined to the basal half of the cells. However, these nuclei are larger and much more hyperchromatic than in the above examples. Thus, this example has the uniformity of a low-grade dysplasia but other changes that resemble those in high-grade dysplasia. (**b**) Another example of the border between low- and high-grade dysplasias. There is prominent crowding of tubules beneath the surface that vary in size but not in shape. The nuclei are a mixture of elongated and round with variable stratification that is basal in the tubules but nuclear stratification is full thickness on the surface and in the middle. However, there is little nuclear hyperchromatism and pleomorphism, and mitoses are not prominent. As with Fig. 10.4b above, the background in this example looks low-grade with the emergence of high-grade features, especially full-thickness stratification on the surface

10.2 High-Grade Dysplasia

High-grade dysplasia is not a single entity but it is a group of epithelial changes characterized by architectural abnormalities such a crowding of subsurface tubules and cytologic changes that generally include nuclear enlargement, pleomorphism, numerous mitoses, and full thickness nuclear stratification, and these changes are more advanced (*ie*, more obvious histologically) than in low-grade dysplasia. The more these changes occur together in an epithelium, the easier it is to make the high-grade dysplasia diagnosis. There are two significant problems in the high-grade dysplasia area. The first is differentiation of the lowest end of high grade from the highest end of low-grade dysplasia. This was dealt with somewhat unsatisfactorily in the last two images of Fig. 10.2. The second problem is identifying subtle changes that indicate that there is adenocarcinoma invading the lamina propria. These will be dealt with in Fig. 10.4. The images in this figure cover only a minute fraction of the high-grade dysplastic spectrum.

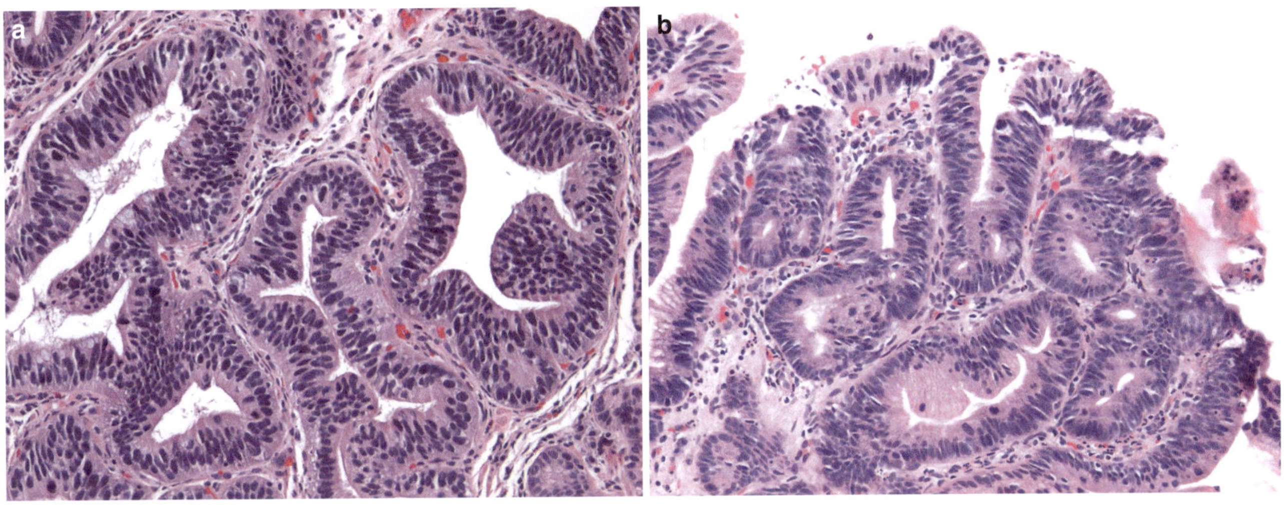

Fig. 10.6 (**a**) Easy to diagnose high-grade dysplasia has cells with little if any cytoplasmic differentiation, enlarged hyperchromatic nuclei leading to a high N:C ratio, full-thickness nuclear stratification. These cells line irregularly shaped and crowded tubules. (**b**) The tubules are much the same size but their orientation is not uniform. The lining cells are columnar with hyperchromatic nuclei and vary from elongate to round. Mitoses are numerous. Nuclear stratification varies from basal to full thickness especially toward and on the surface. Some cells toward the base have lots of cytoplasm but this is lost toward the surface

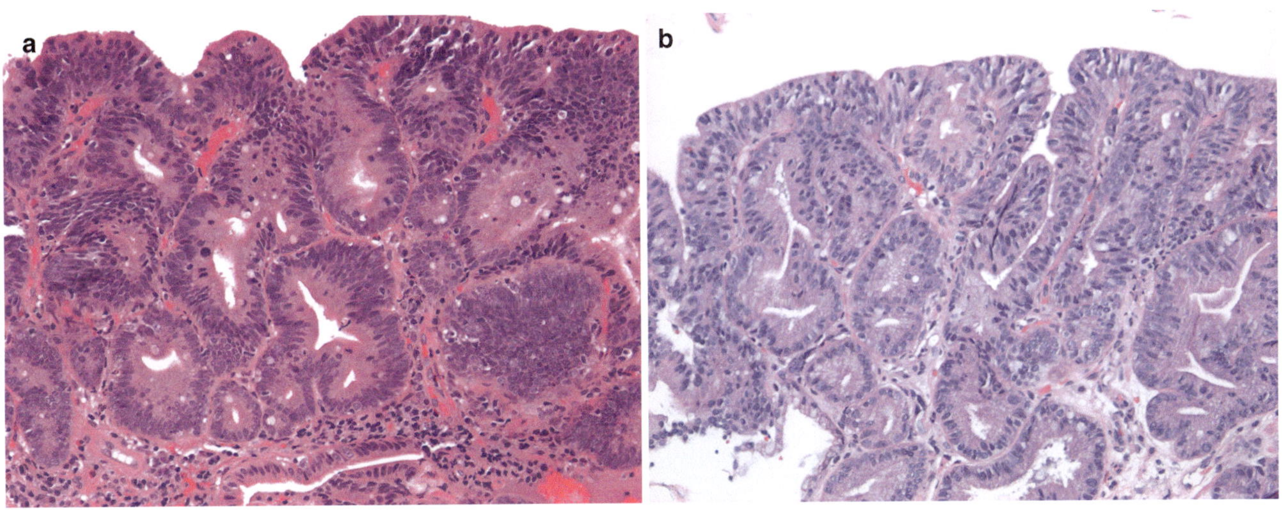

Fig. 10.7 (**a**) Dark epithelium with undifferentiated cytoplasm with hardly any maturation except for a few goblet cells lines these crowded tubules. The nuclei are hyperchromatic and stratified with full-thickness stratification on the surface. Mitoses, some of which are on the surface, are easily found. (**b**) Another example with crowded superficial tubules lined by epithelium with little cytoplasmic maturation. Here the nuclei are not so hyperchromatic, possibly because the hematoxylin was weaker, but many of the nuclei are round with prominent nuclei. Nuclear stratification is full thickness superficially

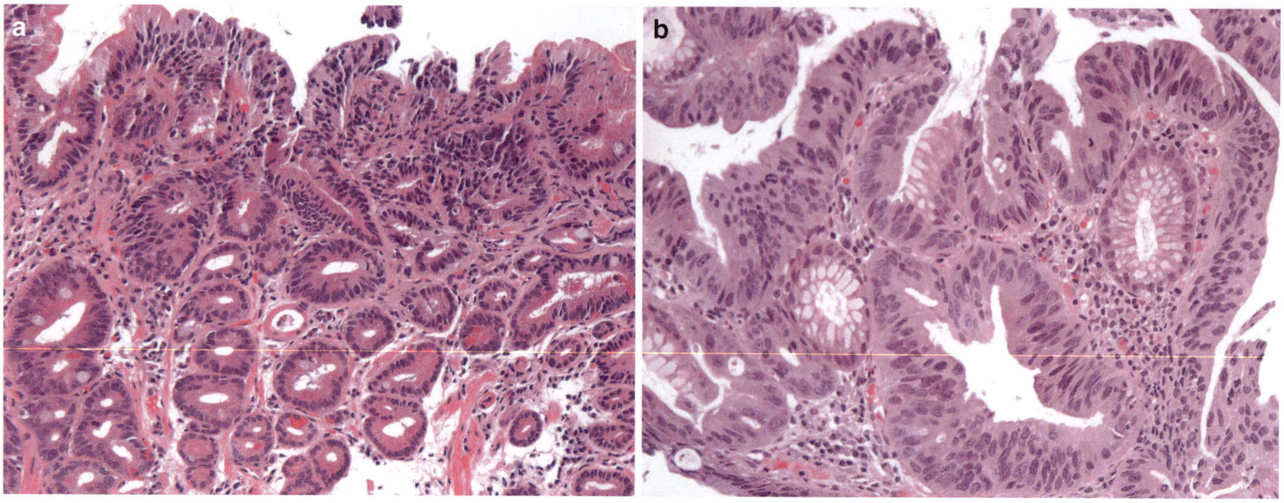

Fig. 10.8 (**a**) Superficial high-grade dysplasia. Here the cells lining the tubules toward the bottom have goblet cell and Paneth cell maturation and small basal nuclei. Near the middle of the image, the tubules become closer together, goblet and Paneth cells are lost, and the nuclei are larger, more elongated, and stratified, with full thickness stratification on the surface. Mitoses are easily found. (**b**) The mixture of high-grade dysplastic and nondysplastic epithelium. Much of the epithelium lining the tubules and covering the surface has features similar to those pictured in Figs. 10.6, 10.7, and 10.8a, even with some surface mitoses. However, two superficial tubules and a short stretch of surface epithelium have no dysplastic features. The cells have apical mucus and small basal uniform nuclei

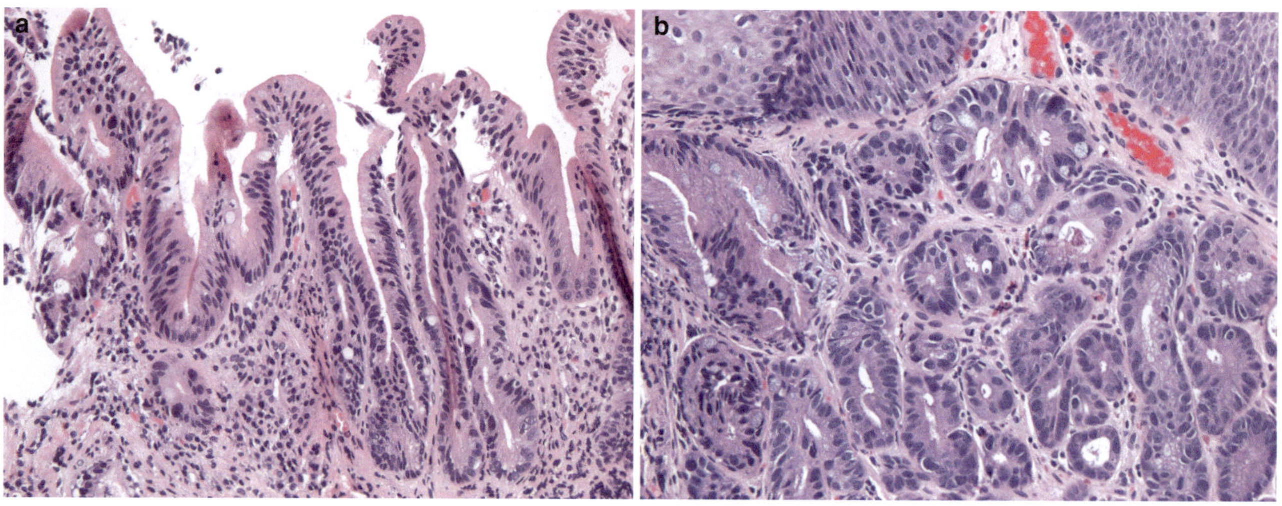

Fig. 10.9 (**a**) A patch of high-grade dysplastic epithelium on the surface and extending into a few long tubules. The surface epithelium has large, hyperchromatic, and focally fully stratified nuclei mixed with more differentiated epithelium with goblet cells and small basal nuclei. The abnormal epithelium involves the superficial half of a few adjacent elongated tubules. One separate tubule (*right*) has cells with some very large hyperchromatic nuclei. This was the only patch of high-grade dysplasia in multiple biopsies. This raises the issue of how much epithelium with high-grade features is required to make a confident, high-grade diagnosis. Because there is no rule, each pathologist must make the decision independently. (**b**) Beneath the squamous epithelium is a cluster of tubules with high-grade epithelium that has large, hyperchromatic, pleomorphic nuclei, and a vaguely cribriform architecture. This is likely to be given a variety of diagnoses, anywhere from indefinite for dysplasia to high-grade dysplasia. When dysplasias involve the surface epithelium, diagnosis is much easier than when they are covered by either nondysplastic Barrett's epithelium or metaplastic squamous epithelium

10.3 High-Grade Dysplasia with Changes Suspicious for Invasive Adenocarcinoma in the Lamina Propria

In a few studies, in biopsies of Barrett's mucosae, certain histologic changes superimposed on high-grade dysplasia were found to be associated with invasive adenocarcinoma in resected specimens. However, these changes by themselves were not convincing for a carcinoma diagnosis. We refer to them as "changes suspicious for carcinoma." It appears that the more of these changes that are present in a biopsy, the more likely that there is a carcinoma nearby or even at the base of a superficial biopsy. The microscopic diagnostic criteria for the most incipient of lamina propria invasion are not defined. Perhaps single cells or small clusters of neoplastic cells in the lamina propria separate from the dysplastic tubules qualify for the minimal criteria. Readers of this section may take exception with our diagnoses and call some of these outright "invasive carcinoma."

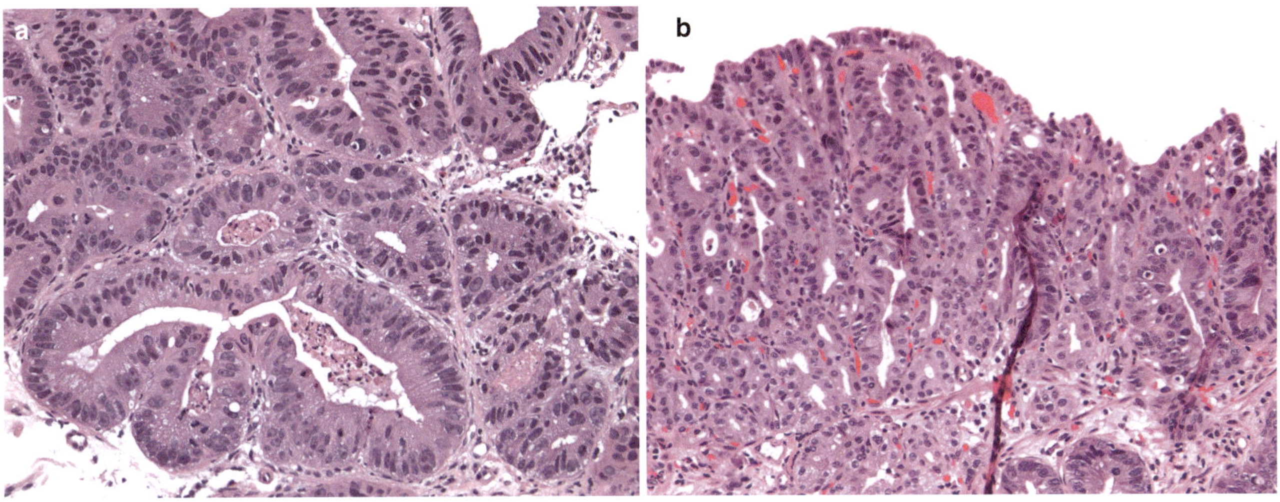

Fig. 10.10 (**a**) Tubules, generally with simple architecture, lined by high-grade dysplastic epithelium, two of which contain necrotic debris. We suggest that dysplasia alone does not lead to necrosis, whereas necrosis is a common finding in carcinomas. (**b**) Complex superficial crowded tubules. Although the tubules extending downward from the surface are parallel and of relatively uniform size, some have a vaguely cribriform architecture and have compressed the lamina propria to the point where in places it is not even recognizable

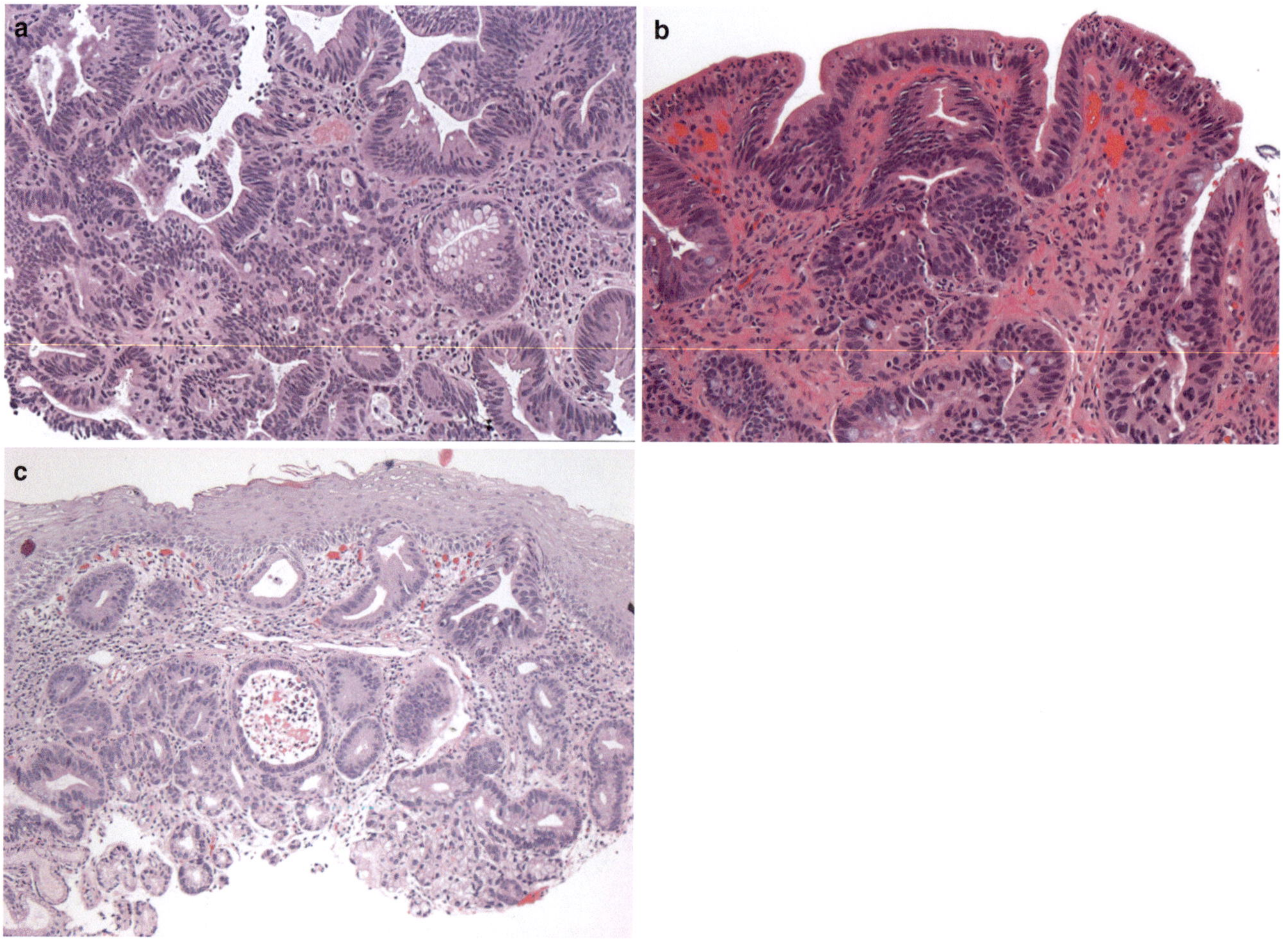

Fig. 10.11 (**a**) Complex tubular architecture. In the center, beneath the surface, there is a tubule lined by dysplastic epithelium that has an obvious cribriform architecture. Other cribriform but less complex tubules are found in the upper and middle-left side of the field. (**b**) Neutrophils in clearly dysplastic epithelium. The surface dysplastic epithelium contains numerous neutrophils. A few neutrophils are also present in the epithelium lining the tubule on the right, which also has a cribriform architecture at its base. (**c**) A mixture of features suspicious for adenocarcinoma occurring beneath an intact squamous epithelial surface. The dilated tubule in the middle contains necrotic debris. At the lower right is a complex tubular cluster with cribriform architecture. Another complex tubule abuts the base of the squamous epithelium, raising the possibility that it is in the process of invading that epithelium

10.4 Indefinites for Dysplasia

Indefinites for dysplasia are marked by changes that may seem almost like low-grade dysplasia and also almost like regenerative epithelium but are not convincing for either. Trying to illustrate a convincing indefinite for dysplasia is almost a guarantee of failure, since it has no criteria, is virtually not reproducible, and never looks the same on more than one viewing. Furthermore, all pathologists are likely to have their concepts of indefinite, and it is impossible to argue about the diagnosis. My concept of indefinite for dysplasia is epithelium that looks like dysplasia but lacks one or more aspects that I cannot define, and this lack prevents my making the dysplasia diagnosis. Perhaps we and the patients would be better off if we got rid of the indefinite concept entirely. The images in Fig. 10.5 are taken from consult cases that were sent to us with the diagnosis of indefinite.

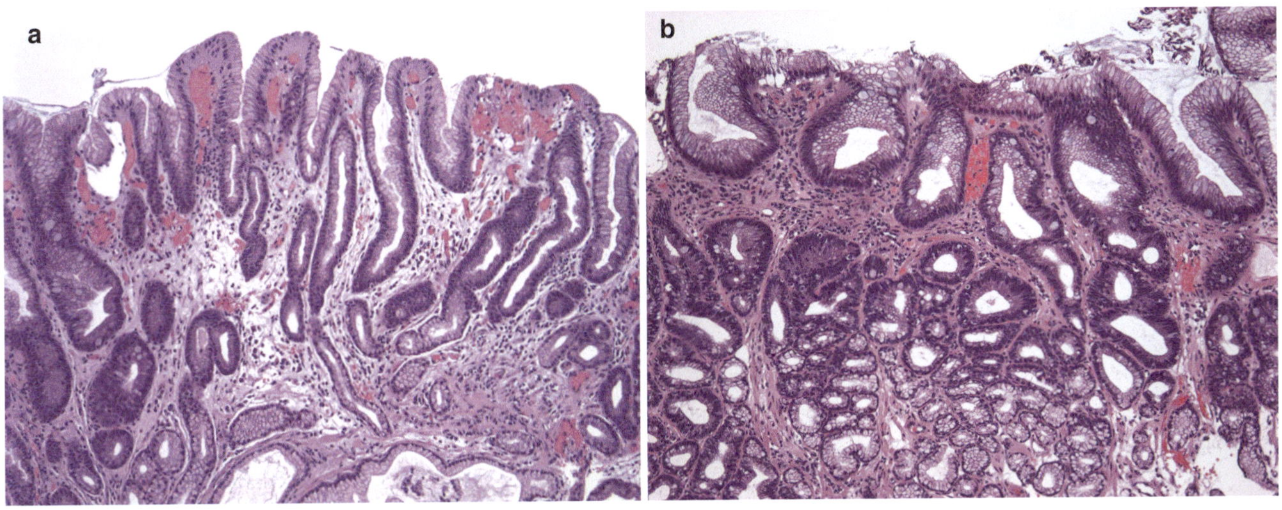

Fig. 10.12 (**a**) These long tubules are dark in the center and toward the base because of larger nuclei and less cytoplasm, and they are lighter toward the surface because of smaller nuclei and more cytoplasmic mucin. Small patches of surface epithelium also demonstrate the full-thickness stratification of enlarged hyperchromatic nuclei. (**b**) Crowded dark tubules between the deep mucus glands and the superficial intestinalized tubules. These dark tubules are lined by cells with large elongated nuclei with partial thickness stratification and little cytoplasmic mucin. This would be a satisfactory low-grade dysplasia if these tubules were placed beneath the surface epithelium and if the surface were to contain the same epithelium. The changes are actually occurring in the proliferative zone of Barrett's mucosa. In our experience, this basal clustering is very common. We do not know the cause but it is possibly a proliferative zone response to continued surface injury

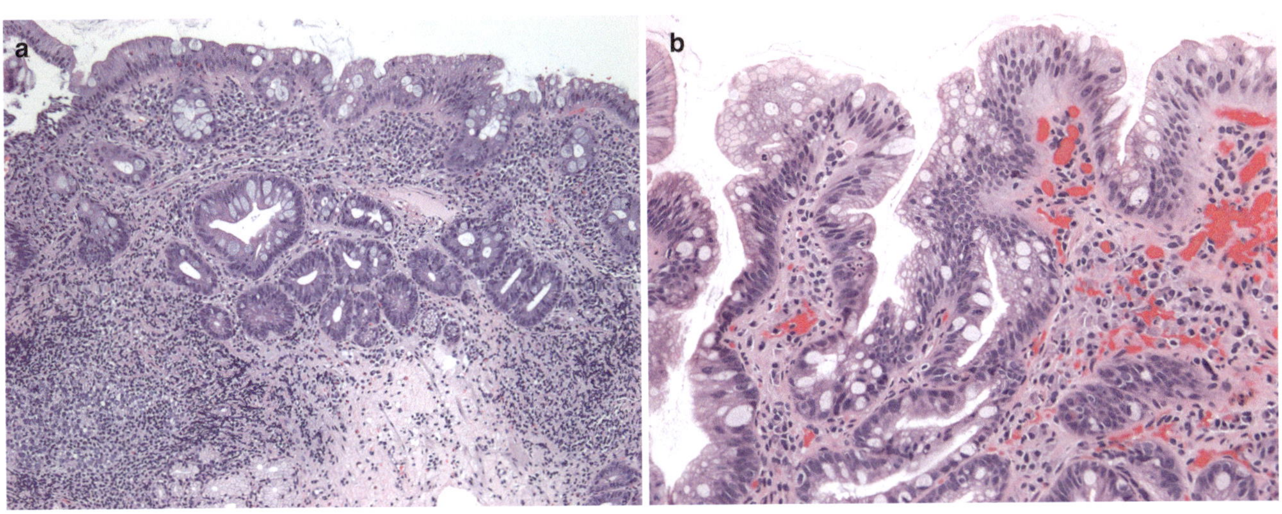

Fig. 10.13 (**a**) This is somewhat similar to Fig. 10.13b but there is much more lamina propria inflammation and the deep clustered tubules in the proliferative zone are even darker and more proliferative. However, there is clear cut loss of these changes and cytoplasmic differentiation toward the surface. (**b**) Full-thickness nuclear stratification on the surface. The nuclei are small, remarkably uniform, and have smooth contours. Such stratification is one of the findings in dysplasia, but this type of change is extraordinarily common in Barrett's mucosa. We do not know the cause but we suspect it is a response to surface injury

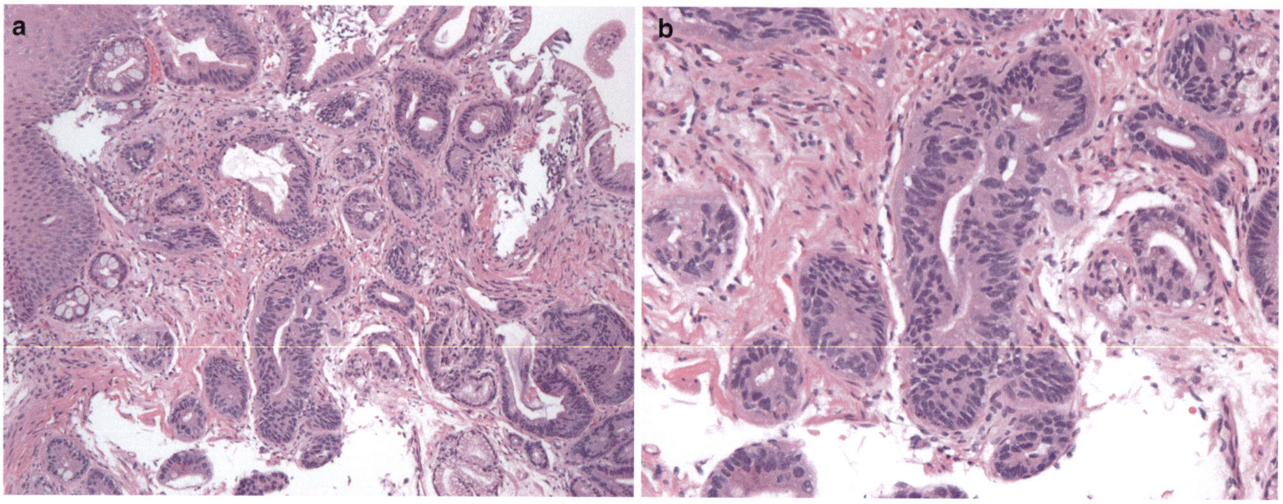

Fig. 10.14 At lower (**a**) and higher (**b**) magnification, this example shows a single long tubule in the center lined by columnar cells with little cytoplasmic mucin and with elongated hyperchromatic nuclei that have full thickness stratification. No other epithelium-lining tubules look quite as impressive. Perhaps this qualifies for what has been termed "basal crypt dysplasia," but we are not convinced it is dysplasia, hence the indefinite designation

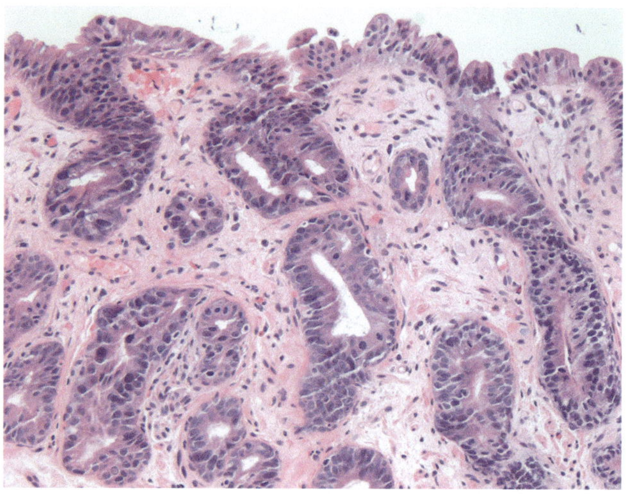

Fig. 10.15 In the toughest of all of these examples, the tubules are separated by abundant lamina propria and are oriented parallel from top to bottom. In fact, they are much the same size, so there is no architectural change. However, the epithelium lining these tubules has enlarged, mostly vesicular nuclei, with a few larger nuclei (*left*). Nuclear stratification is predominantly in the basal half of the cells. Mitoses are easily found but seem more prominent toward the base. The nuclei in the surface epithelium are stratified but they are small and smooth-surfaced. Thus, this example includes some dysplastic cytologic features, but are they enough for dysplasia when the architecture is that of nondysplastic mucosa? So, how about calling this indefinite?

Invasive Adenocarcinoma in Barrett's Mucosa

11

This chapter illustrates the seemingly endless array of cell types and growth patterns that occur in Barrett's adenocarcinomas. Actually, a similar array exists for stomach carcinomas. In contrast, colorectal carcinomas tend to be more uniform, but even in the colon there is considerable heterogeneity.

11.1 Growth Patterns and Cell Types Commonly Encountered in Biopsies

Any esophageal adenocarcinoma is likely to have more than one growth pattern and cell type, but in limited biopsy samples only one pattern or cell type may be present. As a result, it is difficult to define the cell type and growth patterns on small biopsies. The following images include a variety of changes that are often found in invasive adenocarcinomas and some images illustrating depth of invasion.

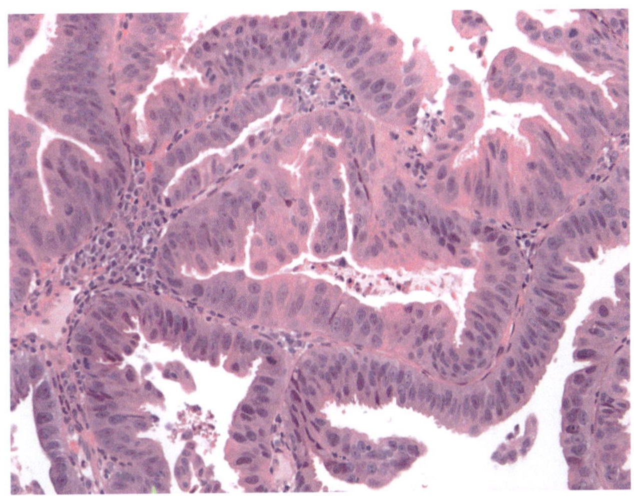

Fig. 11.1 Disorganized tubules. These tubules differ in size, shape, and orientation. Some run across the field whereas others are oriented perpendicularly. This lack of uniform orientation is common in carcinomas. There is no desmopasia suggesting that this carcinoma has not reached the submucosa, where carcinomatous desmoplasia seems to first appear. The tubular epithelium is focally piled up, producing small papillae that project into the tubular lumens

S.R. Owens, H.D. Appelman, *Atlas of Esophagus and Stomach Pathology*, Atlas of Anatomic Pathology,
DOI 10.1007/978-1-4614-8084-6_11, © Springer Science+Business Media New York 2014

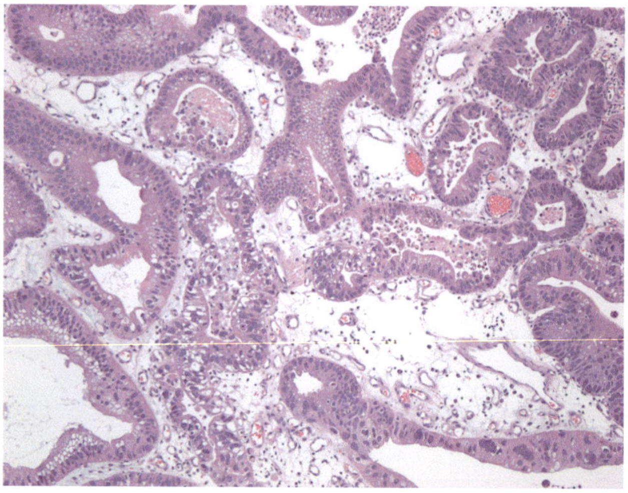

Fig. 11.2 Complex tubules with buds and branches, heading in all directions. This architectural chaos is a typical carcinoma trait

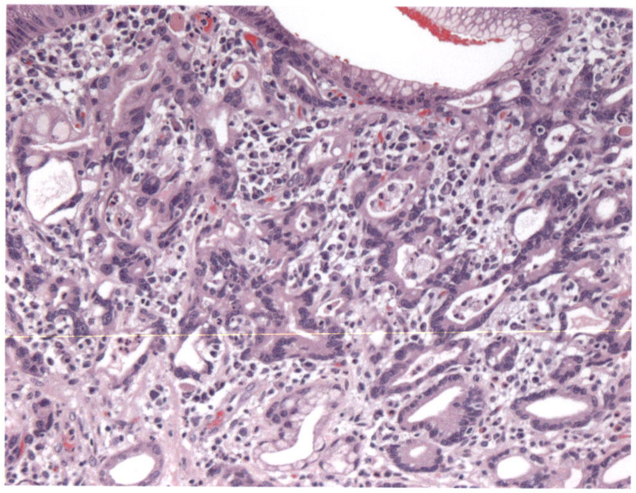

Fig. 11.3 Complex, cribriform, interconnecting branching and budding disorganized tubules

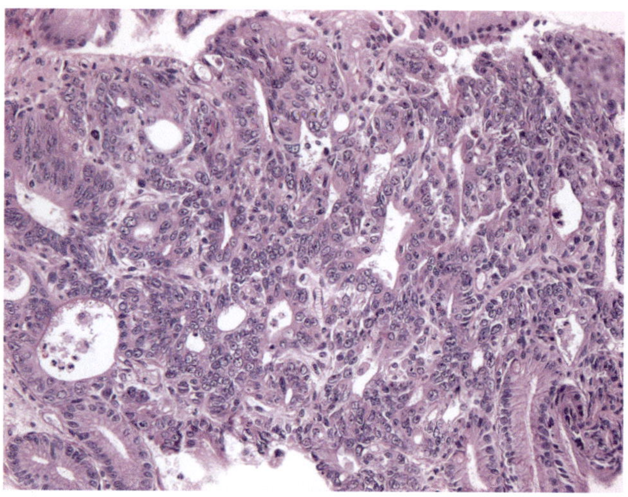

Fig. 11.4 Complex, interconnecting, crowded tubules with loss of almost all lamina propria between them

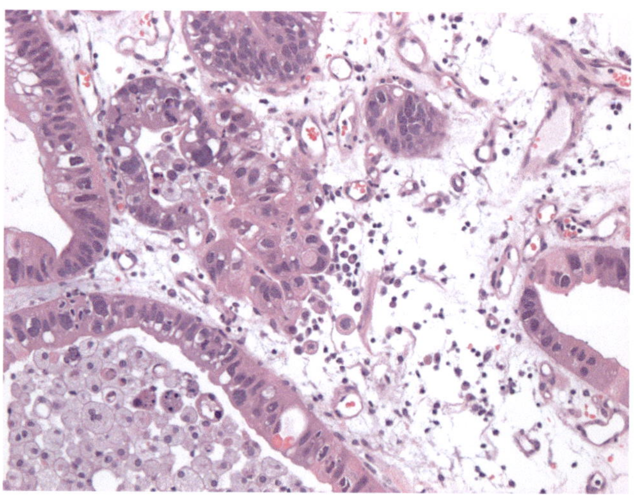

Fig. 11.5 Single cancer cells in the lamina propria next to an architecturally complex tubule. The dilated tubule (*lower right*) is full of necrotic debris and foamy macrophages

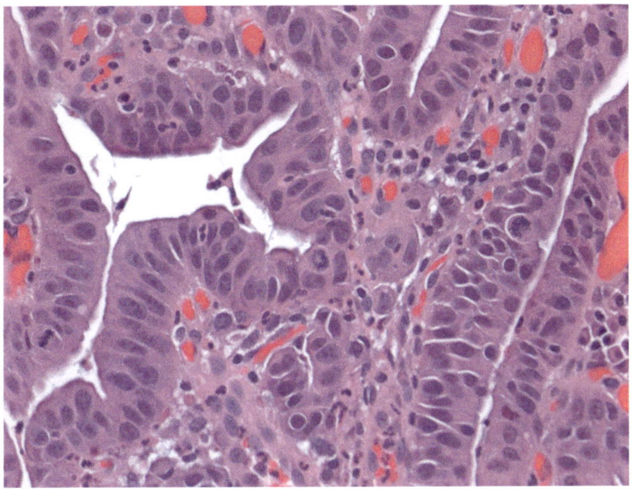

Fig. 11.6 Single cancer cells and a small cluster of such cells in the lamina propria between two dysplastic tubules

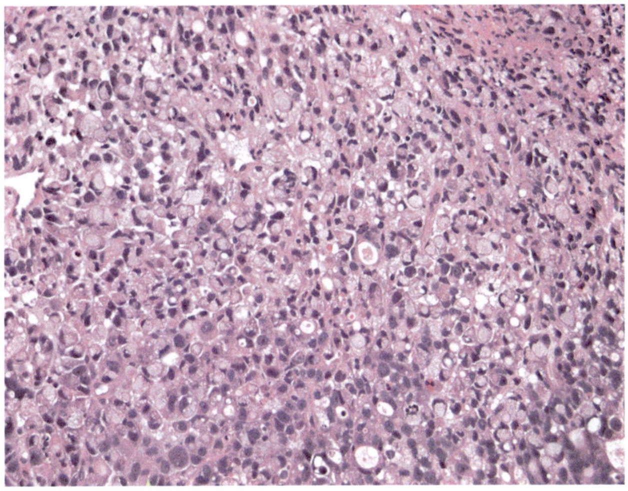

Fig. 11.7 A solid sheet of cells, many of which are signet ring cells

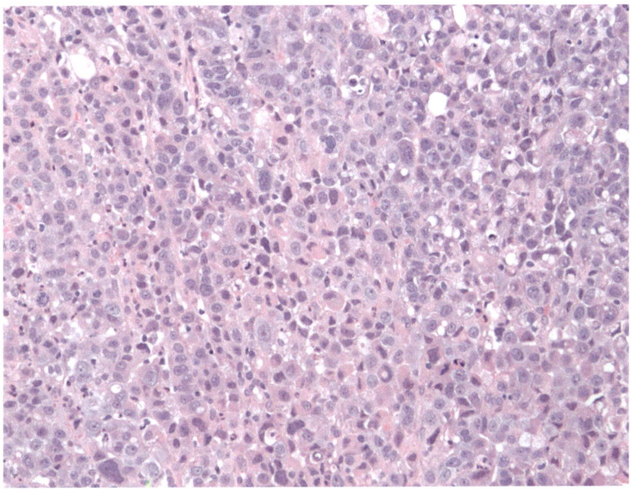

Fig. 11.8 A solid sheet of undifferentiated carcinoma cells. The only hint of adenocarcinomatous differentiation is found in the two small neoplastic tubules at the upper left corner

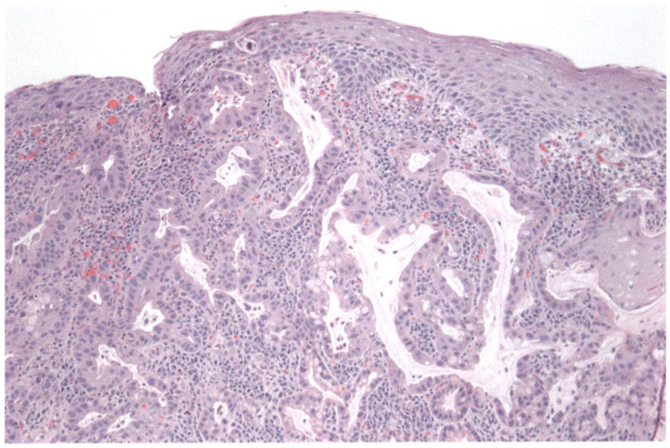

Fig. 11.9 Differentiated adenocarcinoma beneath and invading intact squamous epithelium. The neoplastic tubules have lumens, some of which contain mucus, and they have variable shapes and orientations. Several form complex interconnections. Note the tiny cluster of cancer cells in the squamous epithelium slightly to the left of center

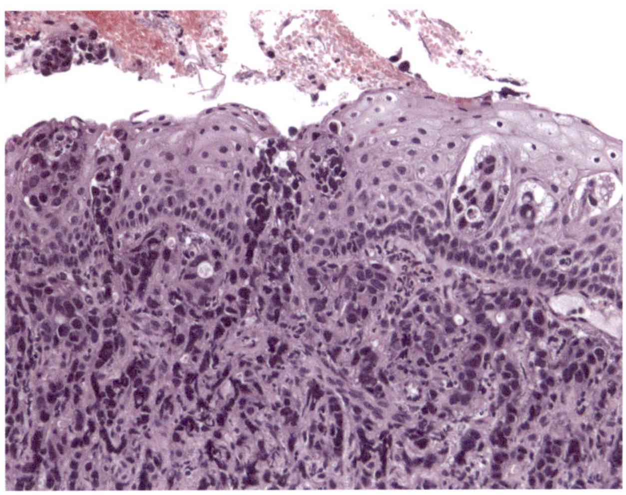

Fig. 11.10 Much less differentiated adenocarcinoma with more obvious invasion of the overlying intact squamous epithelium. In this view, several large nests of carcinoma cells are totally within the squamous epithelium. Esophageal adenocarcinomas commonly invade adjacent squamous mucosa. Some of this may be original squamous mucosa, but some may also be metaplastic. If the squamous epithelium over a carcinoma is thick enough, it is possible that it will hide the carcinoma from the endoscopists's view

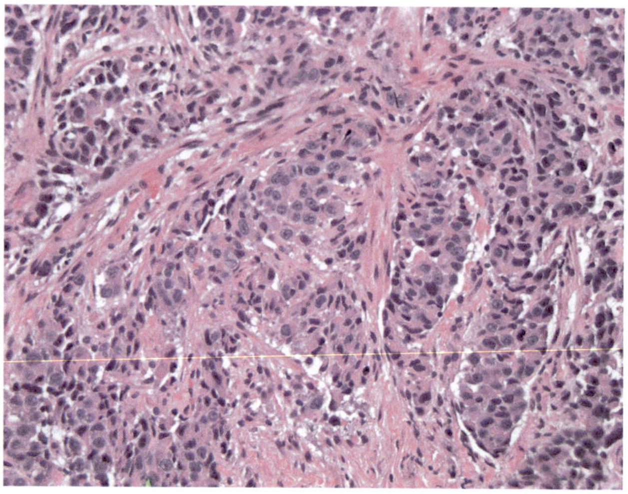

Fig. 11.11 An undifferentiated area of an adenocarcinoma with desmoplastic stroma. In this view, the carcinoma forms cords of undifferentiated cells surrounded by a collagen rich desmoplastic stroma. We think that this desmoplasia indicates that there is submucosal invasion, although we do not have solid data to prove that. There was differentiated adenocarcinoma in other parts of this tumor

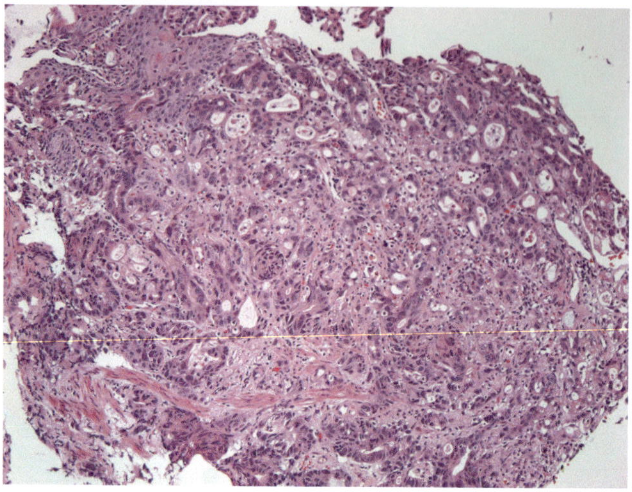

Fig. 11.12 Adenocarcinoma invading through the superficial duplicated layer of muscularis mucosae into the deep layer of lamina propria. Toward the bottom on the left and in the center there are strips of smooth muscle that end abruptly where carcinoma extends through it into a deeper layer. Defining the depth of invasion requires that we remember that Barrett's mucosa comes with a duplicated superficial layer of muscularis mucosae, beneath which is a duplicated lamina propria. Therefore in a biopsy such as this it cannot be assumed that the smooth muscle is the original muscularis mucosae, which is actually likely to be deeper than this layer. As a result, it also cannot be assumed that the carcinoma has invaded the submucosa. It may be no deeper than the deep layer of lamina propria, indicating that it is still confined to the mucosa

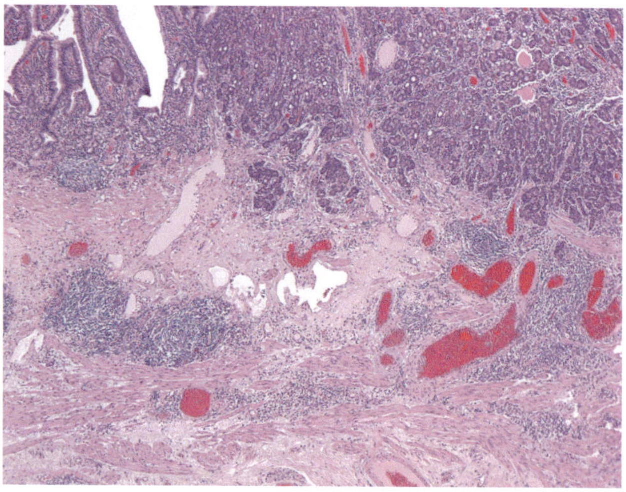

Fig. 11.13 A Barrett's adenocarcinoma invading lamina propria into the superficial duplicated layer of muscularis mucosae. In this field, taken from an endoscopic mucosal resection specimen, there are strips of smooth muscle both at the left and right edges. This is the duplicated superficial muscularis mucosae. The deep or original muscularis mucosae is at the bottom of the image. Small nests of carcinoma extend into but not through this superficial muscle layer

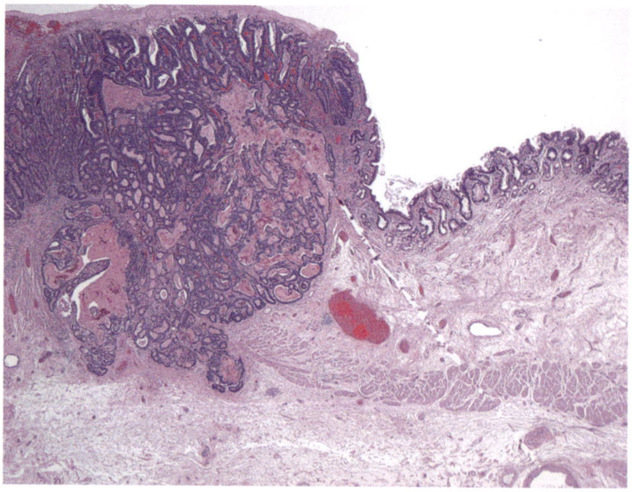

Fig. 11.14 Barrett's adenocarcinoma invading through the deep original muscularis mucosae into the submucosa. This is also from an endoscopic mucosal resection. There is Barrett's mucosa (*right*) beneath which are duplicated muscularis mucosae, the duplicated layer of lamina propria, and the deep original muscularis mucosae. There is an adenocarcinoma (*center*) that has clearly invaded through the deep muscle layer into the superficial submucosa

12 Mesenchymal and Melanocytic Proliferations

Although the esophagus is not exactly fertile ground for mesenchymal proliferations, they do appear every so often in biopsy practice. The most common mesenchymal proliferations are leiomyomas and granular cell tumors. Gastrointestinal (GI)-type stromal tumors are almost nonexistent in the esophagus. By now, virtually every imaginable type of soft tissue tumor has been described in the esophagus. For this chapter, however, it is not worth trying to include all of them. The following figures are from various mesenchymal lumps that we have encountered in our practice, with a few melanocytic proliferations thrown in for the sake of completeness.

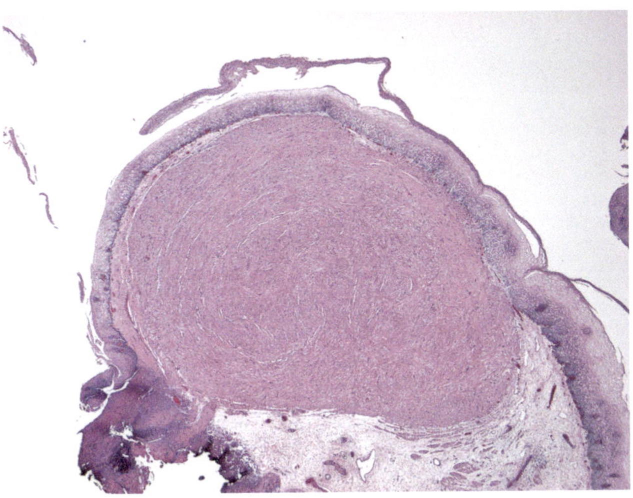

Fig. 12.1 A leiomyoma of the muscularis mucosae that formed an endoscopic polyp. The nodule is well circumscribed and situated immediately beneath a thin rim of lamina propria covered by the squamous epithelium

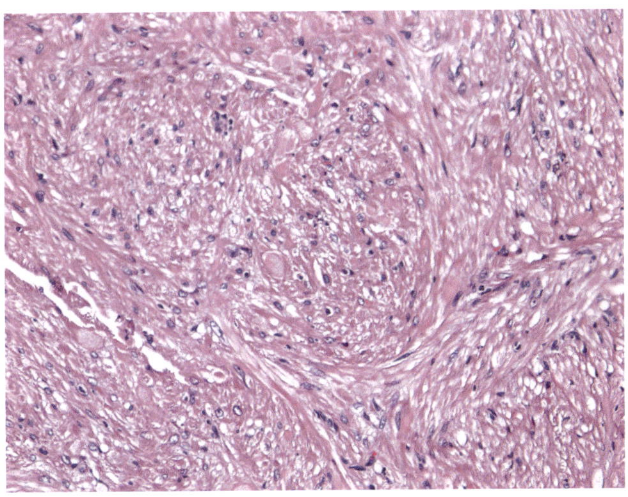

Fig. 12.2 The nodule is composed of large smooth muscle cells arranged in short fascicles. Some cells contain pale cytoplasmic inclusions, which are bundles of actin filaments. This cell type and the inclusions are found in leiomyomas throughout the GI tract

S.R. Owens, H.D. Appelman, *Atlas of Esophagus and Stomach Pathology*, Atlas of Anatomic Pathology,
DOI 10.1007/978-1-4614-8084-6_12,

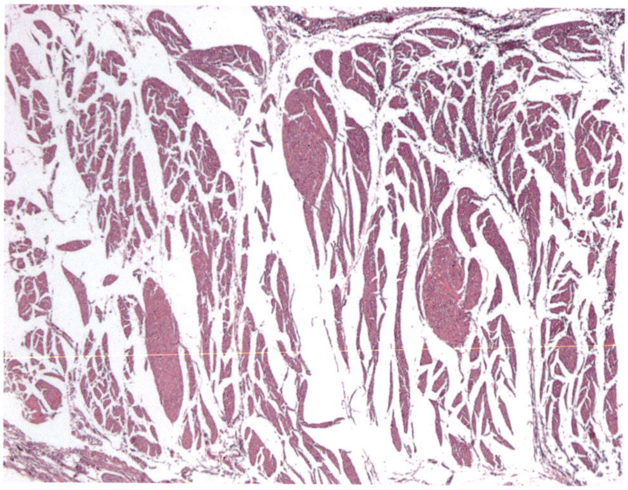

Fig. 12.3 Seedling leiomyomas are small, often microscopic, smooth muscle nodules mostly within the muscularis propria but occasionally in the muscularis mucosae. They were called "seedlings" by Takubo because they were thought to be precursors (seedlings) of larger leiomyomas. In this field, there are three such tiny nodules in the muscularis propria

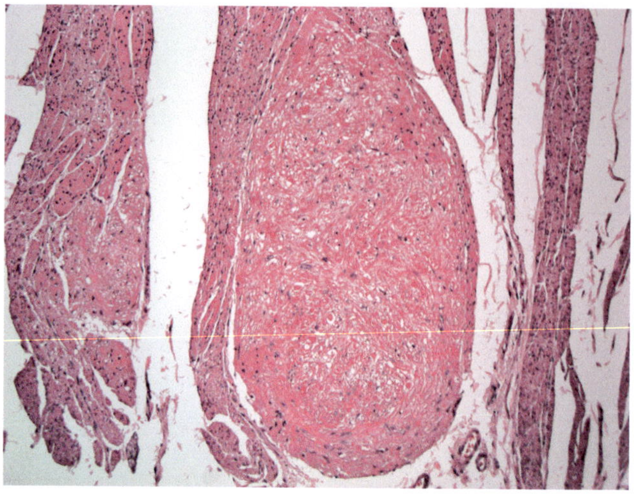

Fig. 12.4 Higher magnification of one of the seedlings. It looks exactly like the leiomyoma in Figs. 12.1 and 12.2, including the cytoplasmic inclusions

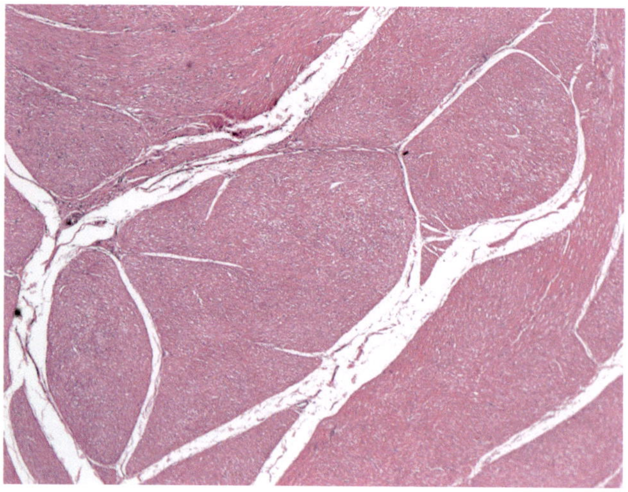

Fig. 12.5 Leiomyomatosis is a peculiar condition in which the muscularis propria seems to have been converted into several discrete muscle nodules that resemble leiomyomas. This can cause obstruction. In children, it may be a component of Alport's syndrome

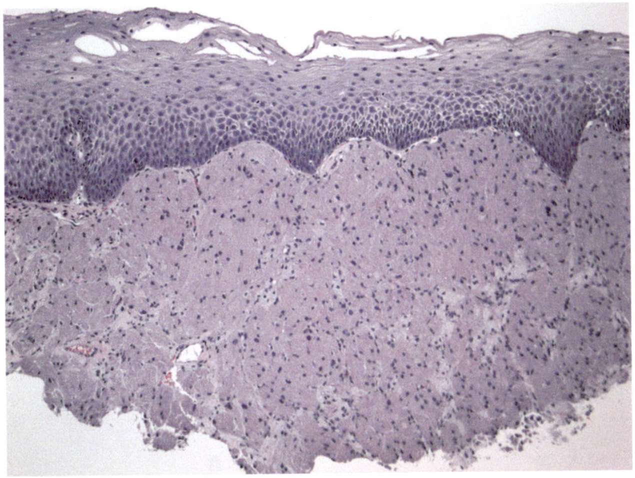

Fig. 12.6 Granular cell tumors are generally small nodules that arise in the lamina propria and push against the basal squamous epithelium. In the esophagus, there may be a small amount of squamous hyperplasia, producing pointed downward extensions as in this view. The pseudoepitheliomatous hyperplasia that so commonly accompanies these benign neoplasms in the skin hardly ever occurs in the esophagus

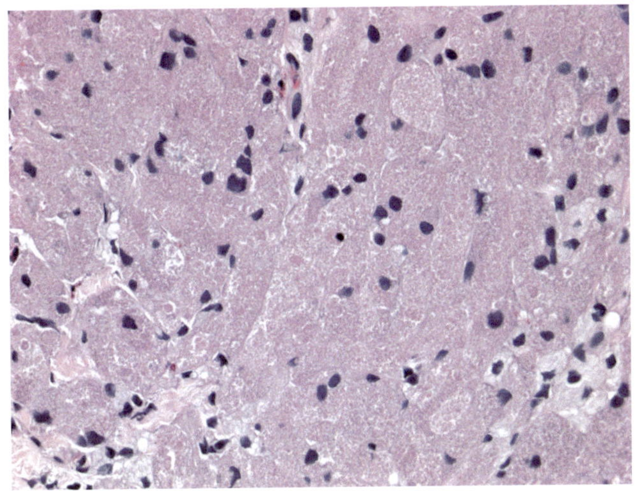

Fig. 12.7 At higher magnification, typical epithelioid and spindled cells with finely granular cytoplasm are seen

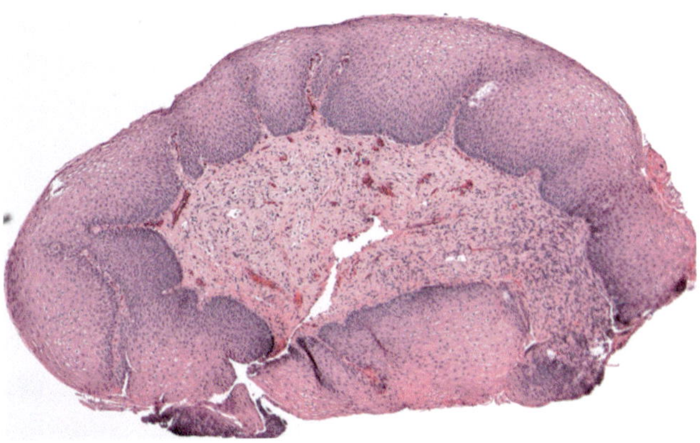

Fig. 12.8 Schwannoma of the lamina propria is a very rare tumor that we have seen a couple of times. This is a small endoscopic polyp characterized by a spindle cell proliferation filling the lamina propria, abutting the essentially normal squamous mucosa, a pattern of growth identical to that in the granular cell tumor in Fig. 12.7

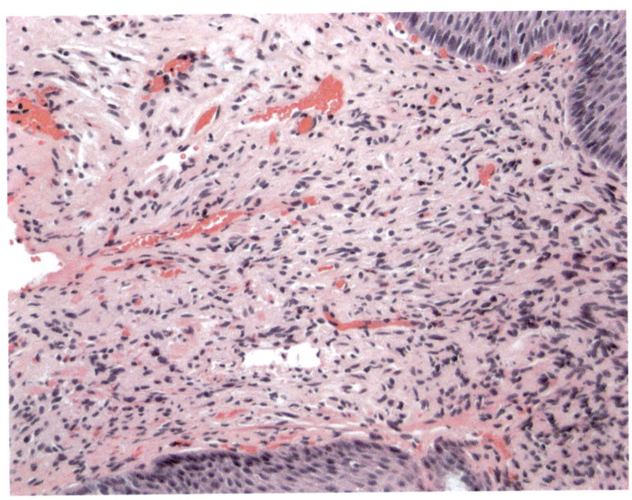

Fig. 12.9 The uniform spindle cells with small dark nuclei form short fascicles with imperfect nuclear palisades. These are S-100 positive, confirming that they are Schwann cells. This may be the equivalent of a granular cell tumor without the granular cytoplasm

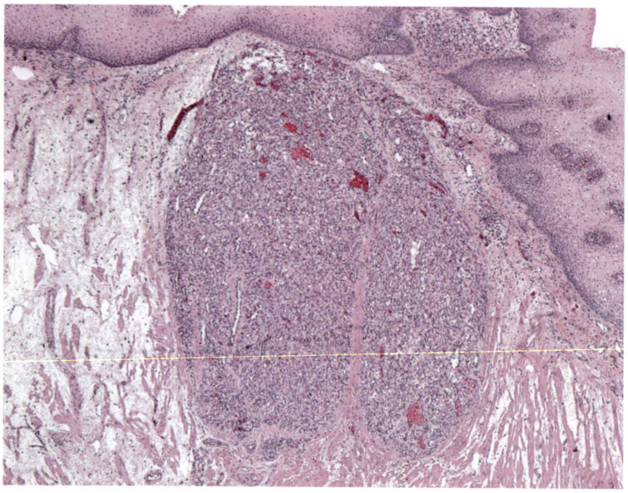

Fig. 12.10 Superficial capillary hemangioma: this very rare tumor presented as an endoscopic polyp. Extending from the muscularis mucosae at the bottom into the lamina propria, almost to the base of the squamous epithelium, is a circumscribed, small vascular nodule with a thin muscle septum extending upward in the middle

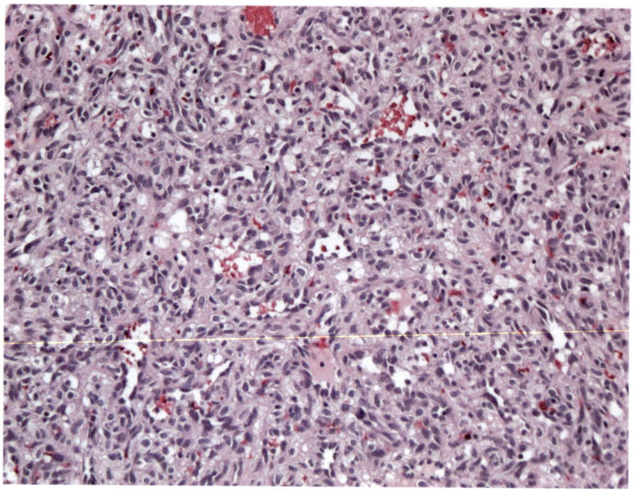

Fig. 12.11 This nodule is composed of uniform small capillaries lined by prominent endothelial cells, surrounded by spindle cells and collagen fibers

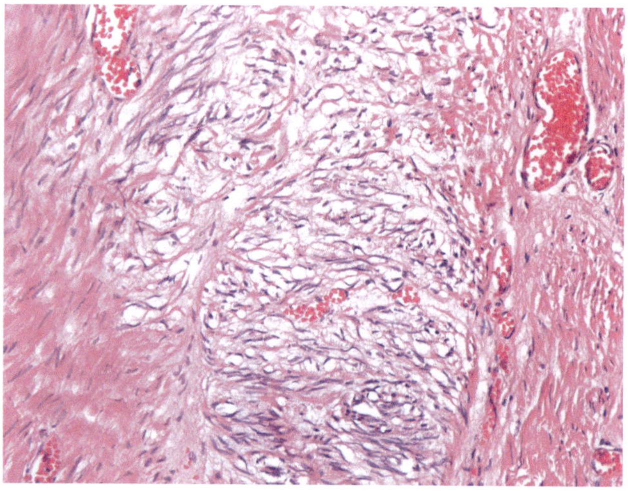

Fig. 12.12 Within the muscularis propria there is a small nodule of plump, vacuolated spindle cells. This is typical of the tiny stromal tumors throughout the gut that are generally found by accident during operations for other reasons. This tiny tumor resembles seedling leiomyomas. It just has a cell type that is characteristic of certain stromal tumors

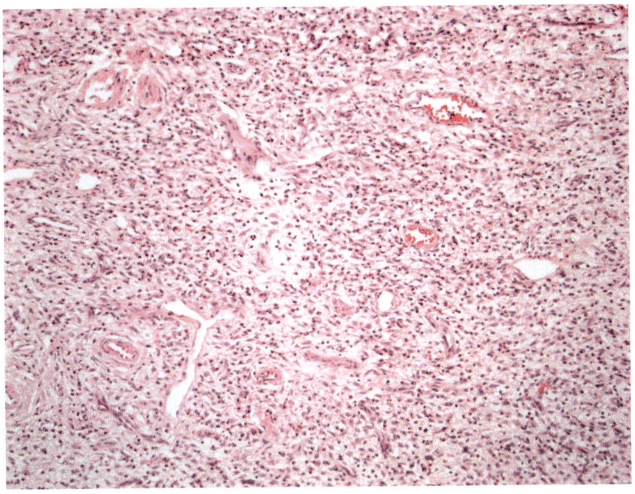

Fig. 12.13 Inflammatory fibroid polyp is a peculiar mixed cellular proliferation that occurs throughout the gut but hardly ever appears in the esophagus. At lower magnification, this mass is composed of cells in an edematous background that also contains many small arteries, veins, and capillaries

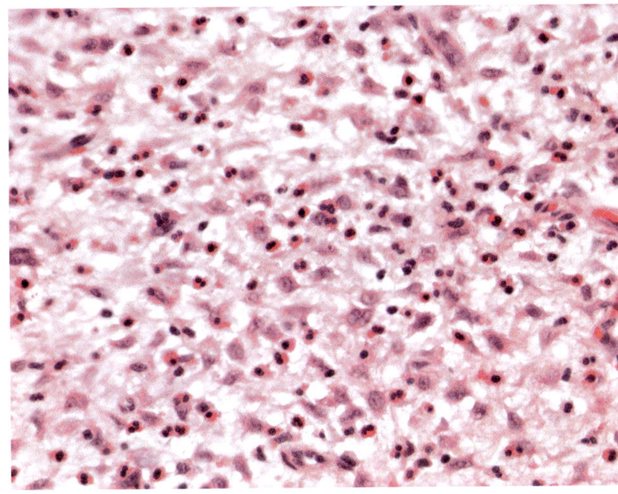

Fig. 12.14 At higher magnification, the cell mixture consists of eosinophils, lymphocytes, and plump spindle and stellate cells, the tumor cells, which may be peculiar myofibroblasts

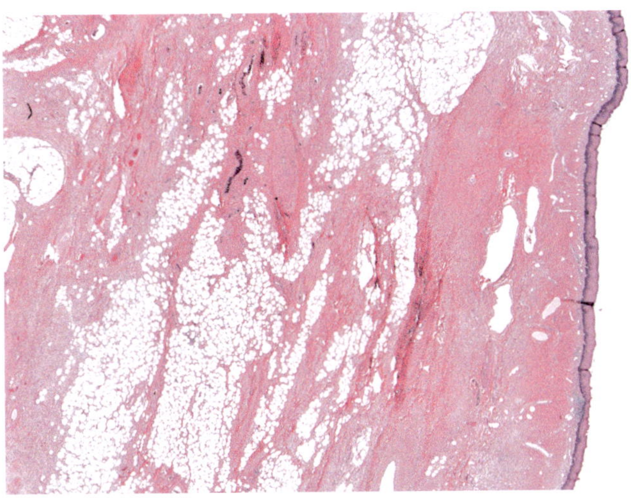

Fig. 12.15 Giant fibrovascular polyps are amazing structures. They arise behind the cricoid cartilage at the esophageal inlet, and they extend distally as smooth-surfaced, banana-like projections, sometimes growing to be as long as the total length of the esophagus. It is most peculiar that something can grow to be this large before it causes obstructive symptoms. Presumably this is due to the slow growth, allowing the esophageal wall to gradually accommodate it. They also tend to be soft, probably because of a large amount of adipose tissue. In this low-magnification view, the squamous mucosa is on the right. The rest of the tissue is the core of the polyp. The abundant adipose tissue accounts for the fact that some of these have been called lipomas or fibrolipomas

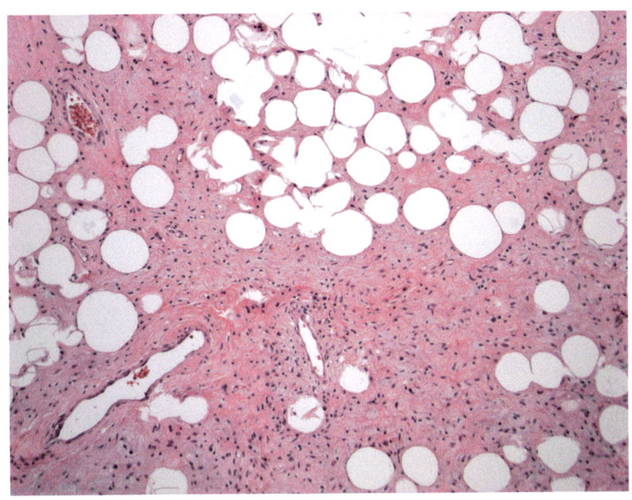

Fig. 12.16 In this closer view, all the components are present including the adipose tissue, the collagen, and the large blood vessels

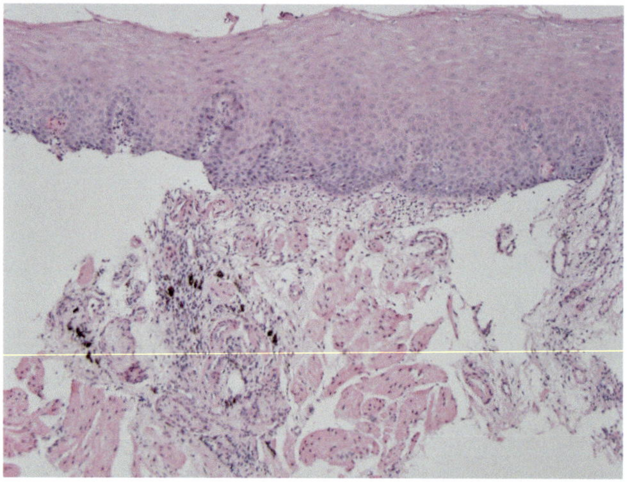

Fig. 12.17 Melanosis. Every so often, an endoscopist will see a small dark spot somewhere in the squamous mucosa. Melanocytosis is a rare condition that may be the precursor of the really rare primary esophageal melanomas. In this low-power view, at the base of the squamous epithelium, there are cells with dark nuclei in the basal layer containing scattered cells with slightly larger more hyperchromatic nuclei. Some may even be pigmented. There is melanin pigment in the lamina propria

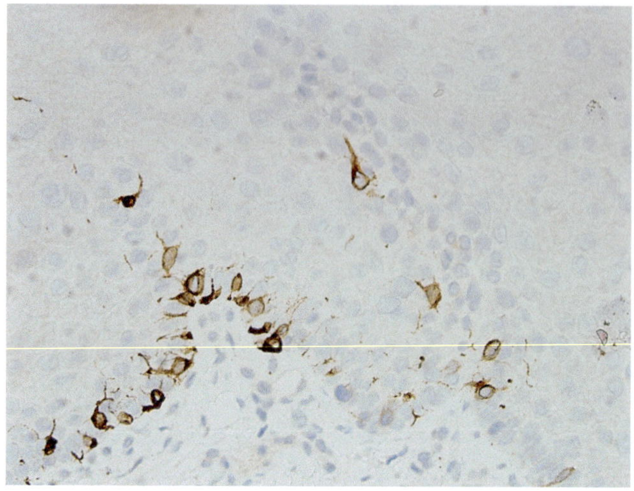

Fig. 12.18 They are proven to be melanocytes with the Melan A antibody stain. Melanocytosis is a rare condition that may be the precursor of the very rare primary esophageal melanomas

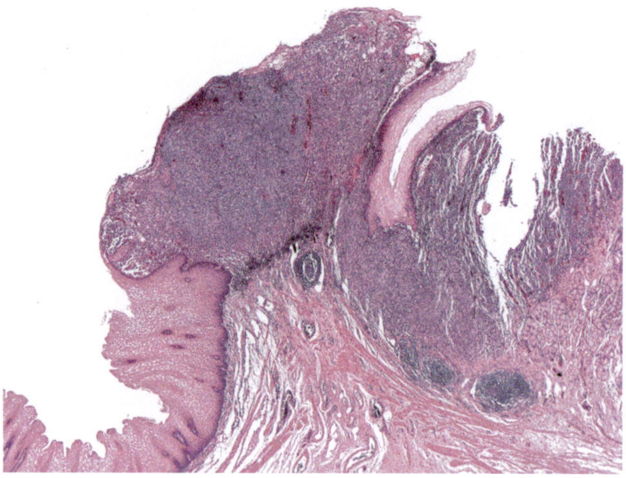

Fig. 12.19 The esophagus is a site of mucosal melanoma, along with the upper aerodigestive tract and the anus. There is nothing special about esophageal melanomas in terms of histologic features. At low power, there is a dark neoplasm that involves the lamina propria and replaces the squamous epithelium

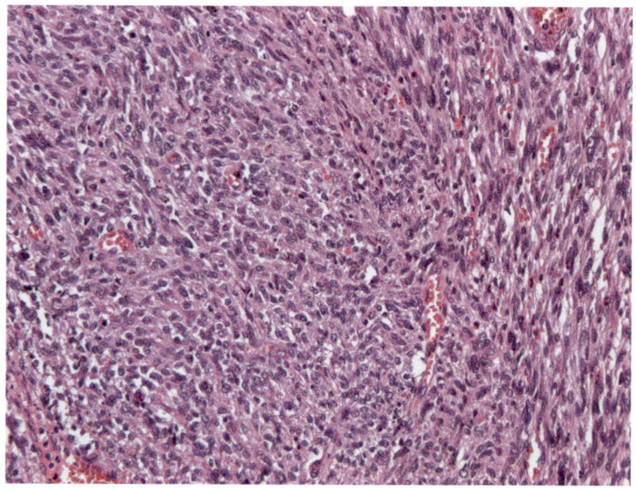

Fig. 12.20 This is a cellular tumor composed of small plump spindle cell, which stains with the usual melanoma markers

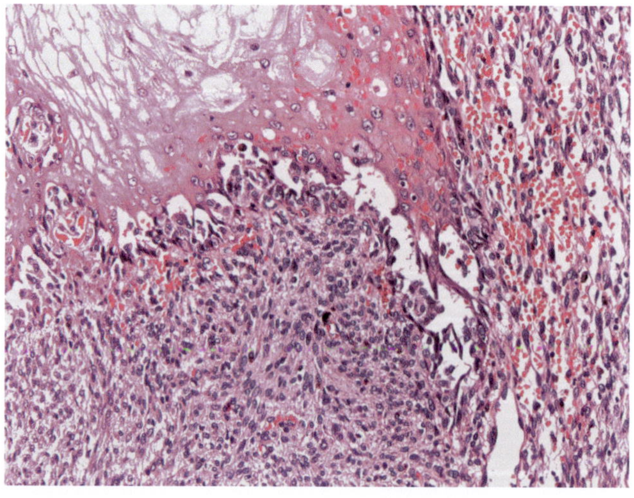

Fig. 12.21 Melanoma markers are not necessary, however, since in this case, there is a prominent junctional component at the edge

Esophageal Odds and Ends

13

The first 12 chapters of this atlas are full of diseases, changes, and aberrations that are relatively easily placed in specific categories. However, some aspects were left out of those chapters, and there were not enough of them to form a specific category (*eg*, malformations of neuromuscular diseases) and warrant additional specific chapter headings. As a result, these odds and ends have been put into a separate chapter, titled appropriately as odds and ends. If readers cannot find something in other chapters, perhaps they can find it here. Regardless, some very odd, very rare things have been left out of this atlas entirely; in other words, they did not even make it into this chapter. For easy discovery by the reader, entities in this chapter have been covered in alphabetical order, beginning with achalasia.

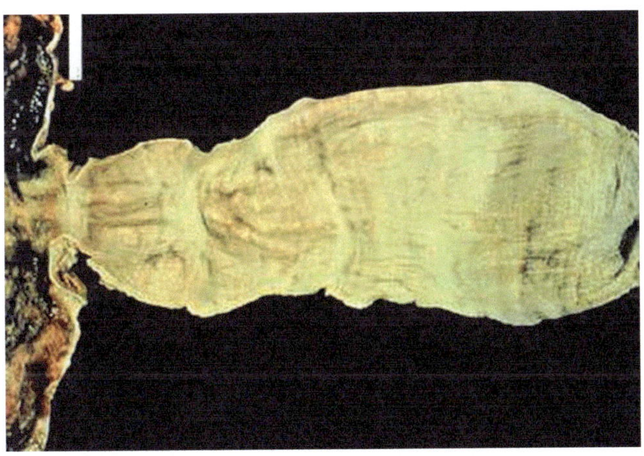

Fig. 13.1 Achalasia is a disease, presumably autoimmune, characterized by destruction of the myenteric plexus leading first to loss of ganglion cells and eventually also to loss of the nerves. This results in loss of peristalsis in the esophageal body and persistent high pressure in the lower esophageal sphincter, causing permanent constriction distally and dilatation from there proximally. Gross view of a resection. Virtually all achalasias look like this, with narrowing or constriction distally and the body dilated. There are coarse, thick longitudinal folds, presumably due to hypertrophy of the muscularis propria

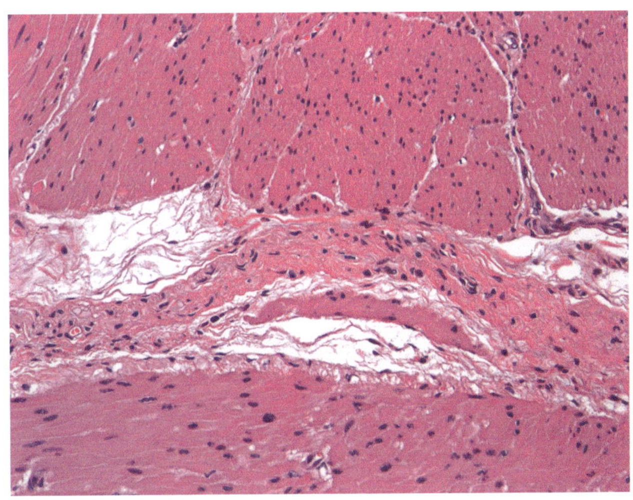

Fig. 13.2 In this section of the myenteric plexus stained with hematoxylin and eosin, there are no ganglion cells. The long structure crossing the center of the field is a myenteric nerve

S.R. Owens, H.D. Appelman, *Atlas of Esophagus and Stomach Pathology*, Atlas of Anatomic Pathology,
DOI 10.1007/978-1-4614-8084-6_13, © Springer Science+Business Media New York 2014

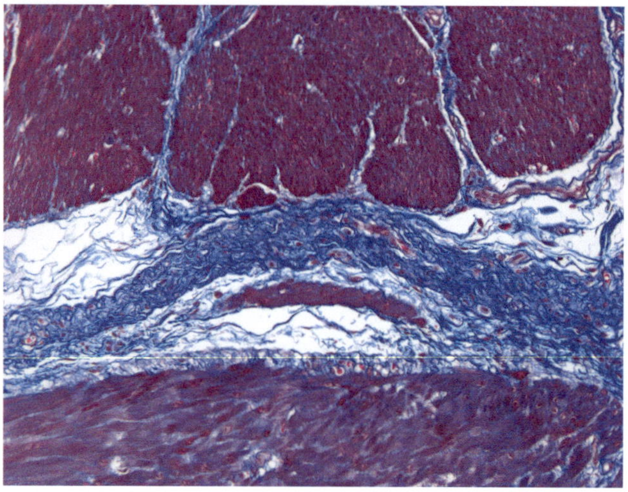

Fig. 13.3 In this trichrome-stained section, myenteric nerves stain blue, indicating that they are full of collagen; in other words, it has undergone fibrous obliteration, the end stage of this disease

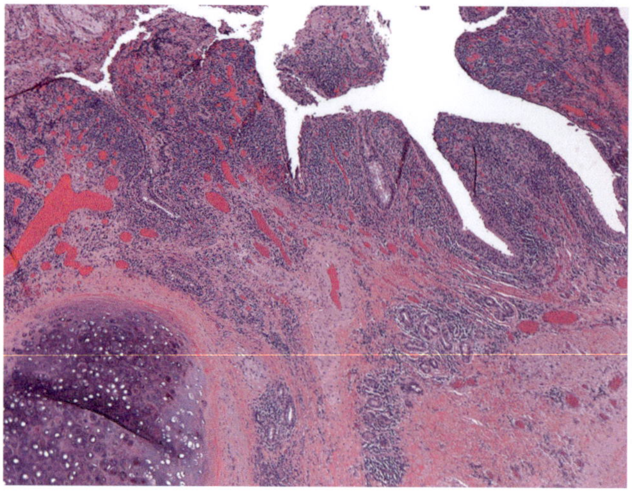

Fig. 13.4 Cysts. There are few cysts in the esophagus, including some that are developmental and some acquired. Only the former are covered in these figures. This cyst is lined by respiratory epithelium that covers stromal projections. It is secondarily inflamed for unknown reasons. Cartilage and respiratory-type glands are present in the wall

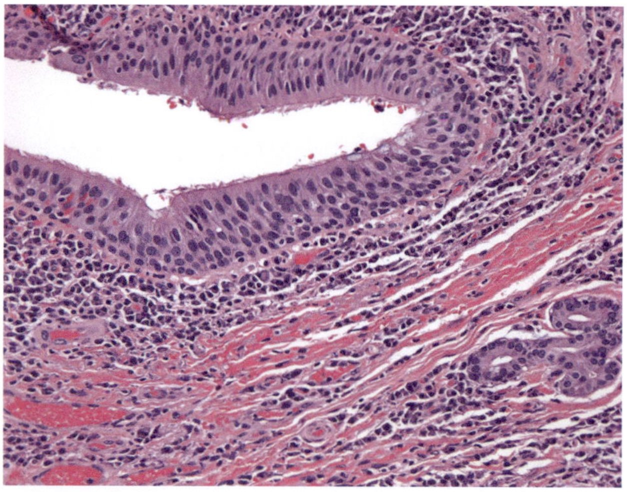

Fig. 13.5 This higher-magnification image brings out the ciliated respiratory epithelium with a few cells that contain apical mucus and the small gland in the underlying stroma. This is a developmental cyst with all the components of bronchial wall; in other words, a bronchogenic cyst

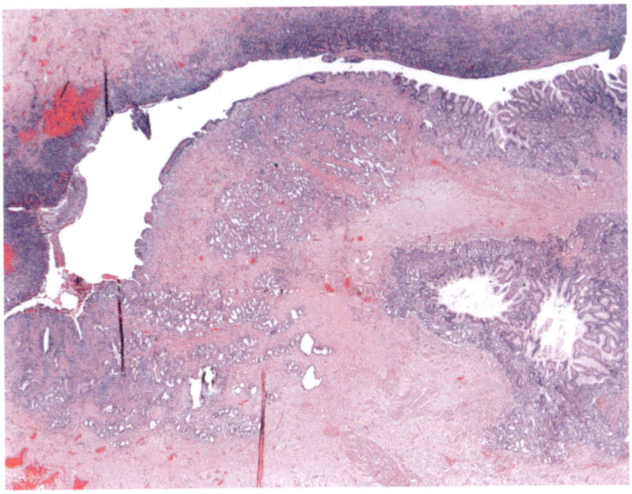

Fig. 13.6 This cyst is different. It is multilocular and lined by gastric mucosa. In this low- power view, the large cyst on the surface is partly ulcerated and inflamed on the left. A smaller cyst is present at the right edge of the image

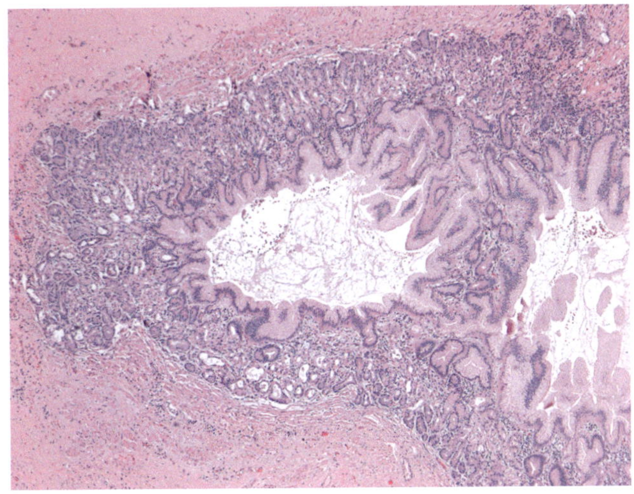

Fig. 13.7 Both the small and large cyst are lined by thin gastric mucosa with both superficial pits and deep glands. This cyst also had a muscularis. Its gastric lining qualifies it as an enteric duplication cyst

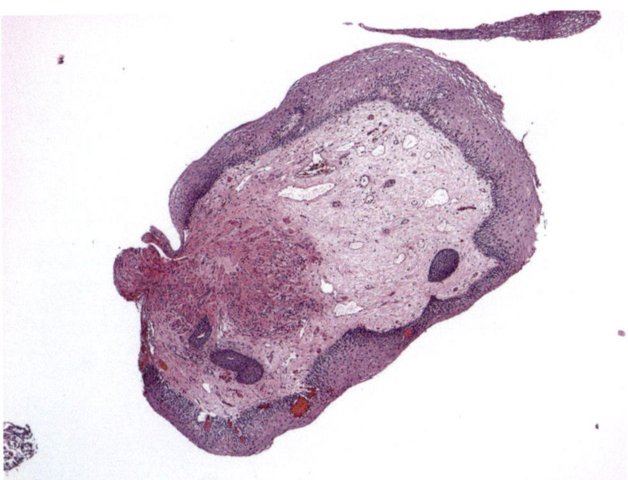

Fig. 13.8 This small polyp has a core of expanded, highly vascularized lamina propria covered completely by normal squamous epithelium. The muscularis mucosae is bunched together at the middle left at the point of attachment to the wall. This is identical to an acrochordon, skin, or anal tag, so it probably deserves the designation of "esophageal tag." Nothing has been written about these very rare polyps, so we know nothing about them, but they are intriguing

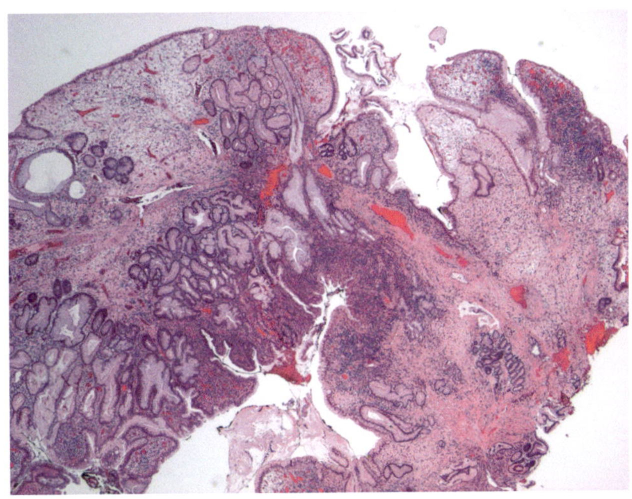

Fig. 13.9 Unusual Polyps. This polyp was found in the proximal esophagus at the inlet. It is dominated by edematous inflamed stroma, actually lamina propria, with numerous irregularly shaped tubules and cysts lined by gastric surface epithelium. The surface contours vary from round and smooth on the left to coarsely villiform on the right. This is a typical gastric-type hyperplastic polyp, but in this case it is arising in ectopic gastric mucosa that is common in the proximal esophagus, an inlet patch. Inlet patches involve risk for all diseases that occur in the stomach because they are tiny foci of stomach in the wrong place

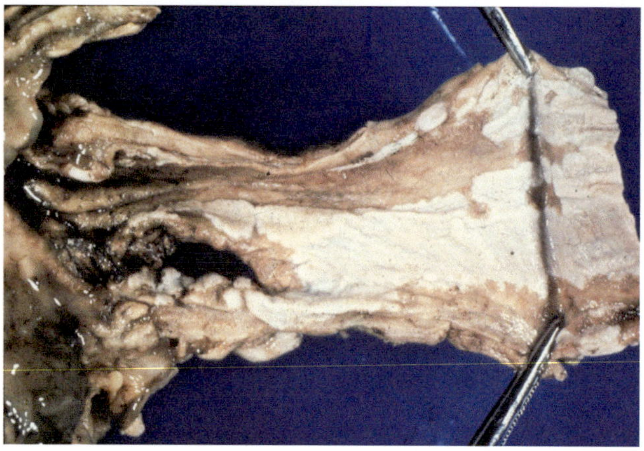

Fig. 13.10 Mallory-Weiss Tear. This is an autopsy specimen. Beginning at the gastroesophageal junction at the lower left, there is a longitudinal tear extending into the lower esophagus. Usually such tears are confined to the mucosa, although this one is much deeper. Such tears were originally thought to be the result of severe prolonged vomiting, especially in alcoholics, but they may occur after a single vomiting episode or an episode of severe coughing, and they can occur in children with a variety of medical conditions, including reflux and portal hypertension

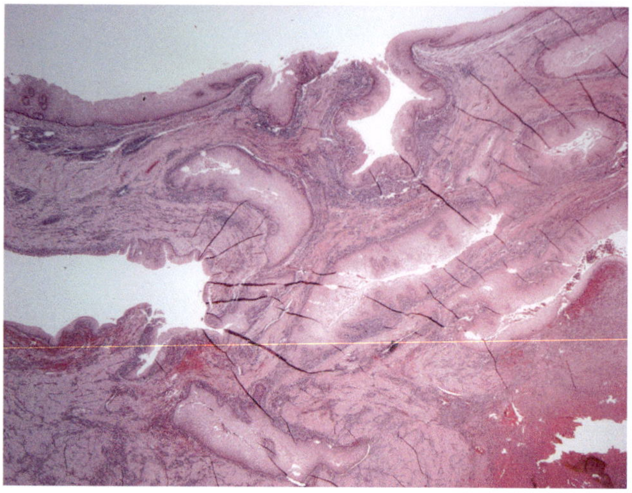

Fig. 13.11 Pseudodiverticulosis. Extending from the surface into the esophageal wall, there are several tracts, some of which are cystic, some of which interconnect. All are lined by squamous epithelium. They are surrounded by a densely inflamed and scarred stroma

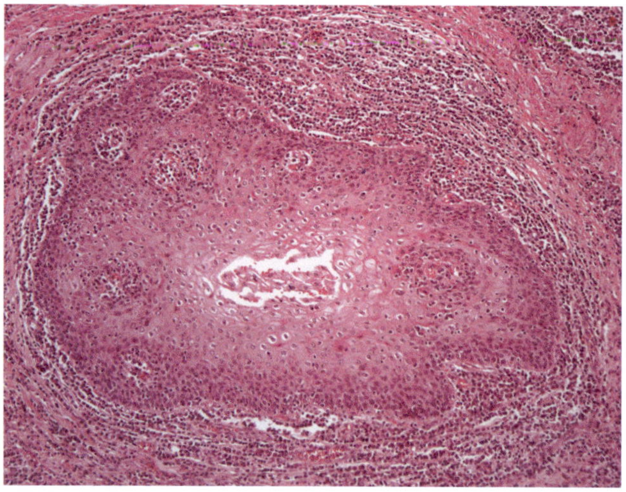

Fig. 13.12 At a higher magnification of one of these cysts, the squamous epithelium matures toward the center, and it is surrounded by a scarred, chronically inflamed stroma. These tracts and cysts are thought to have developed from submucosal gland ducts, which were obstructed, and this led to dilatation and intense chronic inflammation. When large, these cysts can be seen by barium swallow studies in which they look like diverticula (hence the name "pseudodiverticulosis"). It is obvious because of the depth of these tracts and cysts that they will not be seen in biopsies, but they may appear in endoscopic mucosal resection specimens

14 Gastric Cardiac Mucosa

In the seventh edition of the *Cancer Staging Manual* from the American Joint Committee on Cancer published in 2010, the cardia is defined as the proximal 5 cm of the stomach. This is a gross designation that surgeons and many endoscopists use.

This gross definition presumably includes the microscopic cardiac mucosa recognized by pathologists. There is great variability in the amount of cardiac mucosa we possess. Some of us have no more than 1 mm, whereas others have several centimeters. Furthermore, there is variability in the amount of cardiac mucosa from one part of this proximal-most stomach to another in the same individual, so a biopsy from one area may have more cardiac mucosa than a biopsy from another area. Because the length of cardiac mucosa may be so small, if we want to find it, biopsies must be taken across the squamocolumnar junction at the gastroesophageal junction. In fact, most cardiac mucosa that we see in practice comes from biopsies taken from the gastroesophageal junction. Also, since the length of cardiac mucosa is so small, the gross cardia must contain mainly body (oxyntic) mucosa. In general, cardiac mucosa resembles gastric antral mucosa in that it has pit and gland compartments of about equal thickness, and the glands are pure mucous glands. However, it lacks the endocrine cells of the antral mucosa. There is some debate about whether cardiac mucosa is normal or a reflux-induced abnormality, but the fact remains that it exists and we have to deal with it. In general, cardiac mucosa has its own set of normal variants and a remarkable set of peculiarities illustrated in this chapter. Any cardiac biopsy is likely to have several of these changes. It also has dysplasias and carcinomas that are identical to those in Barrett's mucosa, which have been covered in previous chapters.

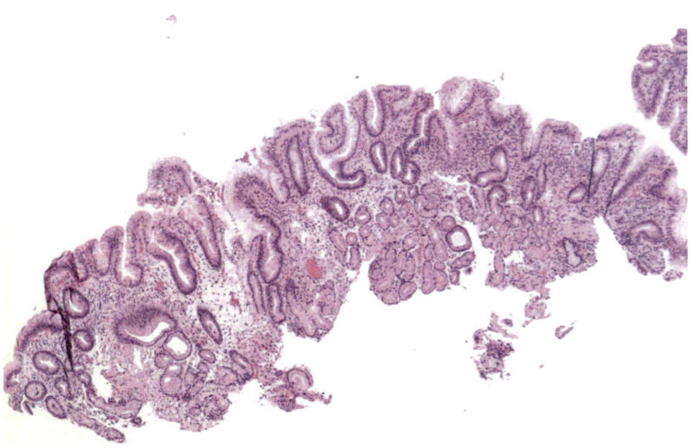

Fig. 14.1 Carditis in a typical cardiac biopsy. This mucosa has long pits, with many that are branched or interconnected. The deep mucus glands are clustered and take up about the same amount of mucosa as the pits. The superficial lamina propria is full of inflammatory cells that are mainly plasma cells. Cardiac mucosa usually has chronic inflammation, some of which may be due to *Helicobacter pylori*, some to reflux, and the rest to unknown influences

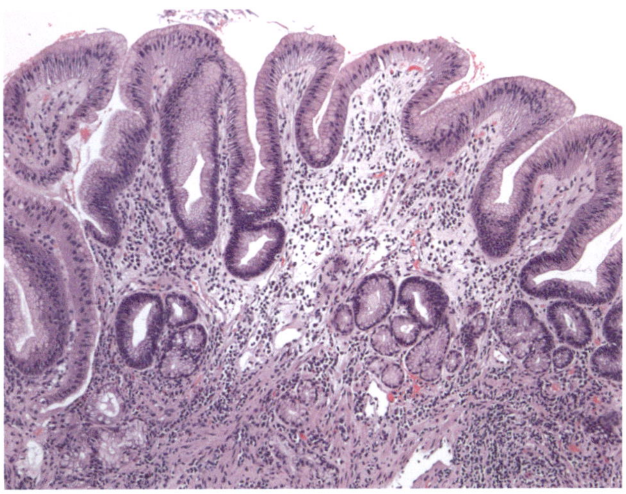

Fig. 14.2 A closer look at the superficial chronic inflammation that is so common in cardiac mucosa

S.R. Owens, H.D. Appelman, *Atlas of Esophagus and Stomach Pathology*, Atlas of Anatomic Pathology,
DOI 10.1007/978-1-4614-8084-6_14, © Springer Science+Business Media New York 2014

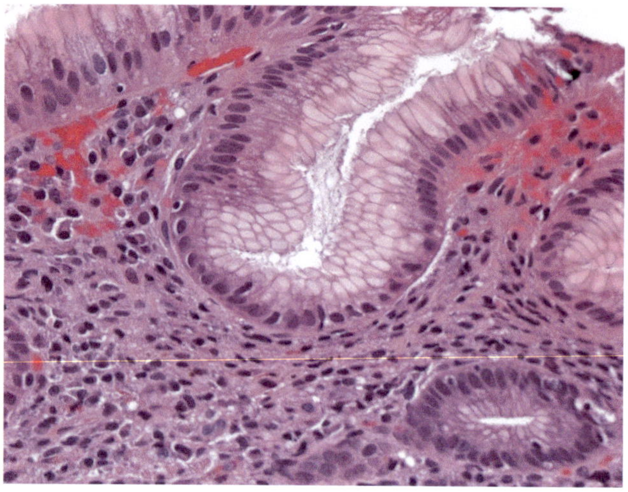

Fig. 14.3 Carditis due to *H. pylori*. Cardiac mucosa is as subject to *H. pylori* infection as any other gastric mucosa. In this field, numerous organisms are in the pit in the center

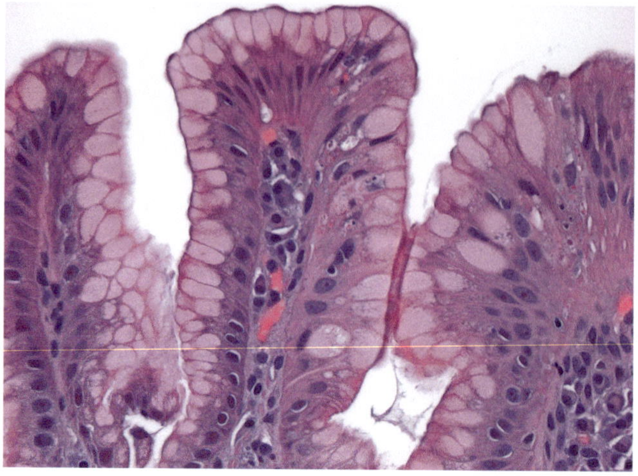

Fig. 14.4 Hypertrophic pit cells. Many epithelial cells covering the surface and lining the superficial pits have huge, bulbous, apical mucous vacuoles. These resemble goblet cells, and, in fact, they have been referred to as "pseudogoblet cells." Their mucin, which is neutral mucin, stains pink in most hematoxylin and eosin (H&E) preparations, whereas goblet cell mucin (an acid mucin) stains blue or gray. Also, these distended surface cells tend to cluster whereas goblet cells are likely to be scattered singly in the epithelium. Cells like this are common in the stomach and in Barrett's mucosa, but they seem to occur with unusual frequency in the cardia. We do not know the cause of this phenomenon

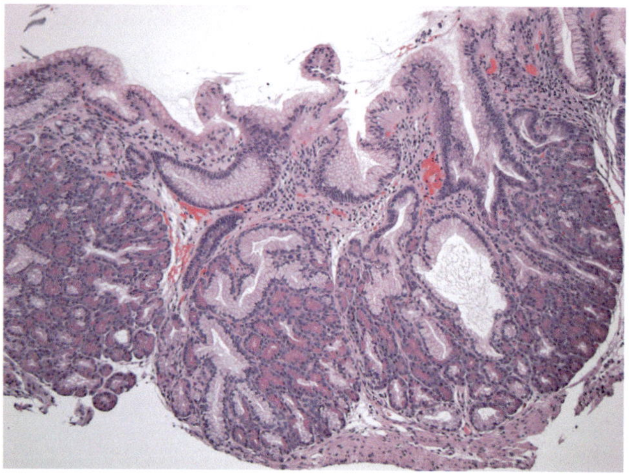

Fig. 14.5 Pancreatic acinar metaplasia. Within this cardiac mucosa with its typical chronic inflammation, there are clusters of deep glands containing cells with dark epithelium

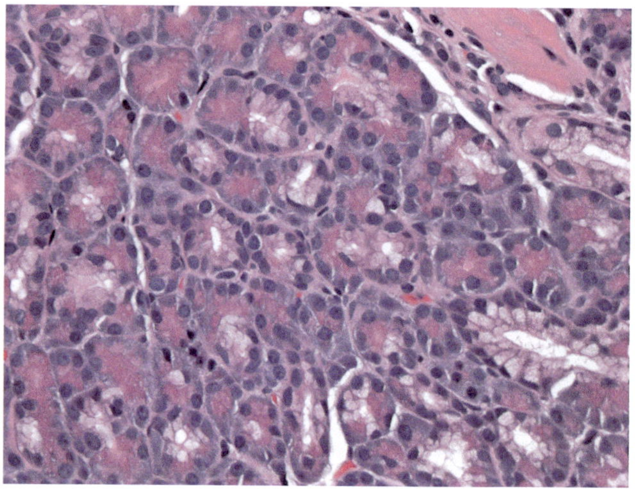

Fig. 14.6 At higher magnification, these dark cells, which are mixed with cardiac gland mucous cells, look like pancreatic acinar cells with finely granular apical cytoplasm and basal nuclei. These cells have been proven to be pancreatic acinar cells; they contain pancreatic acinar enzymes. They have been designated as metaplastic, but we do not know if they really are metaplastic. They are very common in cardiac mucosa and do not seem to be associated with any other change; as such, perhaps this is not a metaplasia but simply a variant of normal

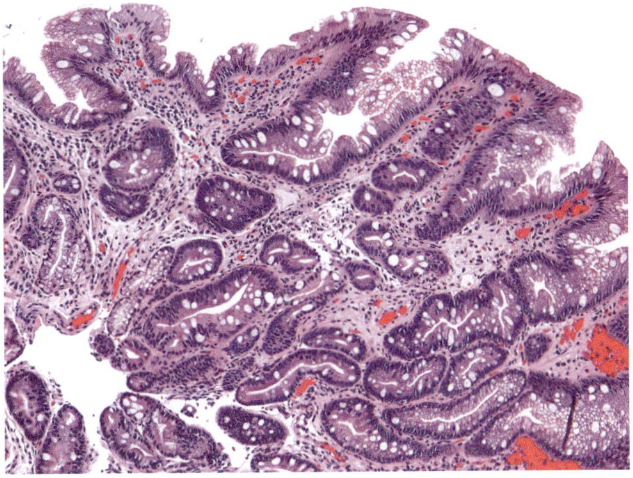

Fig. 14.7 Intestinal metaplasia in the cardia: this columnar mucosa contains numerous goblet cells mixed with gastric type surface cells. This is identical to Barrett's mucosa, but this biopsy came from a focus of erythema in an otherwise normal cardia. The endoscopist did not see anything that even remotely looked like Barrett's mucosa. As a result, the endoscopic requirement for the diagnosis of Barrett's mucosa was not met. No data prove that intestinal metaplasia in cardiac mucosa has a cancer risk, similar to that in Barrett's mucosa. Furthermore, goblet cells in cardiac mucosa are common (44 % of adults in one study). As a result, it may not be a surveillance target

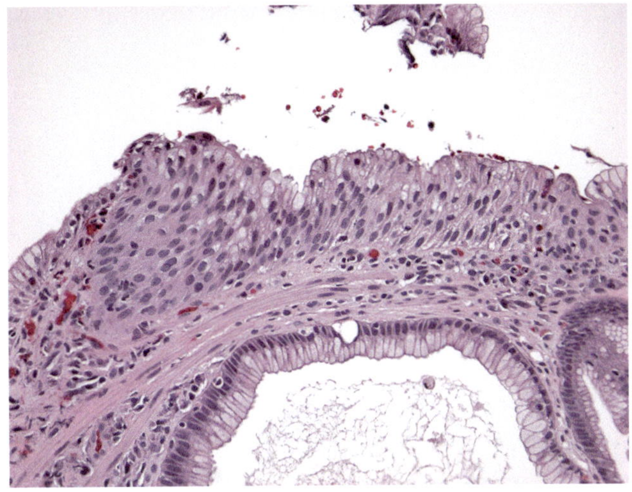

Fig. 14.8 Multilayered surface epithelium. The surface epithelium, at first glance, looks like it might be squamous. It is clearly a stratified epithelium with several deeper layers containing uniform, small, slightly elongated nuclei. The superficial layer or layers have cells with vacuolated apical cytoplasm containing mucus. This multilayered epithelium seems to occur following injury, perhaps more often after reflux injury than other types. Some pathologists suspect that this may be a precursor to Barrett's mucosa, but it is also common in the cardia

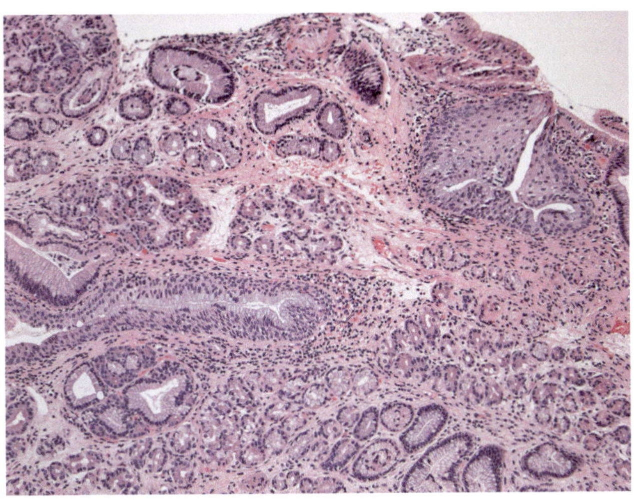

Fig. 14.9 Multiple epithelial types in one field of cardiac mucosa. This biopsy came from an erythematous gastroesophageal junction. It has a delightful mixture of epithelia, including a squamous island (*upper right*) and a tubule coming in from the mid-left edge lined by multilayered epithelium with columnar superficial and basaloid deep cells; pit-like structures lined by mucinous epithelium with basal nuclei; pancreatic acinar cells within a cardiac gland in the middle left; and, toward the base, small glands, some of which are mucus glands whereas others with parietal cells are gastric body-type glands. Furthermore, the lamina propria is inflamed. This seemingly chaotic mixture is common in biopsies taken from cardiac mucosa

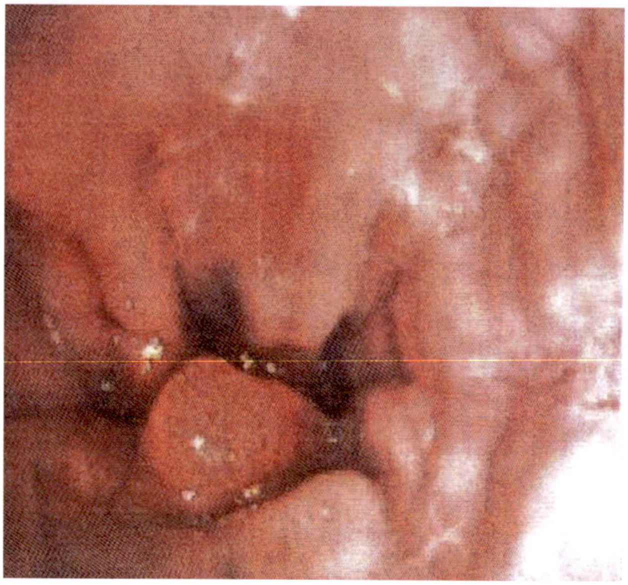

Fig. 14.10 Polyp-fold complex. This is an endoscopic view of a polyp on the top of the proximal-most gastric fold

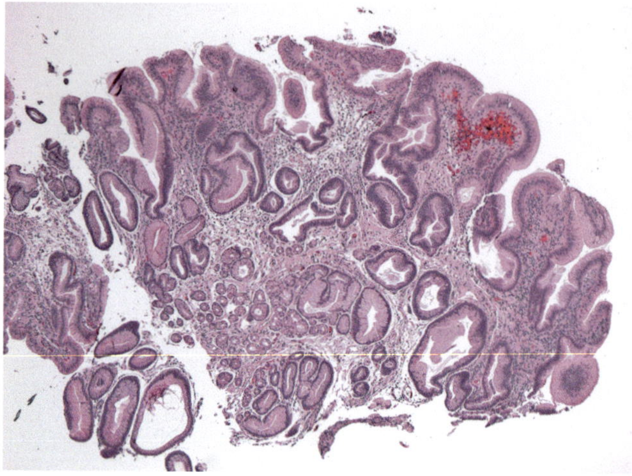

Fig. 14.11 Microscopically, this polyp-fold complex is dominated by vastly expanded and distorted pits. The lamina propria has the typical intense chronic cardiac inflammation and it is also edematous. This combination of changes is similar to what occurs in gastric hyperplastic polyps, and perhaps it is a variant of such polyps. In the cardia, it is a common finding that was originally described in those with chronic reflux, but subsequently it was also found in those without reflux. It is not clear how it develops, but in those with reflux one possibility is prolapse of the proximal gastric fold into the distal esophagus

Suggested Reading

General

American Joint Committee on Cancer. Cancer staging manual. 7th ed. New York: Springer; 2010.

Chandrasoma PT, Lokuhetty DM, Demeester TR, et al. Definition of histopathologic changes in gastroesophageal reflux disease. Am J Surg Pathol. 2000a;24:344–51.

Chandrasoma PT, Der R, Ma Y, et al. Histology of the gastroesophageal junction. An autopsy study. Am J Surg Pathol. 2000b;24:402–9.

El-Serag HB, Graham DY, Rabenack L, et al. Prevalence and determination of histological abnormalities of gastric cardia in volunteers. Scand J Gastroenterol. 2007;42:1158–66.

Lembo T, Ippoliti AF, Ramers C, Weinstein WM. Inflammation of the gastro-oesophageal junction (carditis) in patients with symptomatic gastro-oesophageal reflux disease: a prospective study. Gut. 1999;45:484–8.

Owen DA. Stomach. In: Mills SE, editor. Histology for pathologists. Philadelphia: Lippincott Williams & Wilkins; 2012.

Sarbia M, Donner A, Gabbert HE. Histopathology of the gastroesophageal junction. A study on 36 operation specimens. Am J Surg Pathol. 2002;26:1207–12 (A careful anatomic study detailing how small the cardia is and where it is).

Carditis

Cestari R, Villanacci V, Bassotti G, et al. The pathology of the gastric cardia. A prospective, endoscopic, and morphologic study. Am J Surg Pathol. 2007;31:706–10.

Chen Y-Y, Antonioli DA, Spechler SJ, et al. Gastroesophageal reflux disease versus *helicobacter pylori* infection as the cause of gastric carditis. Mod Pathol. 1998;11:950–6.

Glickman JN, Fox V, Antonioli DA, et al. Morphology of the cardia and significance of carditis in pediatric patients. Am J Surg Pathol. 2002;26:1032–9.

Wieczorek TJ, Wang HH, Antonioli DA, et al. Pathologic features of reflux and helicobacter associated carditis. A comparative study. Am J Surg Pathol. 2003;27:960–8.

Pancreatic Acinar Metaplasia

Doglioni C, Laurino L, Dei Tos AP, et al. Pancreatic (acinar) metaplasia of the gastric mucosa. Histoloy, ultrastructure, immunocytochemistry, and clinicopathologic correlations of 101 cases. Am J Surg Pathol. 1993;17:1134–43.

Wang HH, Zeroogian JM, Spechler SJ, et al. Prevalence and significance of pancreatic acinar metaplasia at the gastroesophageal junction. Am J Surg Pathol. 1996;20:1507–10.

Intestinal Metaplasia

Dixon MF, Mapstone NP, Neville PM, et al. Bile reflux gastritis and intestinal metaplasia at the cardia. Gut. 2002;51:351–5 (Bile reflux, not H. pylori, is the culprit in this study from Leeds).

El-Serag HB, Sonnenberg A, Jamal MM, et al. Characteristics of intestinal metaplasia in the gastric cardia. Am J Gastroenterol. 1999;94:622–7.

Goldblum JR, Richter JE, Vaezi M, et al. Helicobacter pylori infection, not gastroesophageal reflux, is the major cause of inflammation and intestinal metaplasia of gastric cardiac mucosa. Am J Gastroenterol. 2002;97:302–11.

Guelrud M, Herrera I, Essenfeld H, et al. Intestinal metaplasia of the gastric cardia: a prospective study with enhanced magnification endoscopy. Am J Gastroenterol. 2002;97:584–9.

Jung KW, Talley NJ, Romero Y, et al. Epidemiology and natural history of intestinal metaplasia of the gastroesophageal junction and Barrett's esophagus: a population-based study. Am J Gastroenterol. 2011;106:1447–55.

Öberg S, Peters JH, DeMeester TR, et al. Inflammation and specialized intestinal metaplasia of cardiac mucosa is a manifestation of gastroesophageal reflux disease. Ann Surg. 1997;226:522–32.

Oksanen A, Sipponen P, Karttunen R, Rautelin H. Inflammation and intestinal metaplasia at the squamocolumnar junction in young patients with or without *helicobacter pylori* infection. Gut. 2003;52:194–8 (In this Finnish study, age 45 years or younger, intestinal metaplasia, and the squamocolumnar junction seem to be associated with reflux but not with H. pylori).

Peck-Radosavljevic M, Puspok A, Potzi R, Oberhuber G. Histological findings after routine biopsy at the gastro-oesophageal junction. Eur J Gastroenterol Hepatol. 1999;11:1265–70.

van Sandick JW, van Landschot JB, van Felius L, et al. Intestinal metaplasia of the esophagus or esophagogastric junction. Evidence of distinct clinical, pathologic, and histochemical staining features. Am J Clin Pathol. 2002;117:117–25.

Polyp-Fold Complex

Abraham SC, Singh VK, Yardley JH, Wu T-T. Hyperplastic polyps of the esophagus and esophagogastric junction. Histologic and clinicopathologic findings. Am J Surg Pathol. 2001;25:1180–7.

Bleshman MH, Banner MP, Johnson R, DeFord JW. The inflammatory esophagastric polyp and fold. Radiology. 1978;128:589–93.

Ghahremani GG, Fisher R, Rushovich AM. Prolapsing inflammatory pseudopolyp-fold complex of the oesophagagastric region. Eur J Radiol. 1984;4:47–51.

Long KB, Odze RD. Gastroesophageal junction hyperplastic (inflammatory) polyps: a clinical and pathologic study of 46 cases. Am J Surg Pathol. 2011;35:1038–44.

Shepherd HA, Harvey J, Jackson A, Colin-Jones DG. Recurrent retching with gastric mucosal prolapse. A proposed prolapse gastropathy syndrome. Dig Dis Sci. 1947;29:121–8.

Voutilainen M, Juhola M, Farkkila M, Sipponen P. Foveolar hyperplasia at the gastric cardia: prevalence and associations. J Clin Pathol. 2002;55:352–4.

Part II

Stomach

15 Normal Biopsy Anatomy/Histology and General Changes

As was the case with the esophagus section, the first chapter in this section on the stomach illustrates the normal components of the gastric mucosa as we encounter them in biopsy specimens. Our most common "diagnosis" in gastric biopsies is "no significant abnormality," just as it is in the esophagus and elsewhere in the gastrointestinal tract. Indeed, one of the most important things we as pathologists can do for our patients and our clinical colleagues is to render such a diagnosis rather than to describe every minor, clinically unimportant change in our reports, as it allows entire categories of disease to be eliminated from the clinical differential diagnosis.

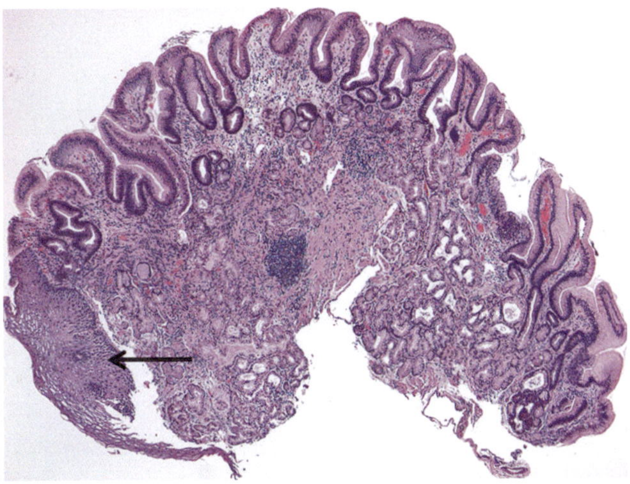

Fig. 15.1 Gastric cardia. The proximal stomach mucosa contains prominent foveolae (pits), beneath which reside mucus-producing glands. The length of this "cardiac" mucosa is variable, and some biopsies will contain a direct transition from esophageal squamous mucosa (*arrow*) to oxyntic mucosa, leading some observers to wonder whether the gastric cardia is actually a metaplastic phenomenon

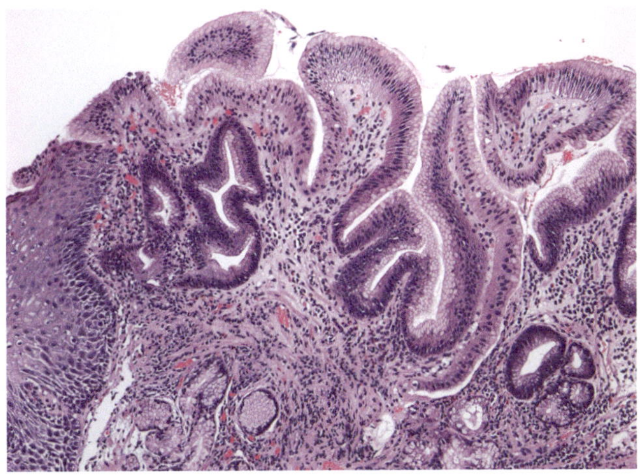

Fig. 15.2 Medium-power magnification of esophagogastric junction. The gastric cardia is very commonly inflamed, with associated reactive epithelial changes in the foveolae. This inflammation occurs so commonly that it need not be mentioned in the biopsy report

S.R. Owens, H.D. Appelman, *Atlas of Esophagus and Stomach Pathology*, Atlas of Anatomic Pathology, DOI 10.1007/978-1-4614-8084-6_15, © Springer Science+Business Media New York 2014

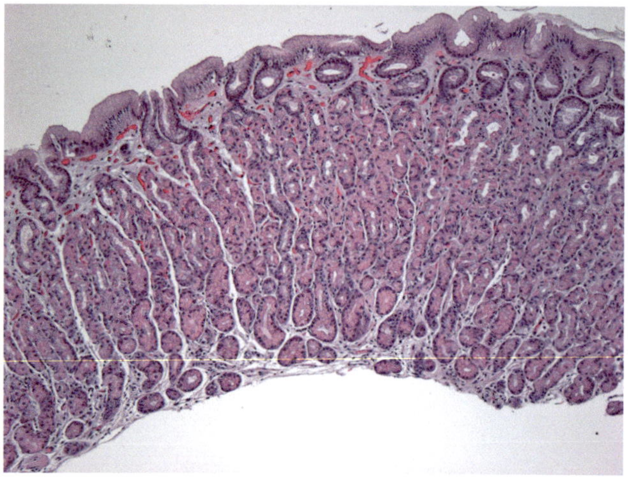

Fig. 15.3 Normal gastric body/fundus mucosa. The mucosa is predominantly occupied by oxyntic glands containing parietal and chief cells, while the pit (foveolar) compartment is fairly short. The glands are arranged back-to-back with relatively little intervening lamina propria

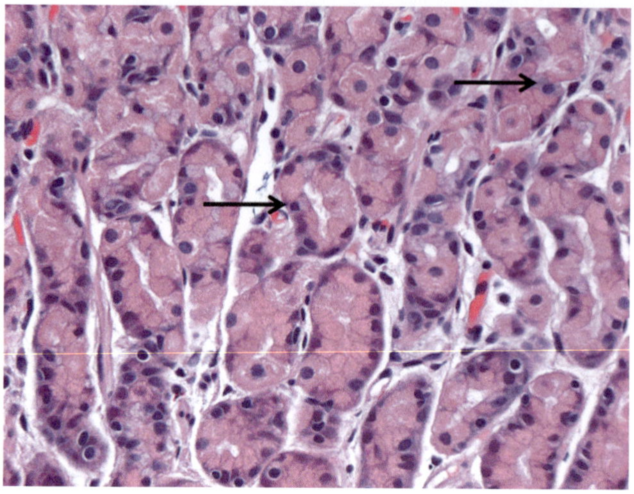

Fig. 15.4 At higher magnification, the eosinophilic parietal cells, which produce gastric acid, and more amphophilic, enzyme-producing chief cells (*arrows*) of the oxyntic glands are more easily seen

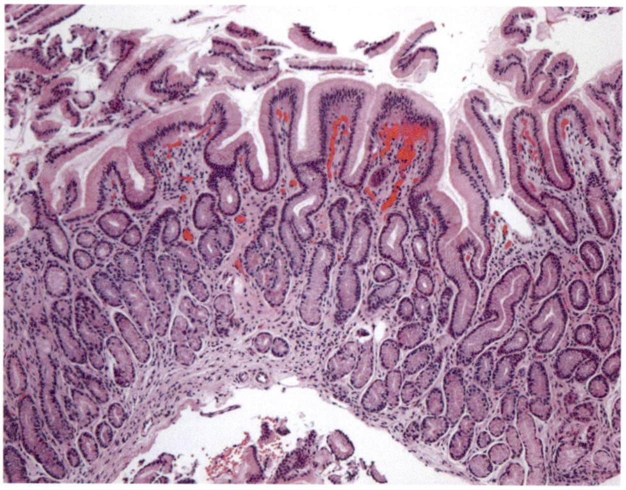

Fig. 15.5 Normal gastric antrum. The antral mucosa contains more prominent gastric pits with foveolar mucin, beneath which lie mucus-producing glands that contain G cells. The lamina propria of the antrum is more prominent than that of the gastric oxyntic mucosa

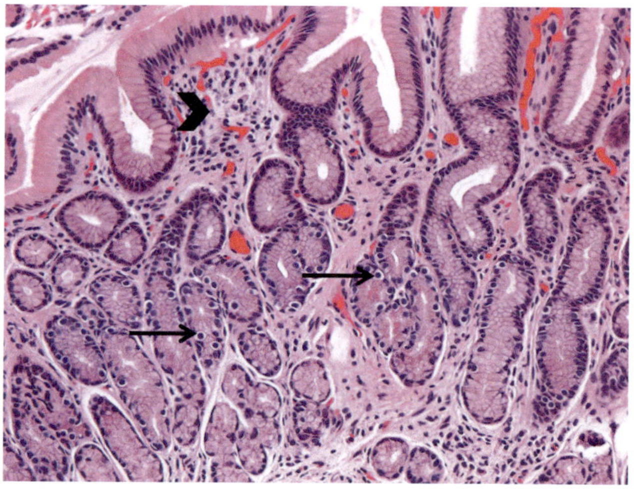

Fig. 15.6 At higher magnification, gastrin-producing G cells with perinuclear halos are easily seen (*arrows*). The antral mucosa commonly contains a few lamina propria inflammatory cells, including plasma cells and small lymphocytes (*arrowhead*)

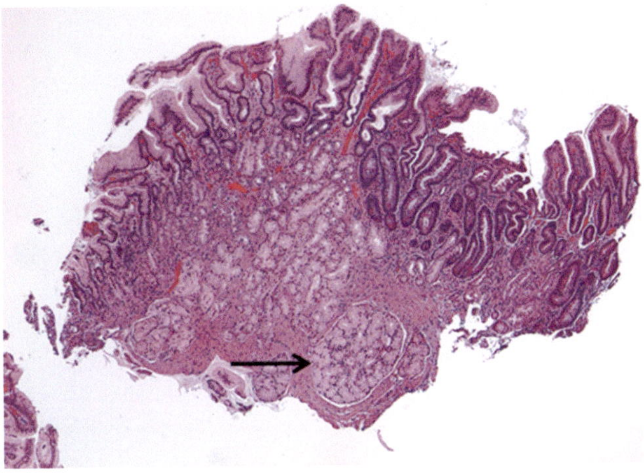

Fig. 15.7 Pyloroduodenal junction. The mucosa of the pylorus is similar to that of the gastric antrum, but the glands do not contain G cells. The mucosal pit compartment is prominent, with abundant foveolar mucin. The right half of the photomicrograph contains the duodenal bulb mucosa, which can have an admixture of foveolar and intestinal surface epithelium. A nest of Brunner glands, with mucus-producing epithelium histologically indistinguishable from pyloric glands, is in the duodenal submucosa (*arrow*)

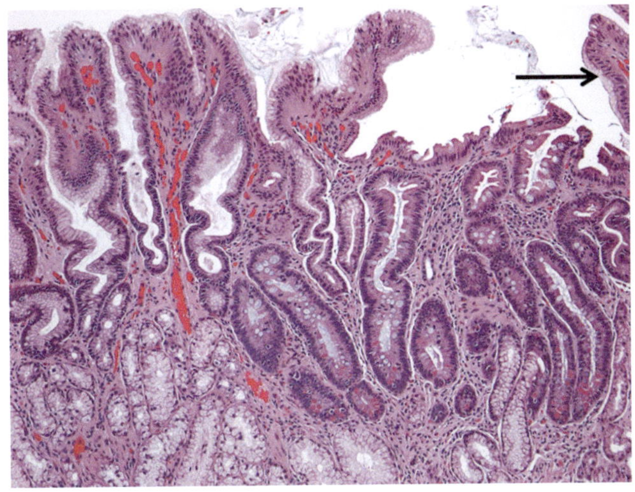

Fig. 15.8 At higher magnification, the junction of intestinal (*right*, containing blue goblet and red Paneth cells) and pyloric (*left*) mucosa is easily seen. Note the normal admixture of intestinal and foveolar (*arrow*) surface epithelium in the duodenal bulb

16 General Microscopic Changes and Findings to Ignore

The second chapter in the stomach portion of the atlas describes general microscopic changes and findings that can be a part of many different clinicopathological conditions. These changes are typically a response to mucosal injury of one sort or another, and they will be encountered again throughout the ensuing chapters. In addition, there are several findings that, while eye-catching, are probably best "ignored" in the context of the pathology report (*ie*, they may be included in the category of "no significant abnormality").

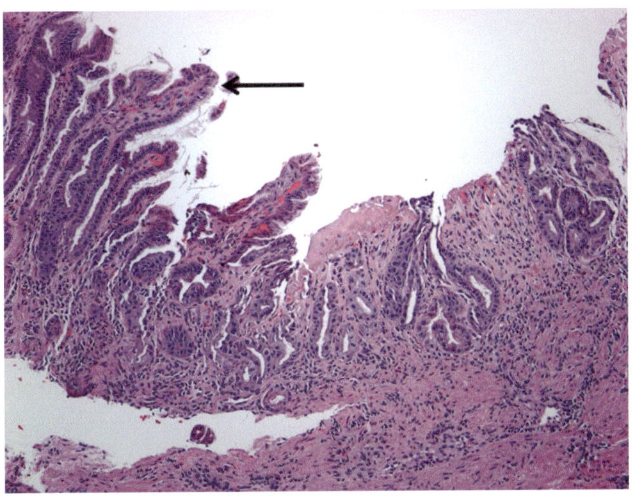

Fig. 16.1 Mucosal erosion. The surface epithelium in this antral erosion has been denuded and the superficial mucosa (including most of the pit compartment) is necrotic. On the surface, fibrinous debris is admixed with a few inflammatory cells, while the underlying glands and adjacent foveolae (*arrow*) are intensely regenerative. Erosions are confined to the superficial mucosa, while ulcers penetrate the full mucosal thickness (*see below*)

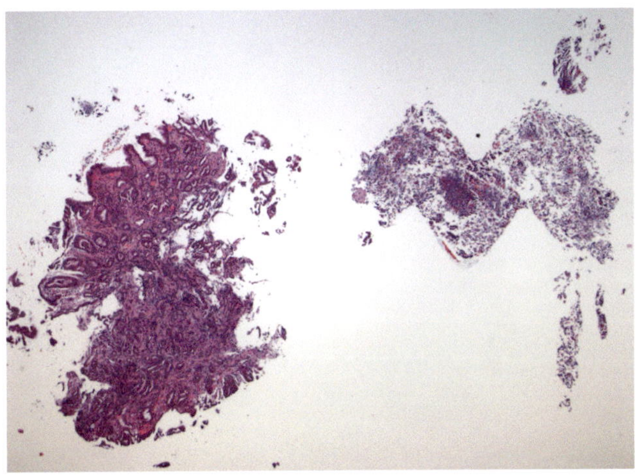

Fig. 16.2 Ulcer. In contrast to erosions, an ulcer penetrates the mucosa. Because endoscopic biopsies are usually obtained from the ulcer edge rather than the base, often only the intensely reactive/regenerative mucosa (*left*) and the ulcer exudate (*right*) are visible on the biopsy section. The presence of the exudate is sufficient to diagnose the ulcer

S.R. Owens, H.D. Appelman, *Atlas of Esophagus and Stomach Pathology*, Atlas of Anatomic Pathology,
DOI 10.1007/978-1-4614-8084-6_16,

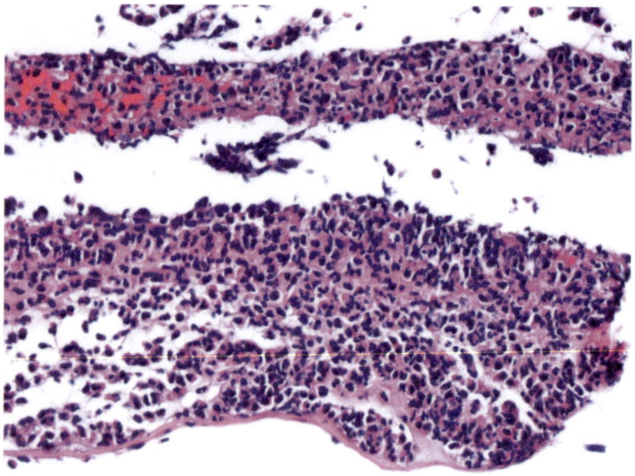

Fig. 16.3 Ulcer exudate. This mixture of fibrinopurulent debris and sloughed epithelial cells characterizes an ulcer exudate. Clumps of eosinophilic fibrin are admixed with inflammatory cells (predominantly neutrophils)

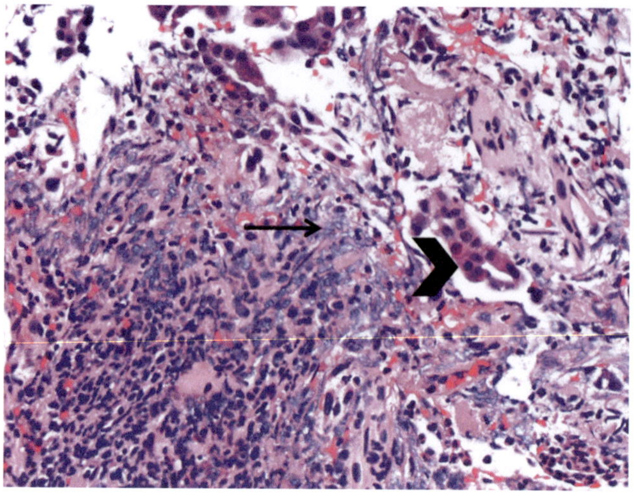

Fig. 16.4 "Peptic smudge." The exposure of cell nuclei from the disrupted mucosa to gastric acid causes a loss of nuclear detail (*arrow*). This "peptic smudge" is often seen in biopsy specimens taken from near ulcers. Note the detached, intensely regenerative-appearing fragments of epithelium suspended in the exudate (*arrowhead*)

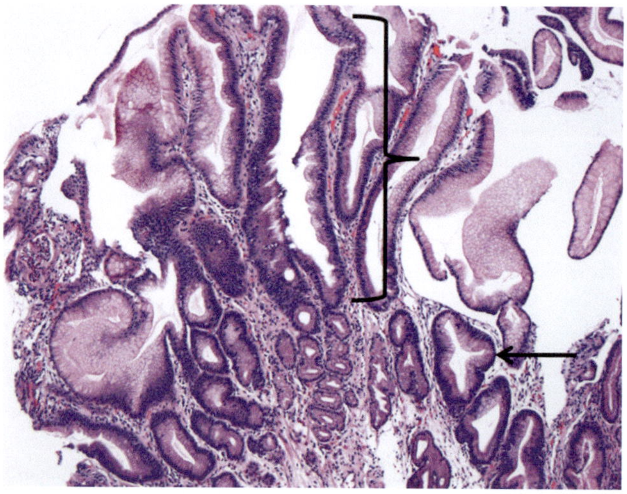

Fig. 16.5 Ulcer edge. Since most biopsies of ulcers sample the ulcer edge, the characteristic foveolar hyperplasia (*bracket*) and hyperchromatic, regenerative-appearing epithelium (*arrow*) of ulcer-edge mucosal changes are commonly encountered in this setting. Even in the absence of ulcer exudate or ulcer bed, one can diagnose "foveolar hyperplasia and regenerative changes consistent with proximity to ulcer" or "ulcer edge changes"

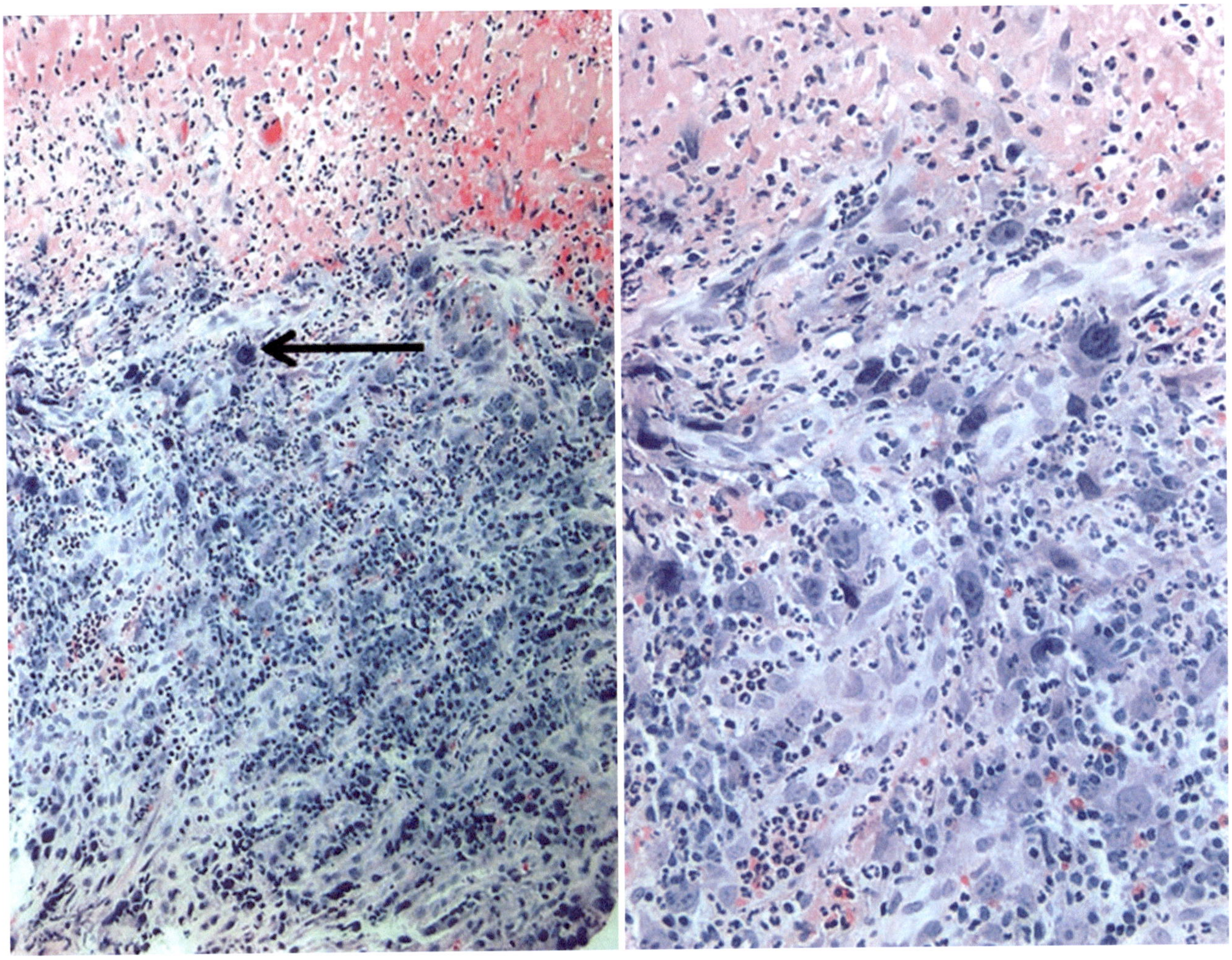

Fig. 16.6 Ulcer bed. If sampled, the base of an ulcer appears in biopsy sections as a loose collection of capillaries with surrounding inflammation (effectively, granulation tissue, seen in *left panel*). In addition, scattered atypical myofibroblasts are commonly seen (*arrow* and at higher magnification in *right panel*). These "ulcerocytes" can have an ominous appearance, mimicking malignancy, but are cytokeratin-negative on immunohistochemistry. They express vimentin and, often, markers of smooth muscle differentiation such as smooth muscle actin

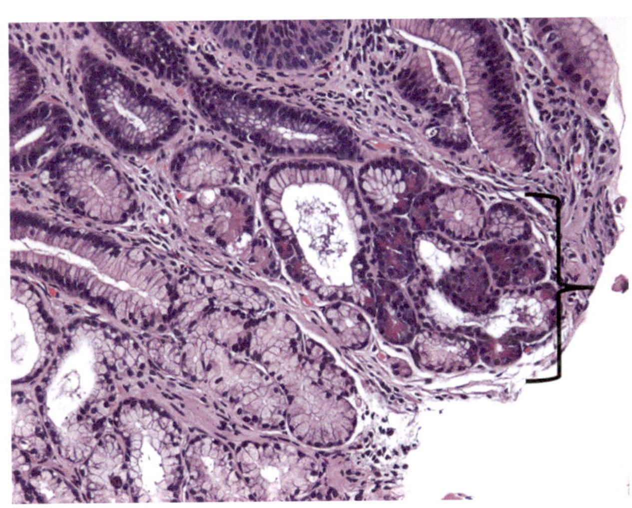

Fig. 16.7 Pancreatic acinar metaplasia (PAM). This common finding in the gastric cardia consists of tight clusters of acini with amphophilic, finely granular cytoplasm, and associated pancreatic ductular structures (*bracket*). It occurs incidentally in the proximal stomach, where it can safely be ignored, as well as in the setting of mucosal atrophy throughout the stomach

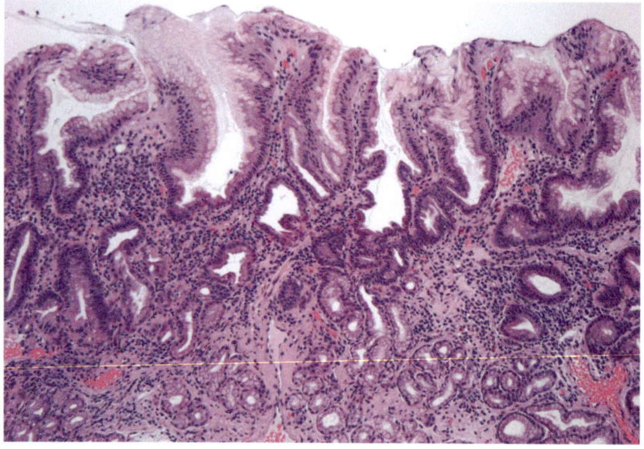

Fig. 16.8 The "ubiquitous" (and idiopathic) chronic carditis. The gastric cardia is so frequently inflamed in biopsy specimens that such inflammation is probably safely ignored in practice. Even a relatively dense plasma cell infiltrate in the lamina propria such as this is most often accompanied by normal mucosa elsewhere in the stomach, as it was in this case. Rarely, *Helicobacter pylori* infection (*see* Chap. 21) will manifest a pangastritis with involvement of the cardia

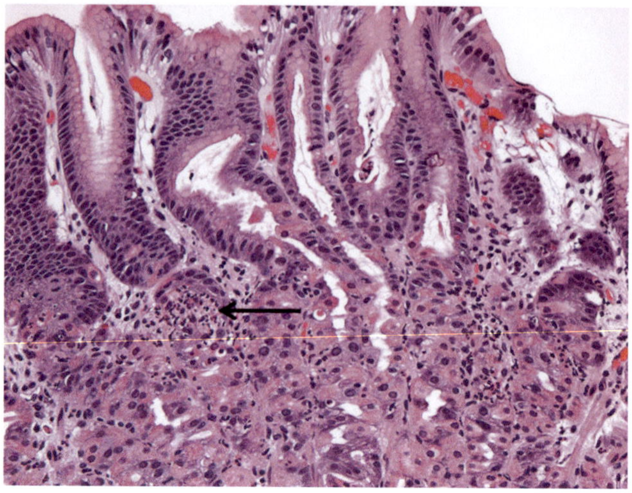

Fig. 16.9 Focal acute gastritis. A collection of neutrophils (*arrow*) infiltrates the mucous neck (junction between foveolar and gland compartments) in this oxyntic mucosa biopsy. There is no background of chronic gastritis. This finding is not infrequent, is of dubious significance, and is probably safely ignored

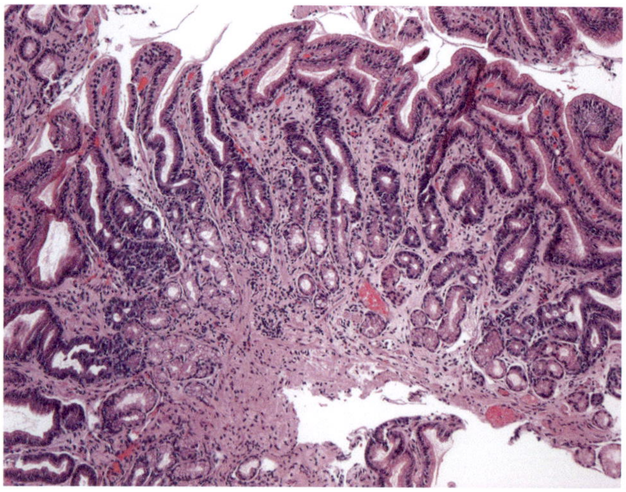

Fig. 16.10 Mild chronic gastritis. This biopsy from the gastric antrum has several abnormalities of no known significance, including mild superficial chronic inflammation, some atrophy of the gland compartment (as evidenced by "packets" of glands with abundant intervening lamina propria), reactive/regenerative foveolar epithelium, and basal lymphoid aggregates with admixed eosinophils. As these findings do not add up to any known disease, the biopsy is probably best regarded as having no significant abnormality

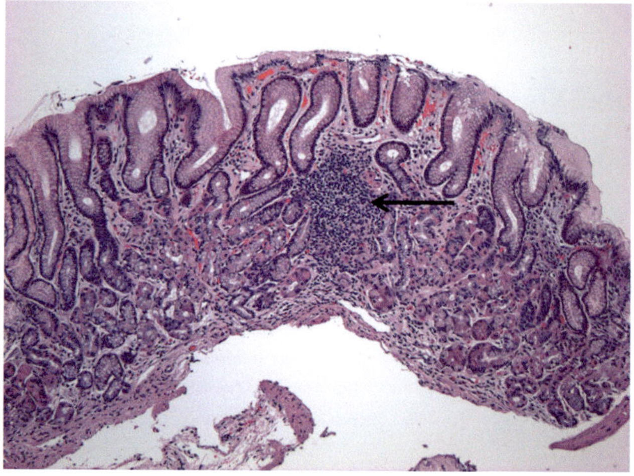

Fig. 16.11 Normal lymphoid aggregate. A circumscribed aggregate of small lymphocytes (*arrow*) in the deep (mid-zone or basal) mucosa is a common incidental finding of no significance. These can be seen throughout the stomach and do not signify any type of chronic gastritis

17 Structural Abnormalities/Heterotopias

This chapter deals with a handful of structural or congenital abnormalities that are important to recognize so that they are not confused with true diseases. Especially when sampled with biopsy forceps, these entities can provide an unexpected—and potentially confusing—admixture of tissue types that could raise the possibility of a neoplasm. Once recognized, they provide a convenient (and clinically reassuring) explanation for the endoscopic finding of a "submucosal mass."

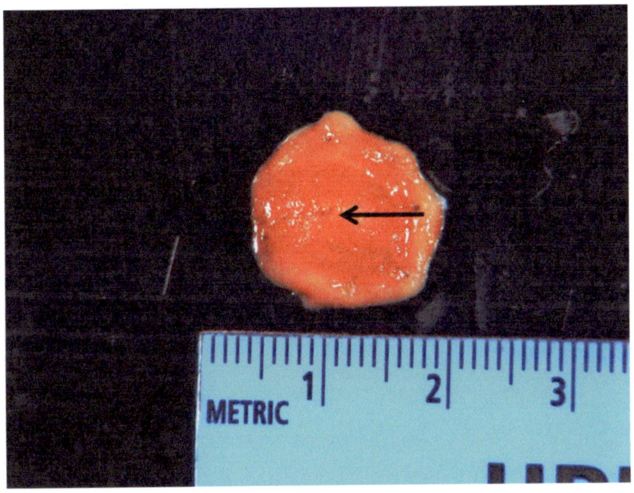

Fig. 17.1 Pancreatic heterotopia. This nodule of heterotopic pancreatic tissue was seen endoscopically as a nodule with a central umbilication (*arrow*). This is the classic endoscopic appearance of pancreatic heterotopia; the central depression is where the associated duct structure opens onto the mucosal surface (*see below*)

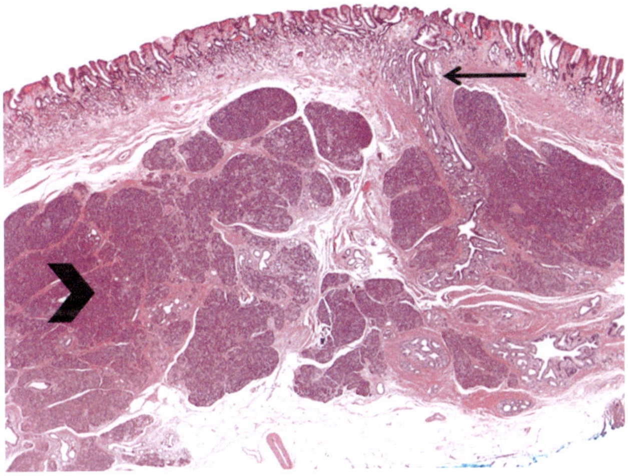

Fig. 17.2 Pancreatic heterotopia. A low-power photomicrograph shows heterotopic pancreatic lobules (*arrowhead*) beneath the overlying gastric mucosa, occupying the submucosa. A duct system (*arrow*) courses up through the mucosa to produce the central umbilication seen in the previous figure. Pancreatic heterotopia is the most common heterotopia in the stomach and occurs most often in the antrum

S.R. Owens, H.D. Appelman, *Atlas of Esophagus and Stomach Pathology*, Atlas of Anatomic Pathology, DOI 10.1007/978-1-4614-8084-6_17, © Springer Science+Business Media New York 2014

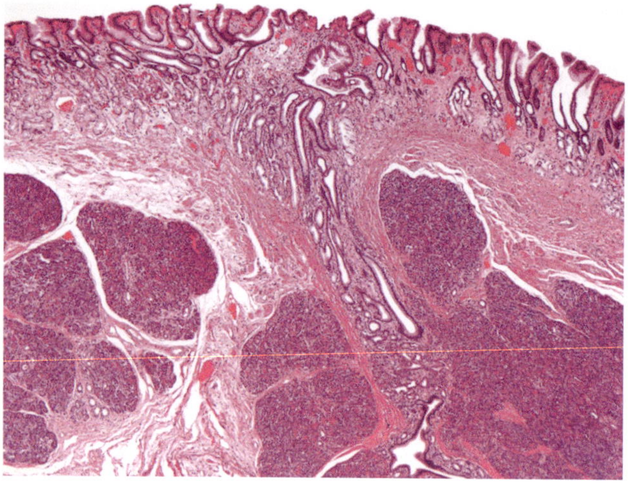

Fig. 17.3 Pancreatic heterotopia. A closer view of the duct leading to the mucosal surface. The acini and ducts are histologically identical to those seen in the normal pancreas. Most cases (~75 %) of pancreatic heterotopia occur in the submucosa and are asymptomatic, although some can involve the muscularis propria and can become inflamed. When both acinar and duct elements are present, the diagnosis is not a challenge, but some cases may be composed predominantly of duct structures and the acini may be difficult to find. Because of the smooth muscle surrounding the duct, such cases can be misinterpreted as adenomyomas or duplications

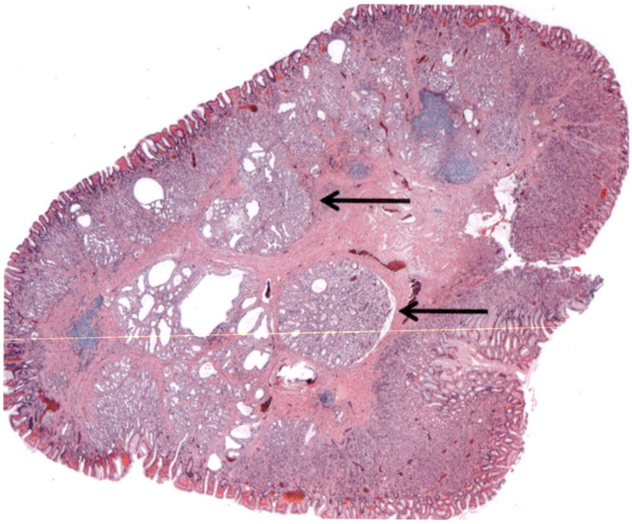

Fig. 17.4 Gastric gland heterotopia. This endoscopically removed polyp contains displaced clusters of gastric mucosa (*arrows*) in the submucosa. The overlying mucosa is unremarkable. At this magnification, it is impossible to distinguish between a congenital heterotopia of gastric glands/mucosa and a displacement secondary to prior mucosal injury/disruption ("gastritis cystica profunda")

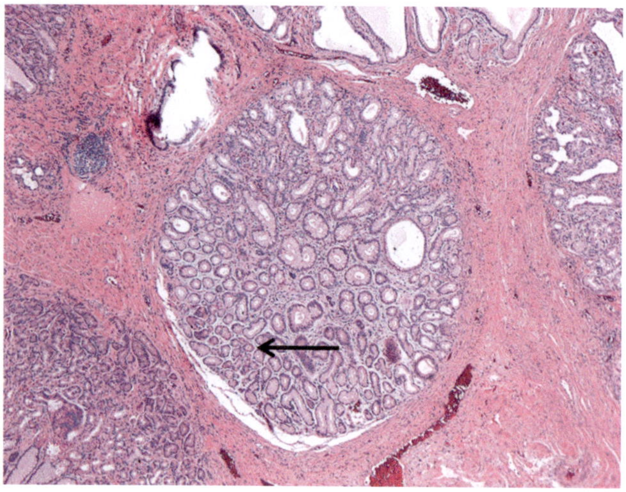

Fig. 17.5 Gastric gland heterotopia. At higher magnification, the nests of heterotopic mucosa are seen to disrupt the fibers of the muscularis mucosae and to be composed of glands at the periphery and foveolar structures in the center of the cluster, all admixed with lamina propria. In contrast to gastritis cystica profunda, the nests in congenital gastric heterotopia usually preserve this orderly mucosal structure and contain at least some oxyntic-type glands (*arrow*)

18 Vascular Abnormalities

Vascular abnormalities in the stomach can all result in upper gastrointestinal bleeding, which often leads to examination by upper endoscopy and, potentially, mucosal biopsies. The venous connection of the stomach to the portal circulation can result in gastric vascular manifestations of portal hypertension (either secondary to liver disease or in noncirrhotic patients). A characteristic mucosal vascular abnormality descriptively termed "gastric antral vascular ectasia" is usually encountered in elderly patients and shares some histological features with portal hypertension and reactive mucosal changes ("reactive gastropathy"; see Chap. 19). Ischemia is a relatively rare cause of mucosal injury in the stomach, and is thus rarely encountered in gastric mucosal biopsies. All of these entities have fairly characteristic endoscopic appearances.

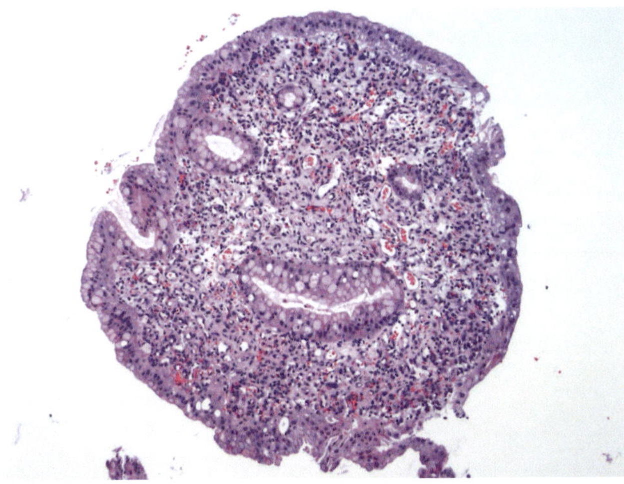

Fig. 18.1 In patients with portal hypertension, mucosal biopsies may contain dilated capillaries without significant inflammation. Endoscopically, these changes are accompanied by a characteristic "mosaic" or "snakeskin" pattern of the mucosa, which appears erythematous. While these dilated mucosal capillaries can be a prominent feature, the vascular changes may be restricted to the submucosa, where venules and veins may be dilated and thick-walled. Thus, a normal-appearing biopsy does not exclude the possibility of PHG in the appropriate clinical and endoscopic setting

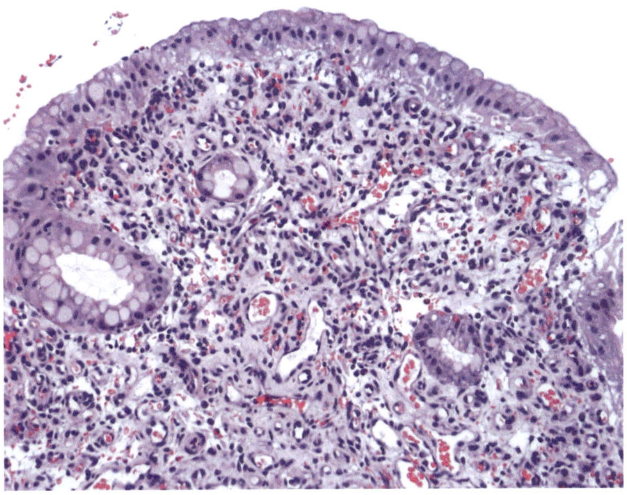

Fig. 18.2 At higher magnification, the dilated and somewhat tortuous mucosal capillaries sometimes seen in PHG are apparent. The lack of significant mucosal inflammation and, importantly, the lack of fibrin thrombi in the dilated capillaries separate PHG from other conditions that can have a similar appearance, such as gastric antral vascular ectasia (*see below*)

S.R. Owens, H.D. Appelman, *Atlas of Esophagus and Stomach Pathology*, Atlas of Anatomic Pathology,
DOI 10.1007/978-1-4614-8084-6_18, © Springer Science+Business Media New York 2014

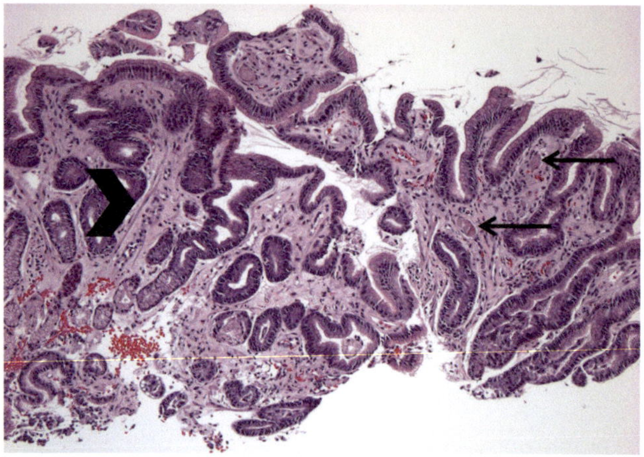

Fig. 18.3 At low power, the mucosa from a patient with gastric antral vascular ectasia (GAVE) has a reactive appearance. With foveolar mucin depletion, elongated and tortuous gastric pits lined by hyperchromatic, regenerative-appearing epithelium, and fine bundles of smooth muscle suggesting mucosal prolapse lying between the pits (*arrowhead*). These background changes are essentially identical to so-called "reactive gastropathy" (see Chap. 19). Superimposed on these features in GAVE are dilated mucosal capillaries, often containing small fibrin thrombi (*arrows*). Endoscopically, these mucosal changes are accompanied by a characteristic appearance of the antrum, with red, linear "stripes" running along the antrum toward the pylorus. This striped appearance has been termed "watermelon stomach"

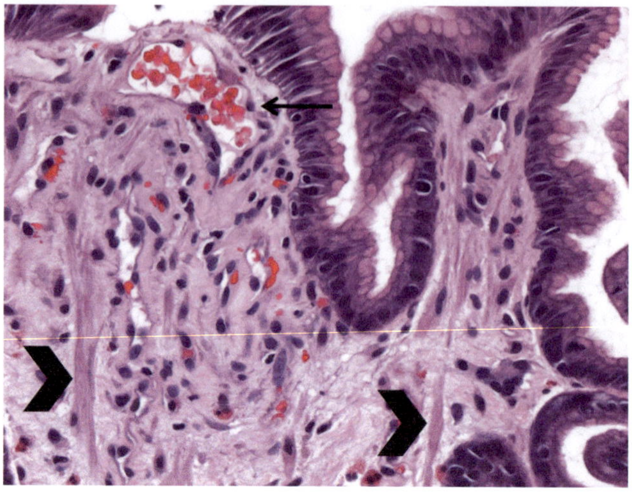

Fig. 18.4 At high magnification, the fine smooth muscle bundles (*arrowheads*) and dilated capillaries (*arrow*) are plainly visible, as are the reactive/regenerative changes of the foveolar epithelium. Note the depletion of foveolar mucin. Occasional capillaries are large enough to rival the cross-sectional size of the gastric pits, although they do not always contain visible thrombi. Although its exact incidence is unknown, GAVE typically occurs in older individuals and may lead to mucosal bleeding

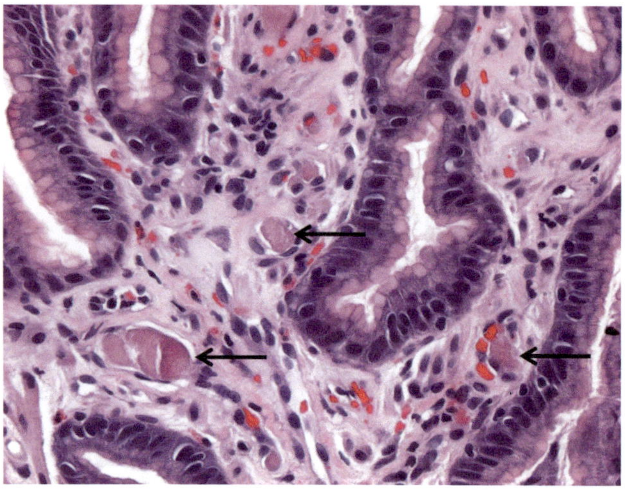

Fig. 18.5 Another high-magnification view of GAVE, highlighting the reactive/regenerative epithelium with hyperchromatic nuclei as well as several fibrin thrombi within dilated capillaries (*arrows*). The etiology of GAVE is uncertain, but it may be an exuberant reactive condition, possibly prolapse-related, with a contribution by age-related degenerative mucosal changes. It is not thought to be caused by portal hypertension

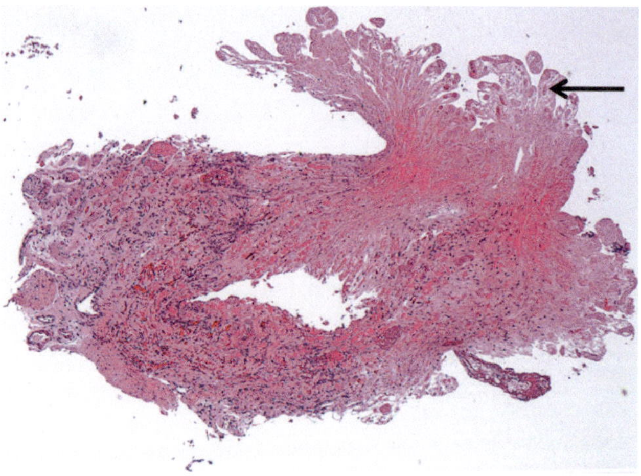

Fig. 18.6 Low-magnification view of ischemic necrosis of the gastric mucosa. Gastric infarction is rare, due to the rich and redundant vascular supply of the stomach. Focal or mild ischemia can cause mucosal erosions or ulcers identical to those described in Chap. 16. In this particular case, the mucosa is almost completely necrotic, with "ghost" outlines of gastric pits on the mucosal surface (*arrow*) and hemorrhage in the deeper mucosa

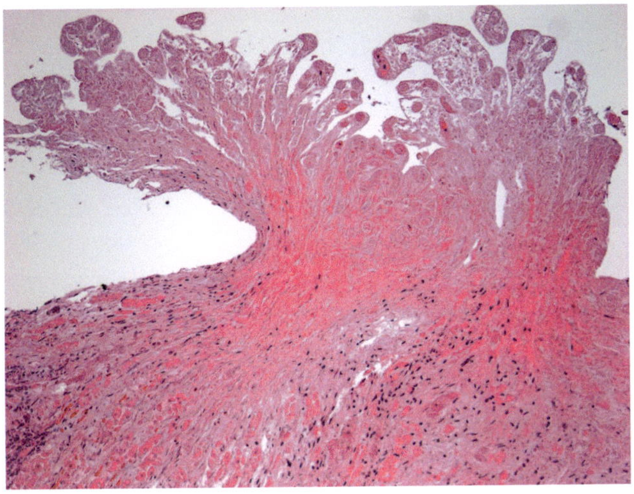

Fig. 18.7 At higher magnification, coagulative necrosis of the mucosal structures is evident. Only congested vessels and scattered inflammatory cells are visible in the deeper mucosa. This patient suffered extensive infarction of the stomach and duodenum due to a dissecting aortic aneurysm

19 Toxic and Medication-Induced Conditions

In our practice, relatively nebulous symptoms such as "dyspepsia" or "heartburn" are common indications for examination by esophagogastroduodenoscopy. Few such patients will present for an endoscopic examination aimed at elucidating the cause of these symptoms without having a tried and failed medical therapy such as proton pump inhibitor (PPI) medications to alleviate their suffering. In addition, many patients seen for such symptoms are on one or more medications unrelated to gastrointestinal disease, and over-the-counter medications are ubiquitous. Finally, other ingested and endogenous substances can affect the mucosa of the stomach, resulting in reactive mucosal changes. Thus, the biopsies that we receive commonly show the effect of one or more medications or toxic substances. Although many types of insult are possible, there is a relatively limited number of ways the mucosa can respond, meaning that intense reactive features to the gastric mucosa can have a variety of causes. In general, these reactive mucosal changes have little in the way of inflammation, leading us to classify most of them as types of *gastropathy* rather than *gastritis*, which will be discussed separately. In addition to the general category of reactive changes, some types of medication- or toxin-induced injury manifest with more characteristic histological findings.

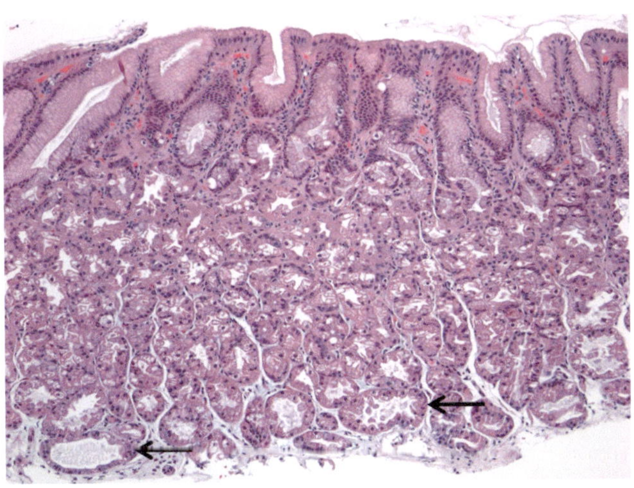

Fig. 19.1 Many biopsies obtained during upper endoscopy will exhibit the effects of PPI administration because most patients attempt at least a trial of such therapies before undergoing an endoscopic examination for upper gastrointestinal symptoms. At low magnification, an overall increase in parietal cell mass can be appreciated in the gastric body/fundus mucosa, with abundant eosinophilic parietal cells crowding the oxyntic glands. A few glands (*arrows*) are dilated, reminiscent of the similar finding seen in fundic gland polyps. *Bona fide* fundic gland polyps (see Chap. 23) may also be found

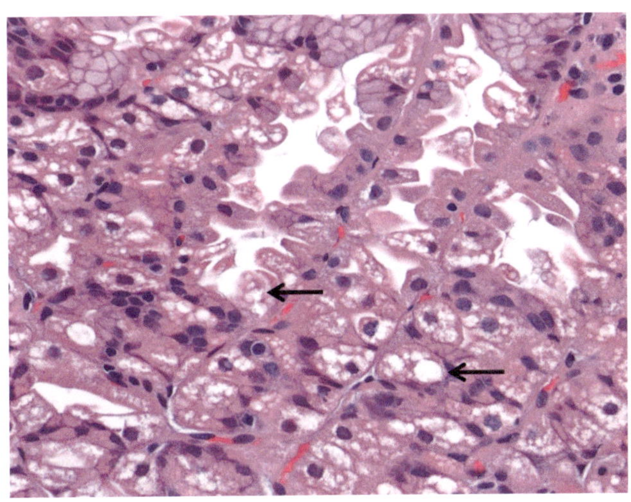

Fig. 19.2 At high magnification, the enlarged parietal cells can be seen to have "snouts" that protrude into the oxyntic gland lumens. In this case, many cells (*arrows*) are also vacuolated, another common finding in the setting of PPI therapy. These changes are so common in the biopsies encountered in our daily practice that we no longer mention their presence

S.R. Owens, H.D. Appelman, *Atlas of Esophagus and Stomach Pathology*, Atlas of Anatomic Pathology,
DOI 10.1007/978-1-4614-8084-6_19,

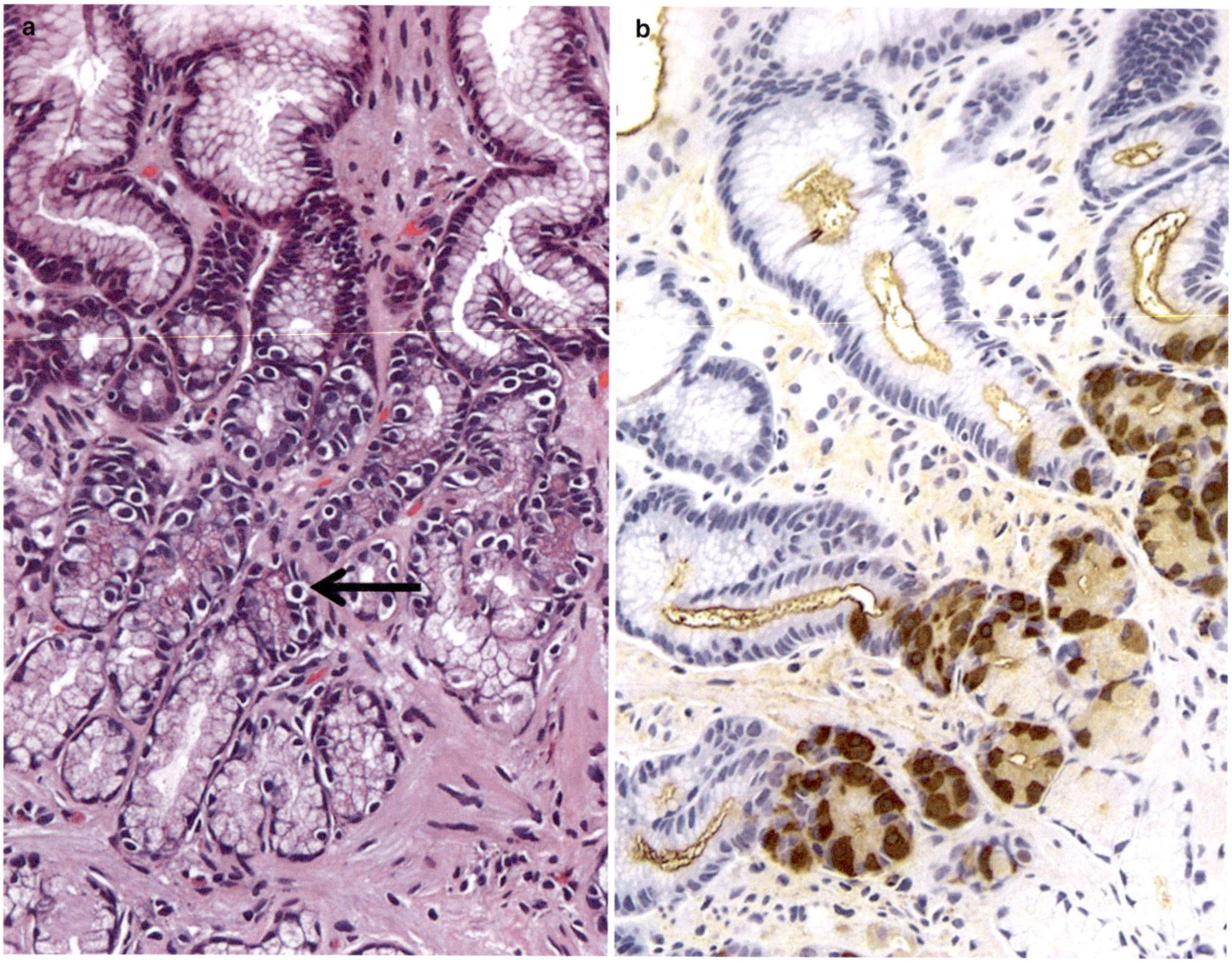

Fig. 19.3 (**a**) In the gastric antral mucosa, PPI therapy can result in hyperplasia of the gastrin-producing G cells (*arrow*). (**b**) These cells are highlighted by a positive gastrin immunohistochemical stain

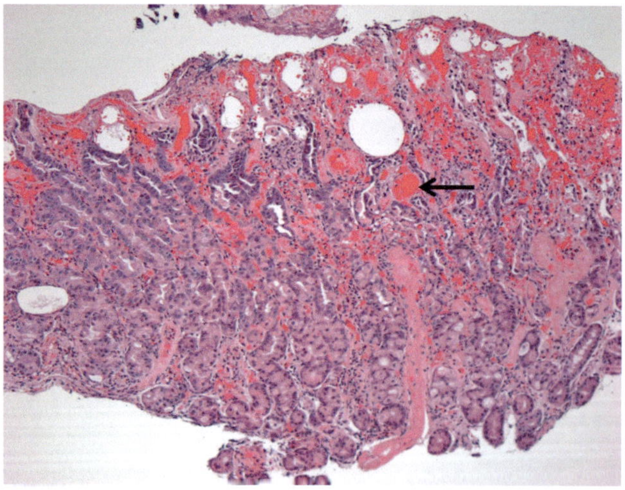

Fig. 19.4 At low magnification, hemorrhagic gastritis is characterized by dilated mucosal capillaries (*arrow*) and collections of extravasated red blood cells, especially in the superficial mucosa. In addition, there is erosion of the surface epithelium. This process is thought to be the result of an imbalance between protective and injurious mucosal influences and can follow ischemic insults, massive trauma, large doses of nonsteroidal anti-inflammatory drugs (NSAIDs), and alcohol binges, among other causes

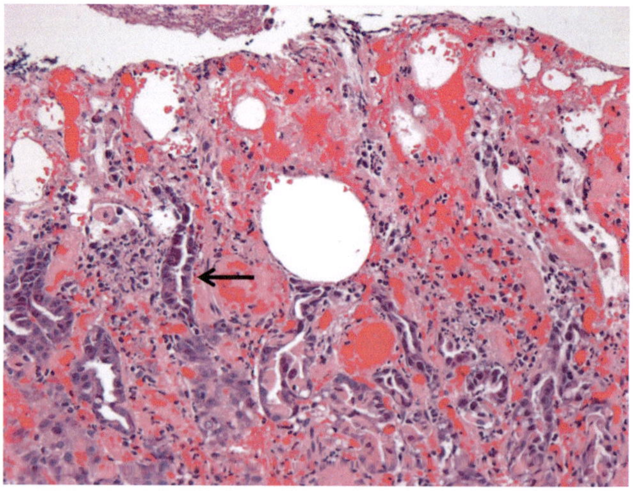

Fig. 19.5 At medium-power magnification, the surface erosion is more easily seen, as are the dilated capillaries and the intensely regenerative appearance of the remaining epithelium (*arrow*). As suggested by the name and the appearance of extravasated blood in the photomicrograph, hemorrhagic gastritis can result in significant blood loss

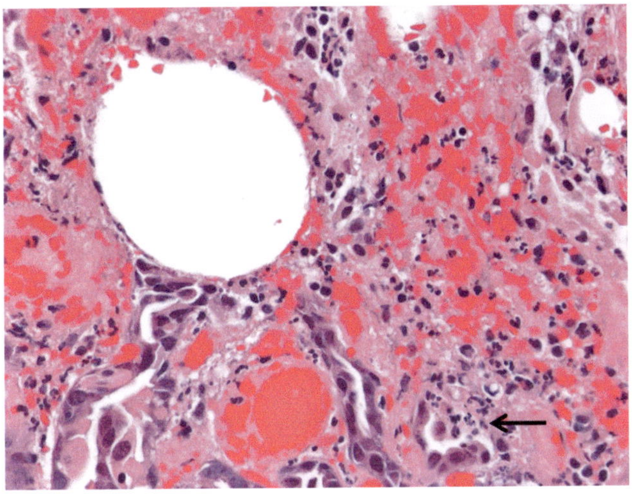

Fig. 19.6 At high magnification, small collections of neutrophils are visible, admixed with fibrin and red blood cells. Hemorrhagic gastritis has a variable amount of acute inflammation, and it is relatively sparse in this case. A few neutrophils infiltrate the reactive epithelium (*arrow*)

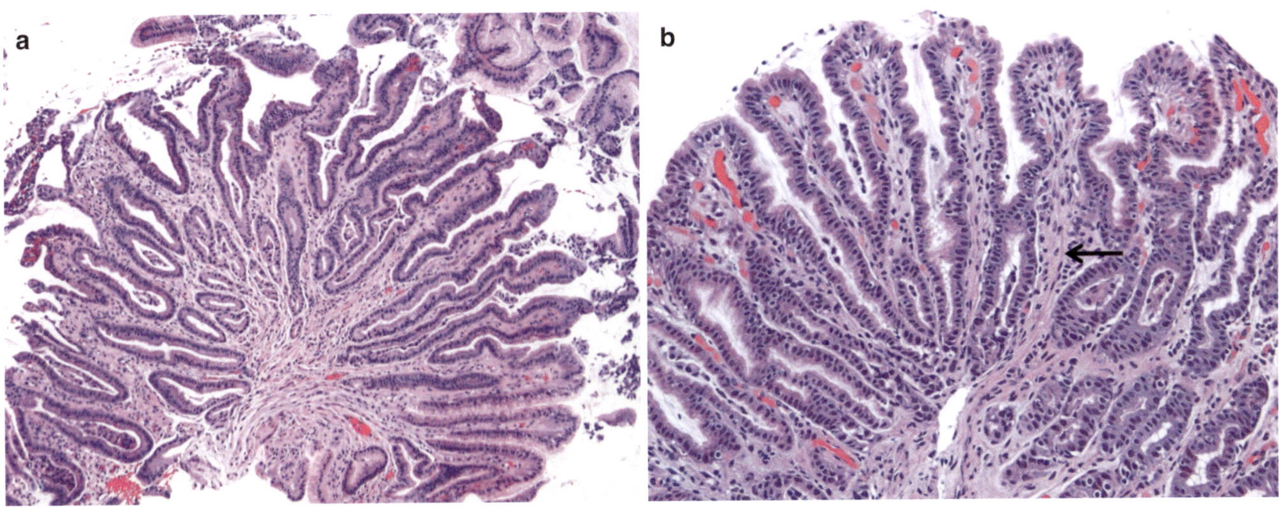

Fig. 19.7 First described in the setting of bile reflux after patients underwent antrectomy for intractable peptic ulcer disease, chemical gastropathy is a common regenerative/reactive pattern of mucosal changes associated with mucosal injury of any cause. In current practice, the most common culprit is NSAIDs, but alcohol, chemotherapy agents, and other toxins can cause a similar appearance. (**a**) The phenomenon, also known as "reactive gastropathy," is characterized by regenerative epithelial changes including mucin depletion and nuclear hyperchromasia, as well as foveolar hyperplasia (elongation of gastric pits) and a characteristic irregularity (serration or "corkscrewing") of the foveolae. (**b**) At higher magnification, the regenerative epithelial atypia is apparent. This should not be mistaken for dysplasia. Additionally, "splaying" of the muscularis mucosae is apparent, with thin smooth muscle fibers (*arrow*) extending into the superficial mucosa between the foveolae

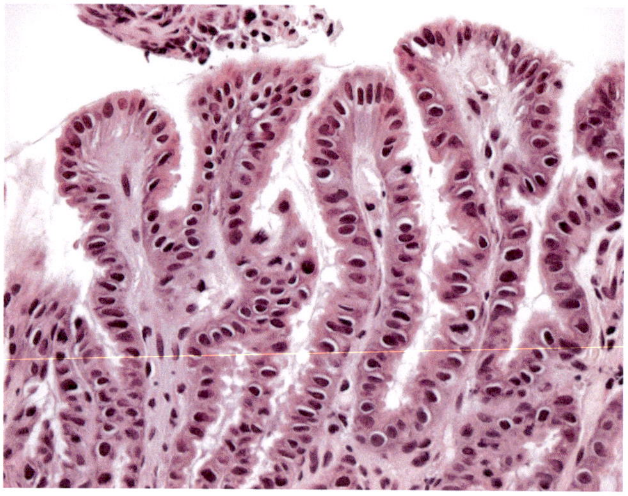

Fig. 19.8 At high magnification, the striking reactive epithelial atypia in this example of chemical gastropathy is easily seen. In the background of irregular foveolae and mucin depletion, one must be careful not to overinterpret this atypia as evidence of dysplasia. While regenerative mucosal changes can accompany inflammatory conditions such as *H. pylori* gastritis, true chemical gastropathy is relatively free of mucosal inflammation, as evidenced by the lack of inflammatory cells in the lamina propria

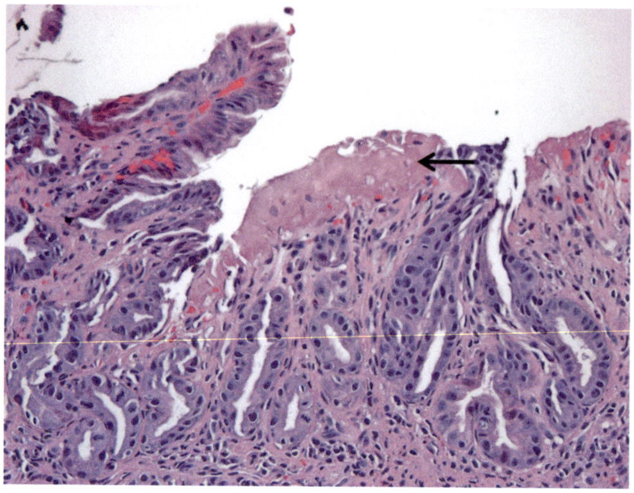

Fig. 19.9 Mucosal erosions may accompany the other changes of chemical gastropathy, particularly when the mucosal irritation is the result of NSAIDs. Here, the reactive atypia and mucin depletion of the epithelium are adjacent to the fibrinous exudate indicating loss of the surface epithelium (*arrow*). Such erosions, as well as ulcers, can occur throughout the gastrointestinal tract of NSAIDs users

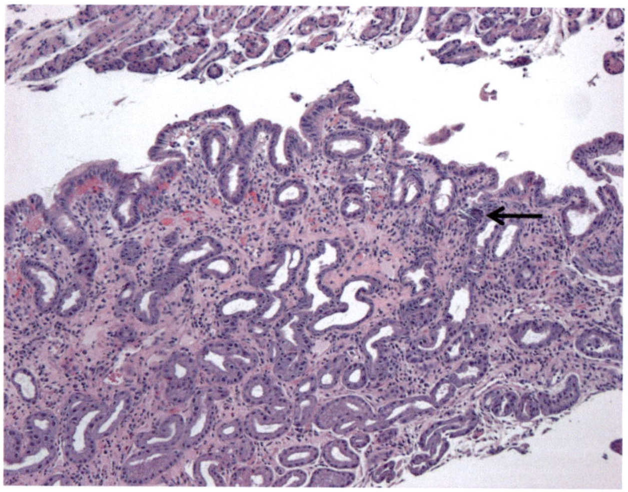

Fig. 19.10 At low magnification, the mucosal injury caused by oral iron pill therapy resembles the changes of chemical gastropathy (*see* Fig. 19.3), with depletion of surface mucin and regenerative epithelial changes. The surface may be eroded as well. The clue to diagnosis is the deposition of pigmented material in the superficial mucosa (*arrow*)

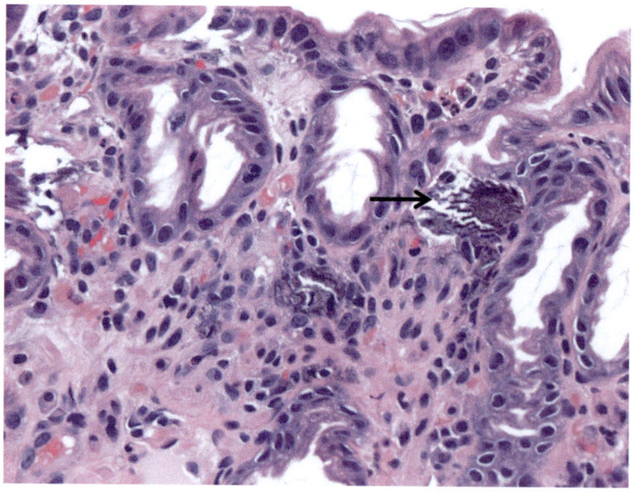

Fig. 19.11 At high magnification, the deposited iron, which most commonly occurs in the setting of oral ferrous sulfate therapy, can be seen in the superficial mucosa. Iron may accumulate in the extracellular matrix of the lamina propria (where it is seen here), as well as in macrophages and/or epithelial cells, and usually has a reddish-brown appearance. Occasionally, it will appear more basophilic, as in this example. It typically has a fibrillar appearance as well (*arrow*)

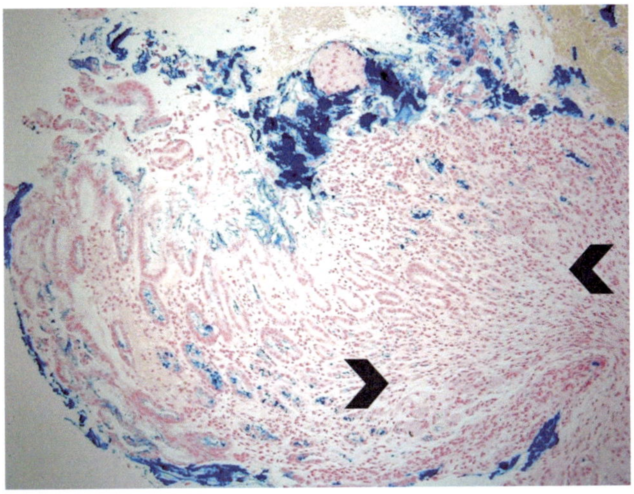

Fig. 19.12 The diagnosis of iron-pill gastropathy can be aided by a careful review of the patient's medication log (when available) as well as with a cytochemical stain for iron such as Prussian blue. Note the characteristic deposition of exogenous iron in the superficial mucosa, whereas the deep mucosa (*arrowheads*) is essentially devoid of iron. In contrast, accumulation of endogenous iron, such as in primary hemochromatosis, also involves the deep mucosal glands and lamina propria

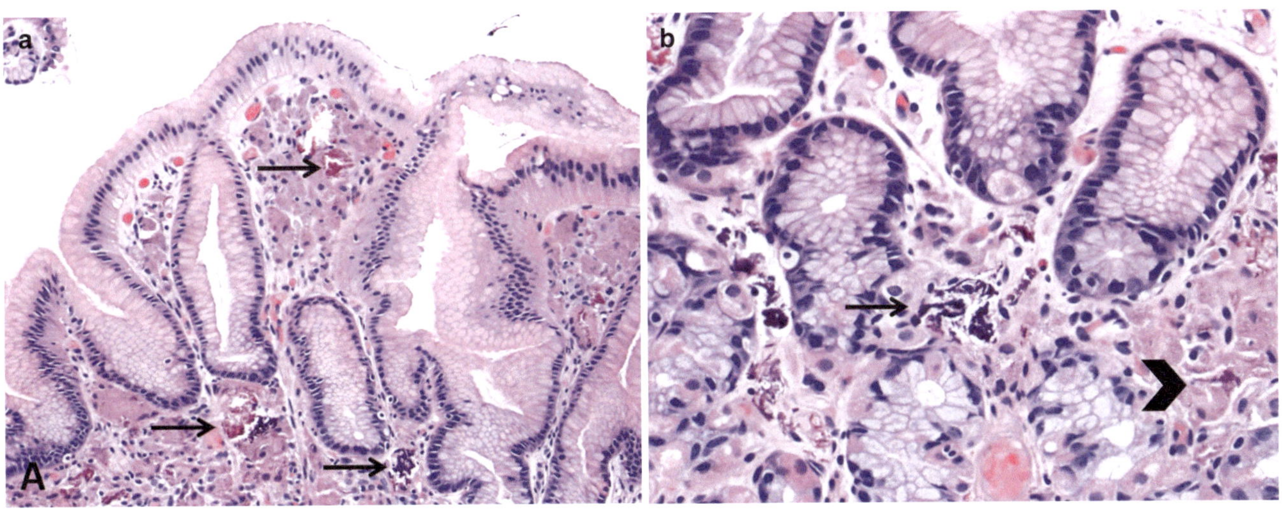

Fig. 19.13 Mucosal calcinosis can be associated with iatrogenic situations and/or derangements in calcium metabolism, often in chronic renal failure patients and/or those with solid organ transplants. (**a**) Crystalline deposits of calcium (*arrows*) are found in the lamina propria, typically in the more superficial mucosa. (**b**) Calcium deposits are often surrounded by macrophages and have a red-purple hue (*arrow*). In addition, finely granular deposits of calcium may be found within macrophages and can mimic viral inclusions such as those seen in cytomegalovirus infection (*arrowhead*)

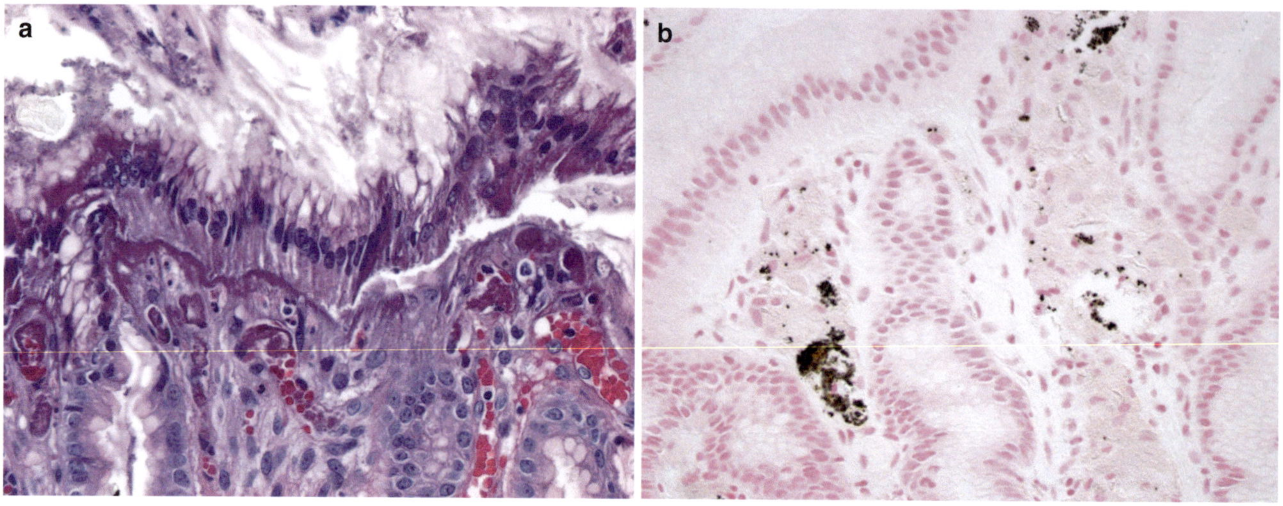

Fig. 19.14 (**a**) In the very superficial mucosa, calcinosis has been particularly associated with aluminum-containing antacid therapy and sucralfate therapy. Mucosal calcium deposits have also been associated with mucosal injury/necrosis (dystrophic calcification) or systemic hypercalcemia (metastatic calcification). (**b**) The diagnosis of mucosal calcinosis can be aided using a von Kossa cytochemical stain, which stains the calcium deposits very dark brown or black

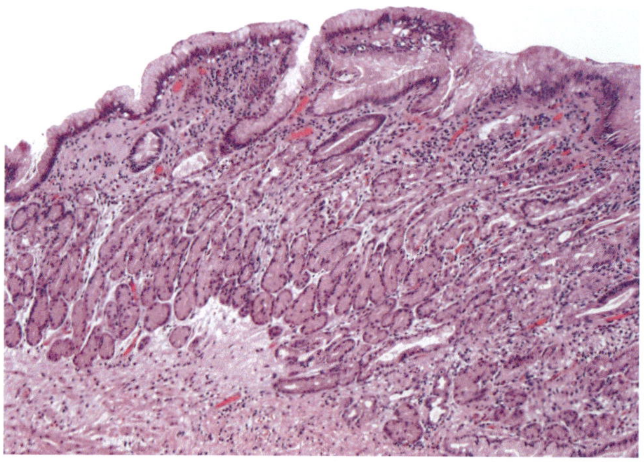

Fig. 19.15 In patients who have received adjuvant or neoadjuvant chemotherapy, it is common to encounter histological findings indicative of mucosal injury, corresponding to the clinical phenomenon of "mucositis." Such patients commonly have reactive-appearing mucosa with evidence of epithelial injury, but minimal mucosal inflammation (unless an infectious process is superimposed). These reactive changes are characterized by epithelial damage and regeneration, with enlarged and atypical epithelial cells

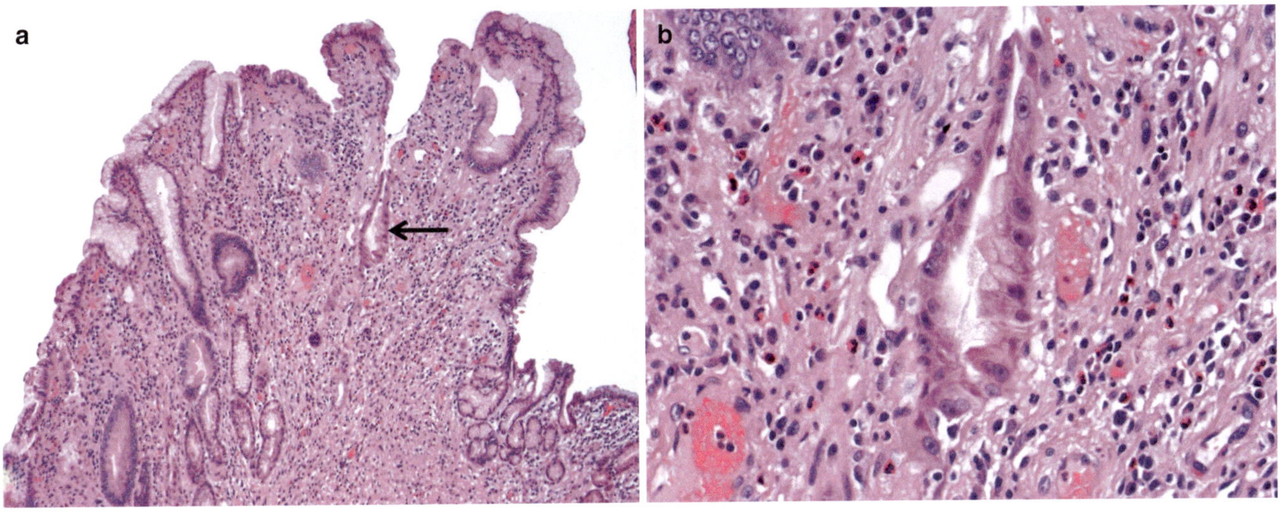

Fig. 19.16 (**a**) At higher magnification, the reactive epithelial atypia is more apparent, with enlarged and hyperchromatic nuclei that can mimic epithelial dysplasia. One particularly regenerative-appearing gastric pit (*arrow*) is lined by large, eosinophilic epithelial cells. (**b**) At high magnification, the symmetrical enlargement of these reactive epithelial cells is apparent. Several have one or more prominent nucleoli

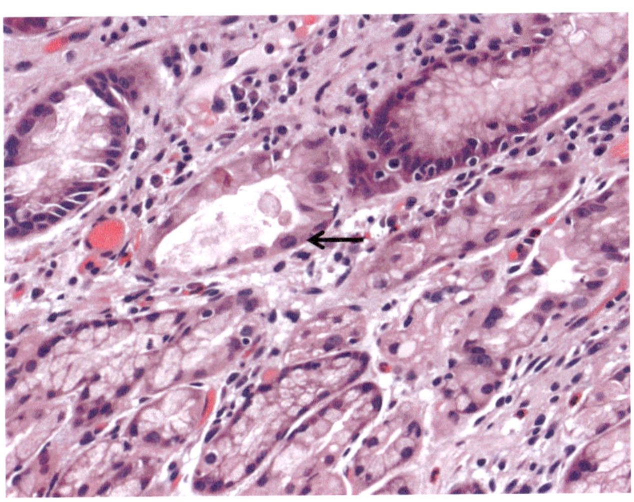

Fig. 19.17 Some of the gastric glands damaged by chemotherapy agents are dilated and contain necrotic luminal debris. Enlarged and hyperchromatic nuclei (*arrow*) can resemble viral inclusions, an important differential diagnosis in patients who are immunosuppressed secondary to therapy

20 Noninfectious Inflammatory and Systemic Diseases Affecting the Stomach

Like the rest of the gastrointestinal (GI) tract, the stomach is affected by a variety of inflammatory and systemic diseases that may or may not have primary manifestations elsewhere in the body. Some of these, like autoimmune atrophic gastritis, involve relatively specific changes in the stomach, while others, like lymphocytic gastritis, are a single morphologic manifestation that can be caused by a variety of different conditions. Thus, this chapter presents a bit of a potpourri of diseases and histological patterns that provide interesting (and sometimes striking) microscopic appearances but which do not fit well into any of the other chapters in this section.

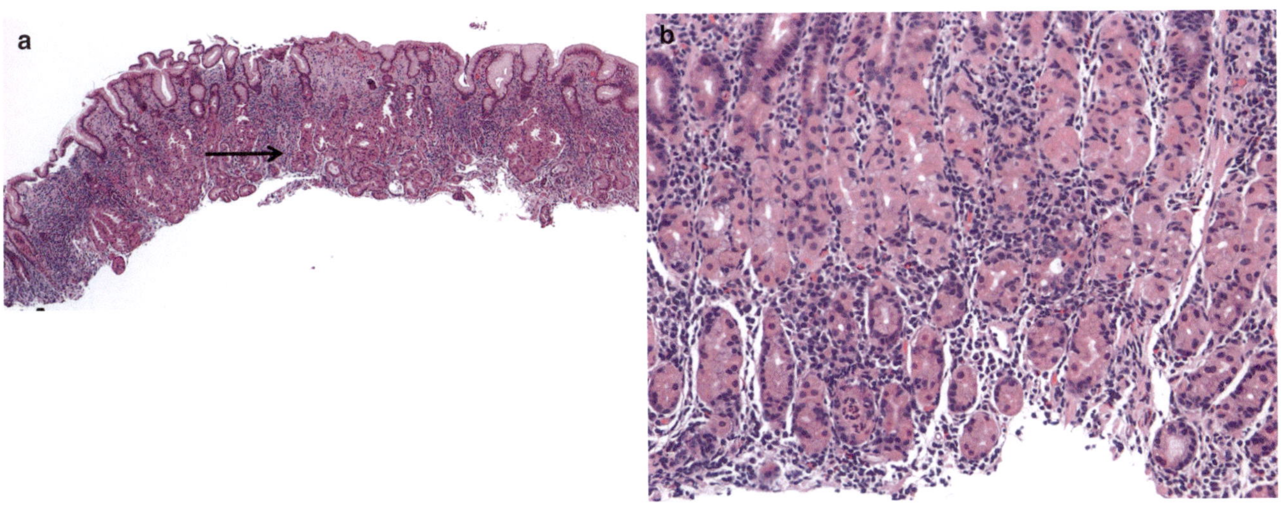

Fig. 20.1 Autoimmune atrophic gastritis (AAG) is caused by autoantibodies directed at gastric parietal cells (specifically at the "proton pump" ATPase and intrinsic factor). Accordingly, there is a mucosal inflammatory process that centers on the oxyntic glands in the gastric body/fundus. (**a**) In the early or active phase of the disease, the parietal cell mass will be relatively intact, but surrounded by a dense lymphoplasmacytic inflammatory population that makes the gland compartment (*arrow*) appear densely cellular and "blue." (**b**) At higher magnification, the plasma cells and lymphocytes can be seen surrounding the oxyntic glands, but the overall structure of the mucosa is basically intact

S.R. Owens, H.D. Appelman, *Atlas of Esophagus and Stomach Pathology*, Atlas of Anatomic Pathology, DOI 10.1007/978-1-4614-8084-6_20, © Springer Science+Business Media New York 2014

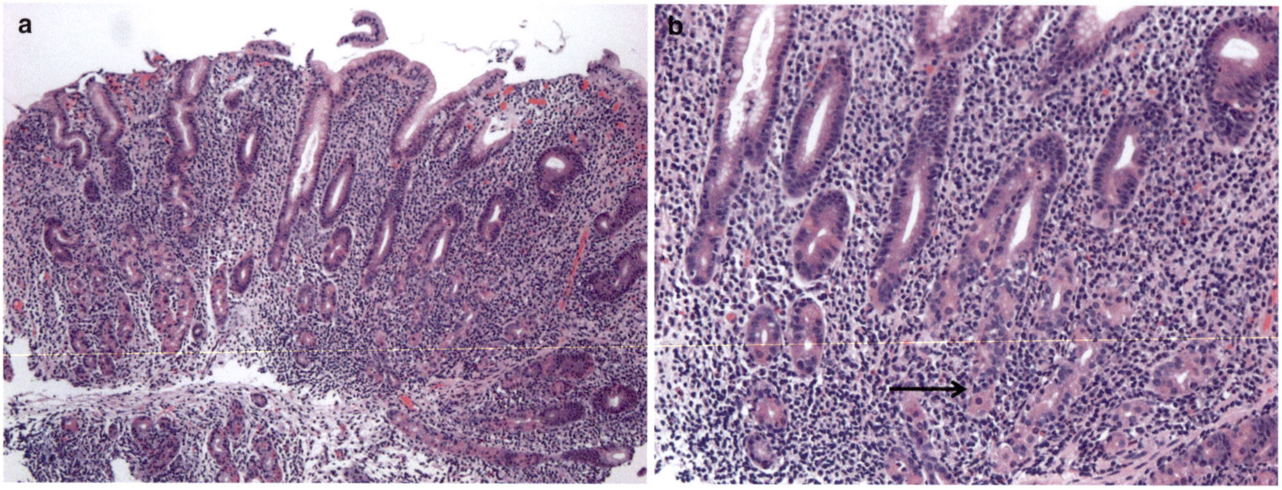

Fig. 20.2 As the disease progresses to the "florid" phase, parietal cell mass decreases and the mucosa begins to become atrophic. (**a**) At low magnification, the dense lymphoplasmacytic inflammation remains very prominent, but the loss of parietal cells is apparent in the lack of eosinophilic staining. At this point, the mucosa may begin to appear thinned or atrophic on endoscopic examination, and areas of metaplasia (intestinal and/or pancreatic) can make an appearance in biopsies of the mucosa. (**b**) The loss of parietal cells is apparent on this higher-magnification photomicrograph, and lymphocytes and plasma cells can be seen surrounding and infiltrating the oxyntic glands (*arrow*)

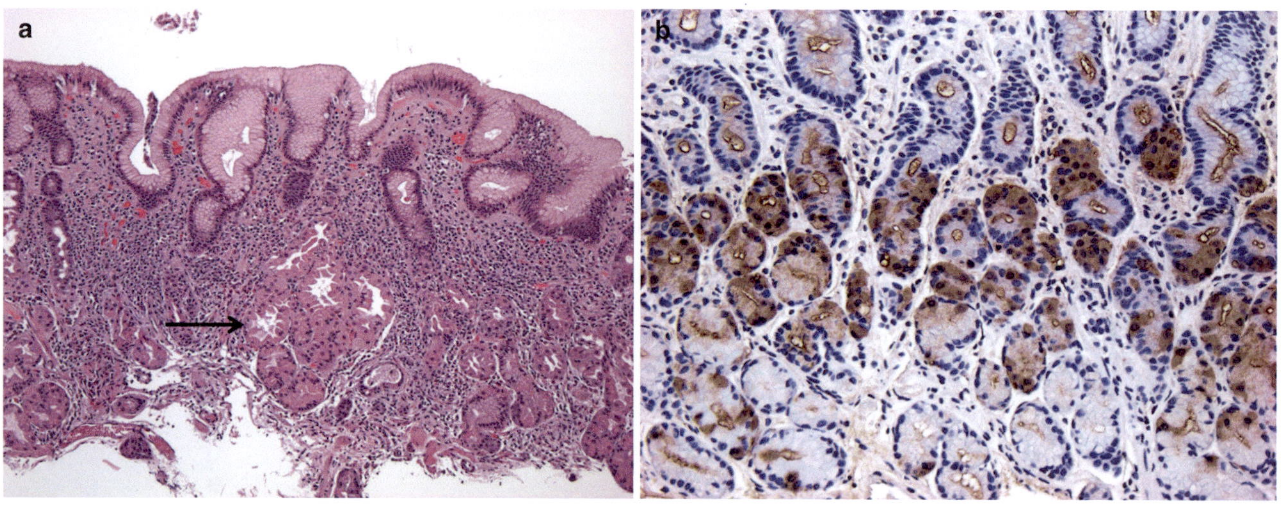

Fig. 20.3 (**a**) The loss of acid-producing parietal cells in the oxyntic mucosa leads to hypochlorhydria, which in turn causes an increase in gastrin production by the G cells in the gastric antrum. This may cause the remaining intact parietal cells to take on a hypertrophic appearance with apical "snouts" similar to that seen in the setting of proton pump inhibitor pharmacotherapy (*arrow*). Areas where residual parietal cells persist can appear endoscopically as nodules or "polyps"; these are, in fact, islands of intact mucosa with hypertrophic parietal cells, surrounded by thinned and atrophic mucosa that has lost its parietal cell mass. (**b**) In the antrum, which is devoid of significant inflammation in AAG, an immunohistochemical stain for gastrin highlights the G-cell hyperplasia

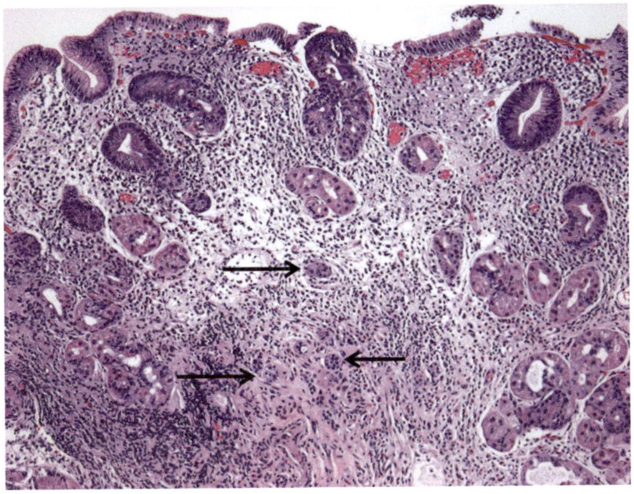

Fig. 20.4 In the fully developed "end" phase of AAG, the mucosa is very atrophic and may be entirely devoid of parietal cells. The residual gastric glands of the body and fundus produce only mucus, and can appear nearly identical to the glands of the prepylorus or antrum, apart from the lack of G cells. This "antralized" mucosa can be proven to be from the more proximal stomach by using a gastrin immunostain, which will be positive in true antral mucosa and negative in "antralized" gastric body mucosa. Hyperplasia of enterochromaffin-like (ECL) cells results from hypergastrinemia, and ECL cell nodules (*arrows*) appear as the mucosa becomes atrophic

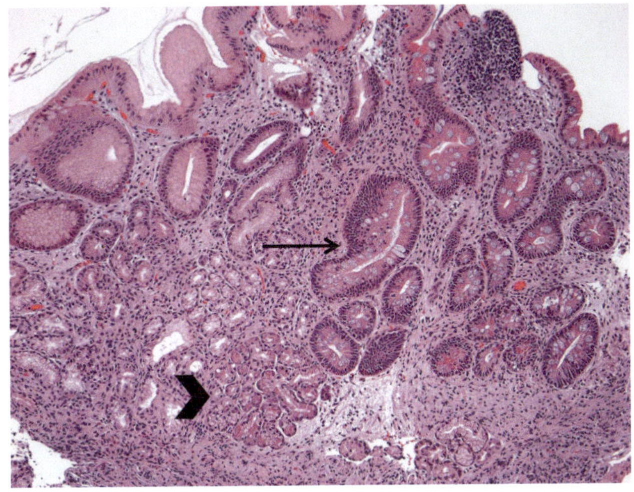

Fig. 20.5 Intestinal metaplasia (*arrow*) and pancreatic acinar metaplasia (*arrowhead*) are hallmarks of mucosal atrophy in AAG. Areas of intestinal metaplasia in the gastric body/fundus can harbor gastrin-positive cells, a potential point of confusion when utilizing immunohistochemistry to determine whether a biopsy was obtained from antral or oxyntic mucosa

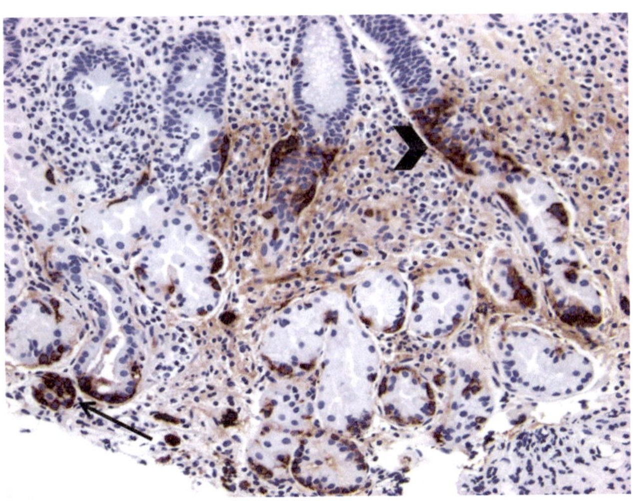

Fig. 20.6 ECL cell hyperplasia in the setting of AAG is both linear (*arrowhead*) and nodular (*arrow*), as highlighted on this chromogranin immunohistochemical stain. The nodules of ECL cells may be seen on hematoxylin and eosin (H&E) staining, but the linear component is more difficult to appreciate. As the hypergastrinemia continues, the ECL cell hyperplasia may result in the development of well-differentiated neuroendocrine (carcinoid) tumors (*see* Chap. 26). Gastric carcinoids arising in the setting of hypergastrinemia caused by AAG are classified as "Type 1" tumors

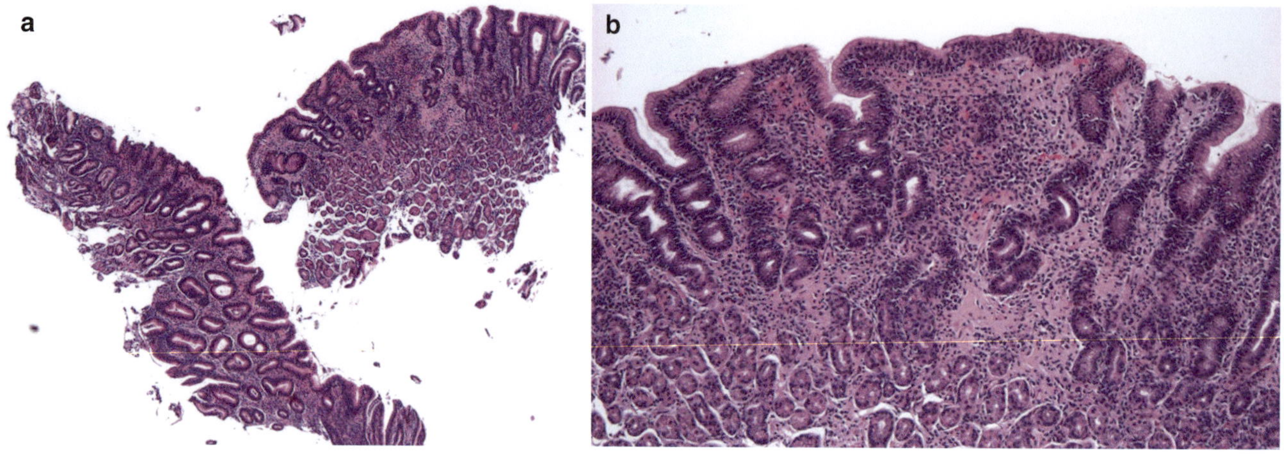

Fig. 20.7 The histologic pattern of lymphocytic gastritis is a common appearance that has a variety of causes. (**a**) At low magnification, there is an impression of some type of gastritis in this case, with a cellular and hyperchromatic appearance to the mucosa. (**b**) At higher magnification, there is a chronic inflammatory infiltrate in the lamina propria but, even at this power, an impression of "too many cells" in the surface and pit epithelium can be gleaned. In addition, the epithelium has a reactive appearance. This histological pattern has been associated with *Helicobacter pylori* infection, celiac disease (a classic association), inflammatory bowel disease, certain drugs, and other conditions

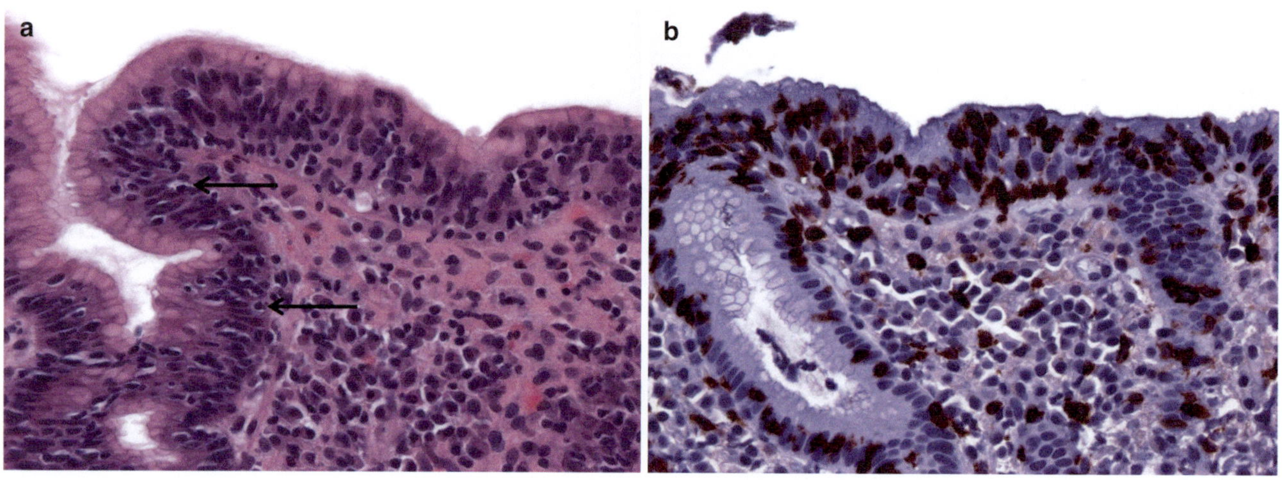

Fig. 20.8 (**a**) At high magnification, many small lymphocytes can be seen infiltrating the surface and foveolar epithelium. Some are surrounded by a clear "halo" (*arrows*). (**b**) Using immunohistochemistry, the intraepithelial cells prove to be CD3-positive T lymphocytes. Most have the cytotoxic, CD8-positive phenotype. Although many observers use a "gestalt" approach to recognize lymphocytic gastritis, it is defined as having more than 25 intraepithelial lymphocytes per 100 epithelial cells

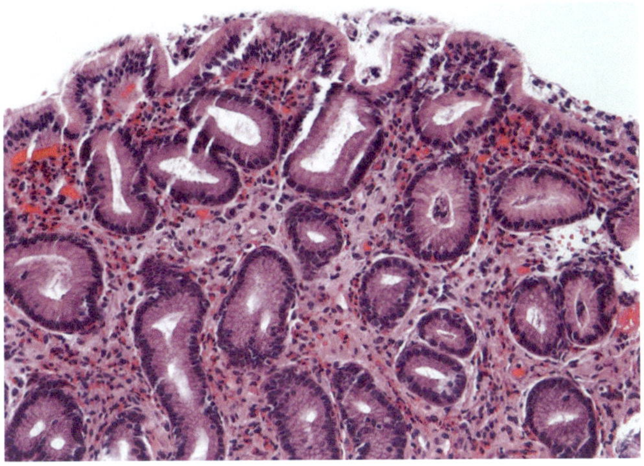

Fig. 20.9 Pathologists struggle with the significance of eosinophils in mucosal biopsies, and the literature contains reports both alleging their significance and suggesting that their number varies seasonally and geographically. Eosinophilic gastritis/gastroenteritis is a recognized disease entity, and can be related to atopic conditions or other hypereosinophilic syndromes. Mucosal involvement has been associated with diarrhea and malabsorption, but the diagnosis depends on ruling out other things that can lead to hypereosinophilia such as parasitic infections. This biopsy contains numerous eosinophils infiltrating the mucosa and is from a patient that had peripheral blood eosinophilia

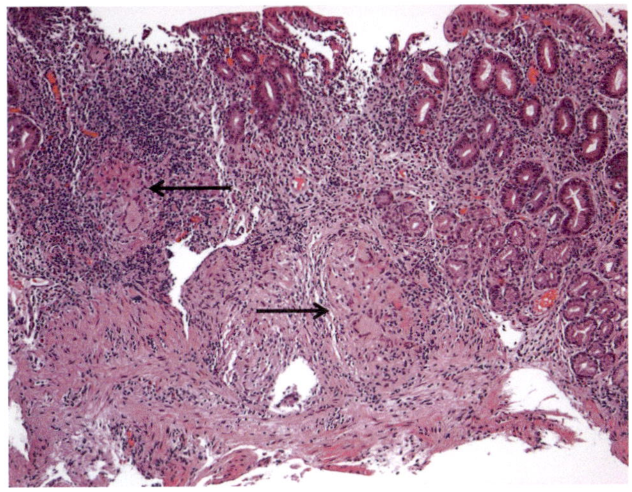

Fig. 20.10 As with eosinophils in mucosal biopsies, mucosal granulomas (*arrows*) can be associated with a variety of conditions such as sarcoidosis, granulomatous infections, Crohn's disease, and foreign body reactions. When all of these underlying conditions have been excluded, the term "granulomatous gastritis" can be applied. In the absence of underlying etiologies, this can be an incidental finding on gastric biopsies obtained in the diagnostic work up of a variety of symptoms

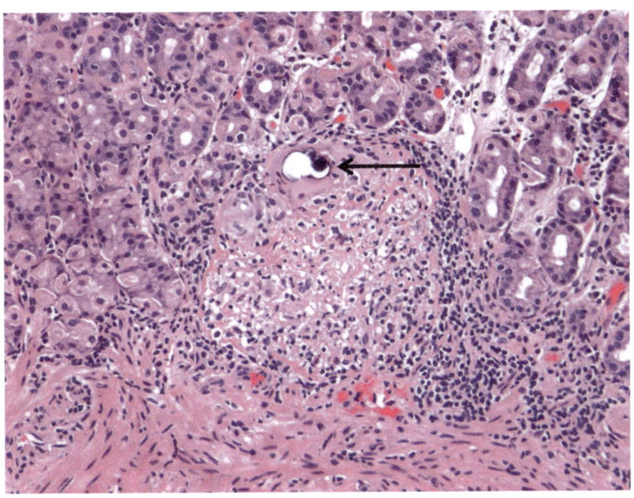

Fig. 20.11 This gastric granuloma was found in a biopsy from a patient with sarcoidosis, and contains a Schaumann body (*arrow*). Note the suggestion on H&E-stained section that the granuloma incorporates bundles of collagen. This is characteristic of sarcoidal granulomas

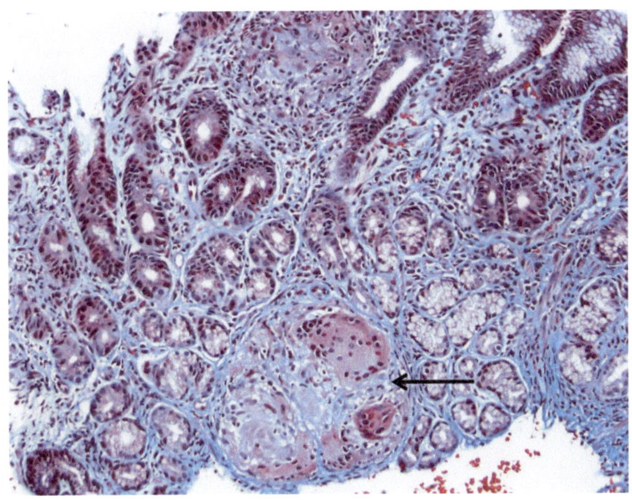

Fig. 20.12 A trichrome stain confirms the presence of collagen (stained blue) in the same granuloma pictured in Fig. 20.11 (*arrow*)

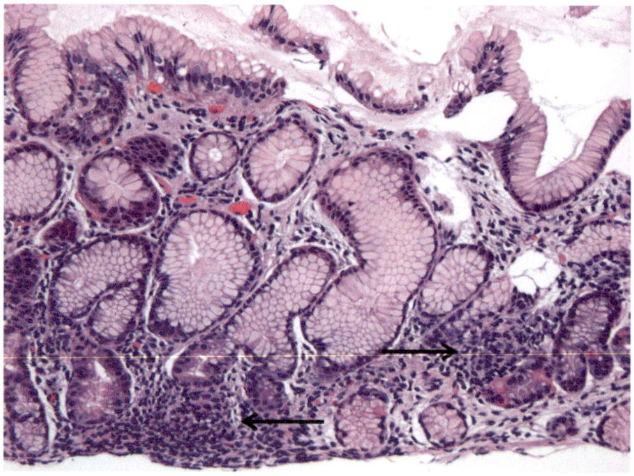

Fig. 20.13 While the ability of Crohn's disease (CD) to affect the entire GI tract from mouth to anus is broadly accepted, the precise nature of upper tract manifestations has been debated in the literature. Furthermore, a few upper tract manifestations of otherwise typical ulcerative colitis (UC), such as diffuse duodenitis, have been reported. The best studied type of gastric inflammation found in inflammatory bowel disease (IBD) patients is so-called "focally enhanced gastritis," which is characterized by clusters of mixed inflammatory cells including macrophages and lymphocytes centered on gastric glands and/or the mucous neck region (*arrows*)

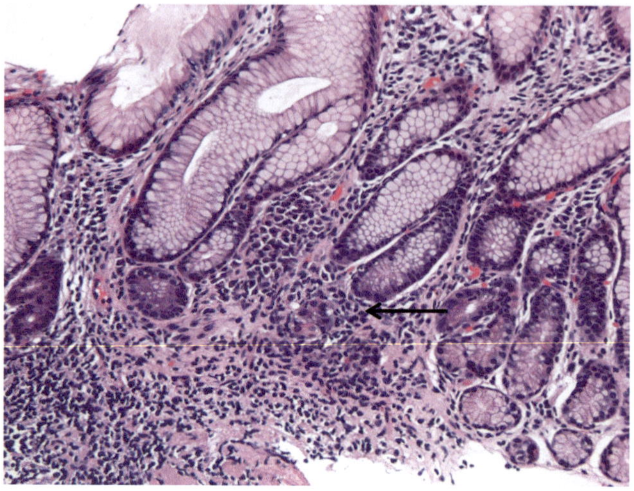

Fig. 20.14 This focus of inflammation (*arrow*) centers on a superficial gland, which is infiltrated by lymphocytes and surrounded by plasma cells and other inflammatory cells. This pattern of focal inflammation has been reported in both CD and UC

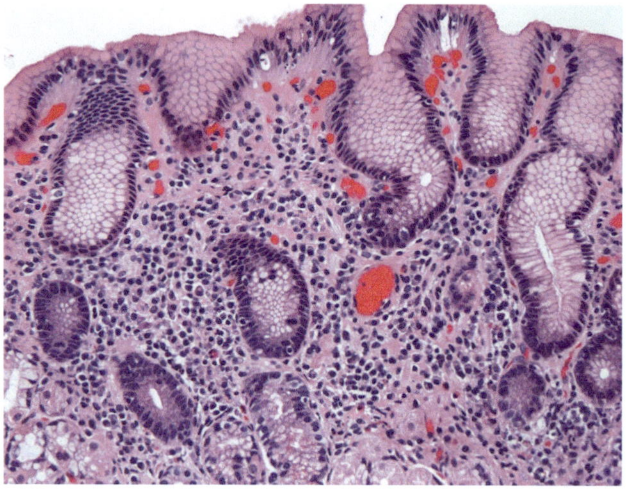

Fig. 20.15 Another type of inflammatory infiltrate reported in UC patients is a superficial plasmacytosis, similar in distribution to *H. pylori* gastritis, but without infectious organisms and devoid of active neutrophilic inflammation

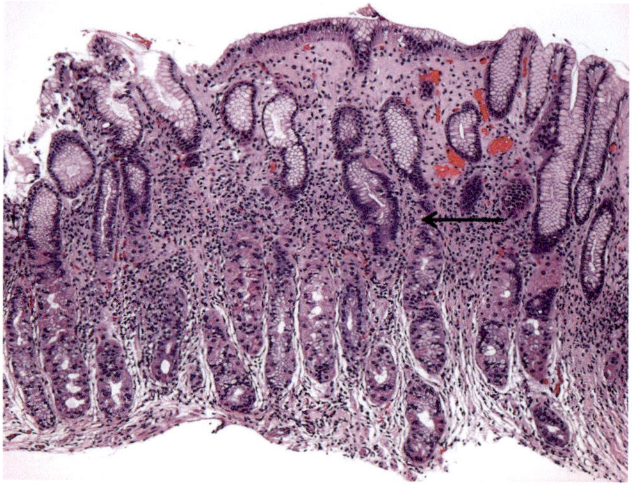

Fig. 20.16 In our practice, we have seen a series of biopsies from patients with a variety of symptoms that contain a gastritis involving the mid-zone (*arrow*) and deep mucosa. The type of inflammation varies, but usually has a lymphoplasmacytic component, and may contain prominent eosinophils

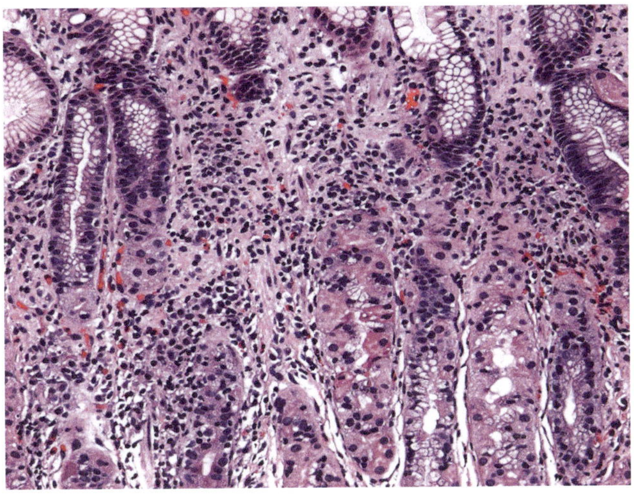

Fig. 20.17 Based on a retrospective study of available clinical information, we could find no unifying set of symptoms, underlying disease(s), endoscopic appearance, or medication history that united these cases of unusual mid-zone and deep gastritis. Importantly, the pattern is not indicative of active or treated *H. pylori* gastritis

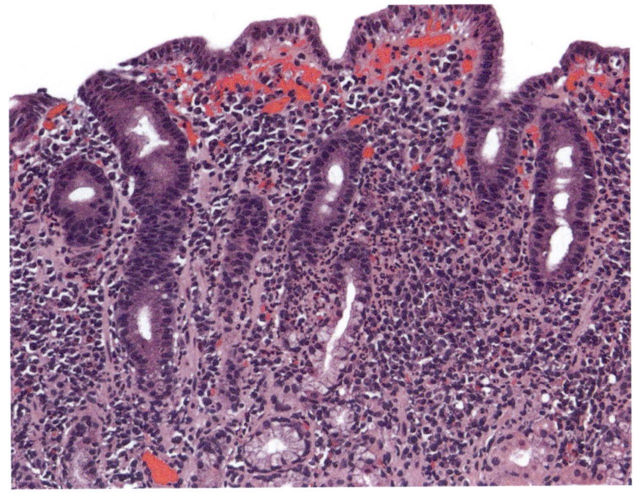

Fig. 20.18 Occasionally, one will encounter an intense gastritis that simply has no name and which defies classification. This particular case had an intensely active and destructive chronic pangastritis that was not associated with *H. pylori* infection or any other known cause. Often, a drug reaction or autoimmune phenomenon will be speculated as a potential cause

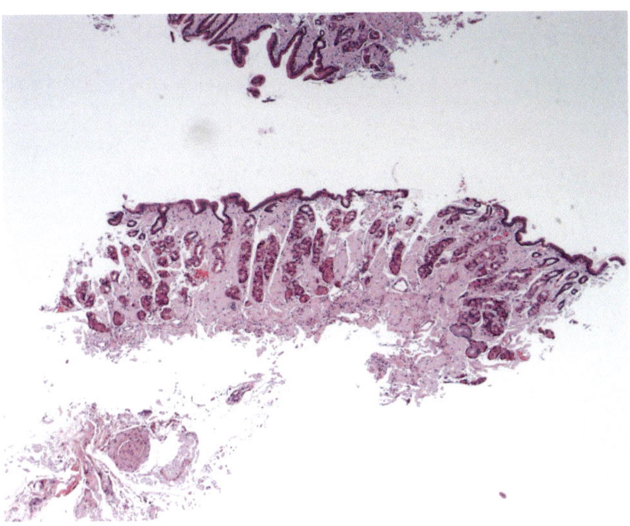

Fig. 20.19 Mucosal and/or submucosal deposition of amyloid can accompany a variety of conditions, including systemic inflammatory conditions, immunoglobulin-producing hematolymphoid neoplasms, hemodialysis, and others. When seen in biopsy specimens, amyloid deposition may be striking, as in this case where it fills the lamina propria with amorphous pink material, or very subtle, only involving submucosal blood vessel walls

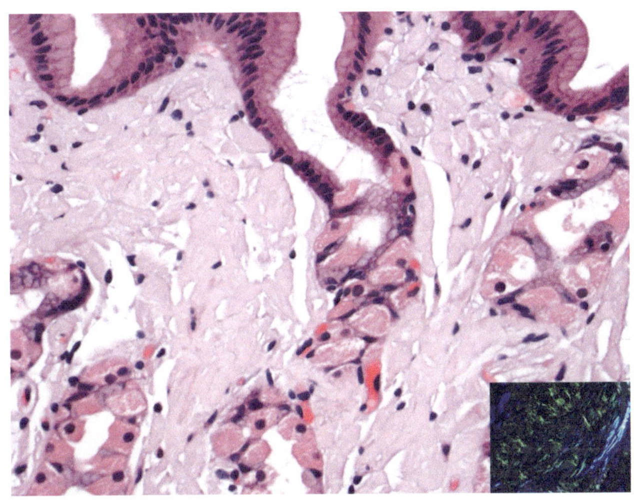

Fig. 20.20 At high magnification, waxy, amorphous amyloid is seen filling the lamina propria and spreading apart the pits and glands in this gastric biopsy. This can lead to mucosal abnormalities visible on endoscopic examination, including ulcers or nodules. The characteristic apple-green birefringence elicited using polarized light and a Congo red stain is seen in the inset

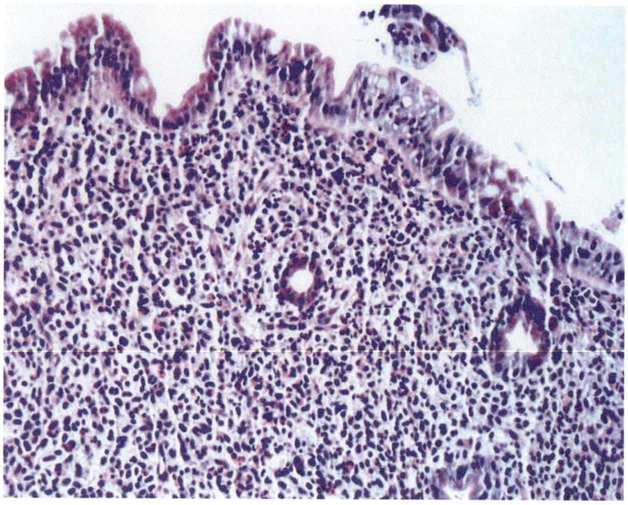

Fig. 20.21 Systemic mastocytosis (SM) is actually a neoplastic proliferation of mast cells, classified as one of the "myeloproliferative neoplasms" (MPN), which can affect many different tissues including the GI tract. Its appearance can be deceiving, and the presence of the neoplastic mast cells can be subtle due to their unusual, spindled appearance and admixture with inflammatory cells. In this case, the markedly expanded lamina propria included plasma cells, eosinophils, lymphocytes, and other cell types that were initially interpreted as some type of inflammatory process

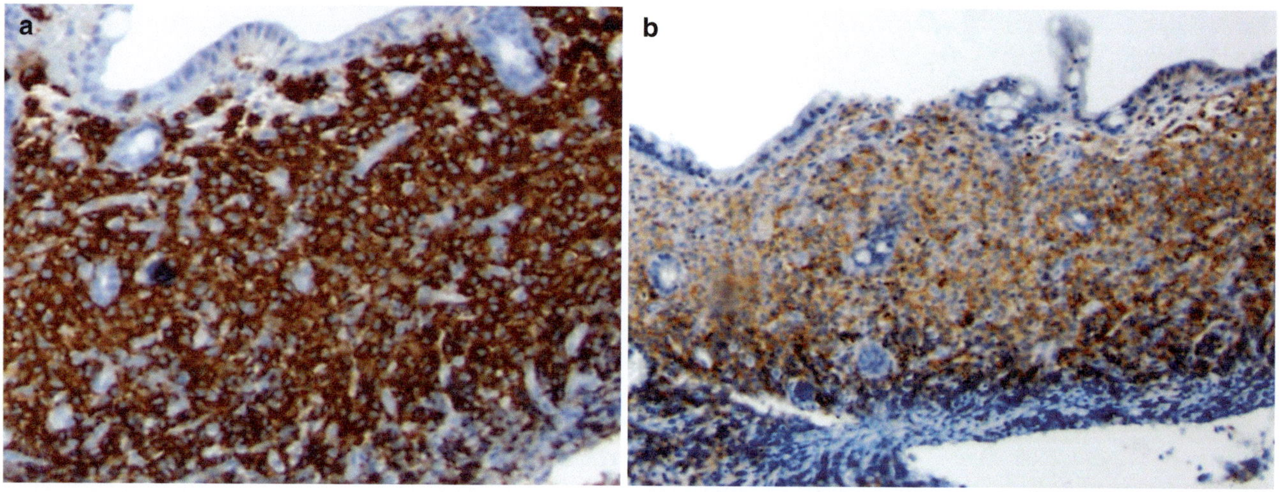

Fig. 20.22 (**a**) Using immunohistochemistry for c-kit expression, the striking number of mast cells in the mucosa is more apparent. A mast cell tryptase stain had a similar pattern. The diagnosis of SM is made using major and minor criteria, but one typical feature is the presence of clusters of more than 15 mast cells. This feature allows separation from other conditions that can have increased mast cells that are individually scattered. (**b**) In addition, the mast cells in SM may have aberrant antigen expression of CD2 and or CD25, the latter pictured here

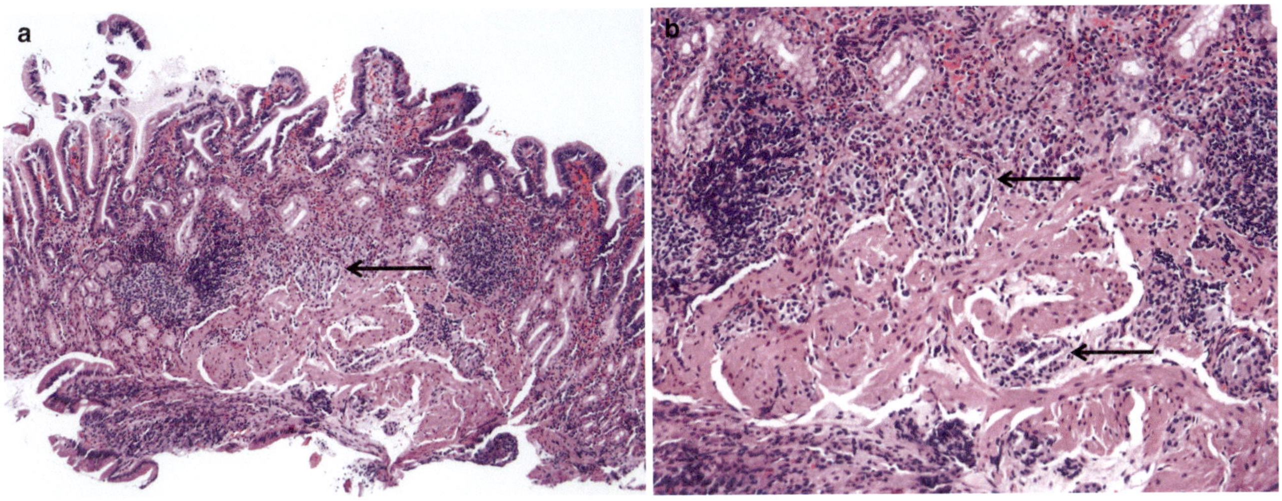

Fig. 20.23 Zollinger-Ellison syndrome is the result of autonomous gastrin production, usually by a gastrin-producing endocrine neoplasm (gastrinoma) somewhere in the gastroenteropancreatic system, but occasionally by primary gastric G cell hyperplasia. This results in fasting hypergastrinemia and excess gastric acid production (hyperchlorhydria), which can lead to intractable gastric and/or duodenal ulcers, as well as gastric mucosal changes. (**a**) This patient had a duodenal gastrinoma (*arrow*). (**b**) At higher magnification, the individual nests of neuroendocrine cells can be seen within and just above the muscularis mucosae (*arrows*)

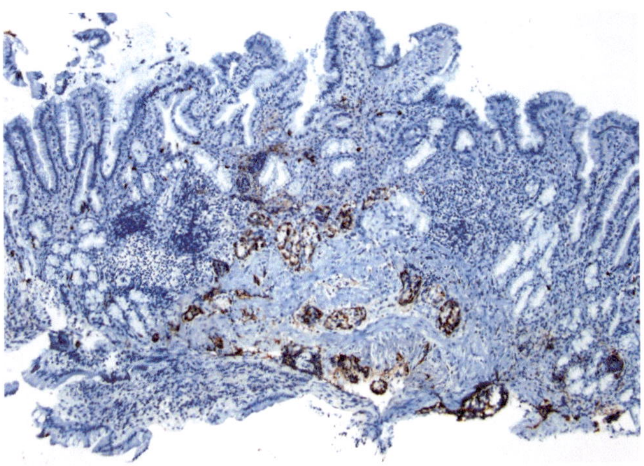

Fig. 20.24 An immunohistochemical stain for gastrin highlights the nest of gastrin-producing neuroendocrine cells

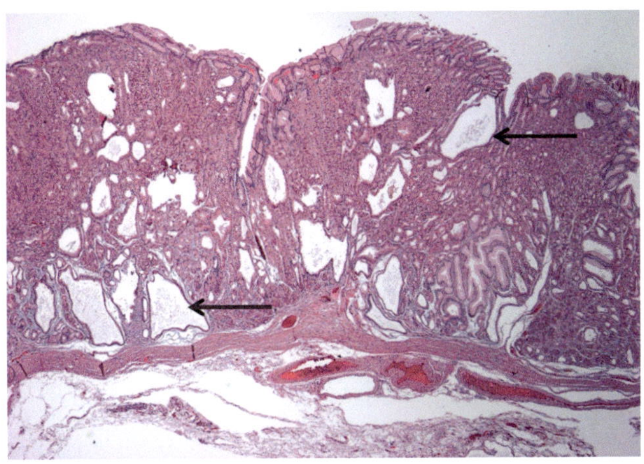

Fig. 20.25 The effects of excess gastrin on the stomach are characterized by hyperplasia of oxyntic glands and overall hypertrophy of the gastric mucosa, which becomes thickened. Note the massive expansion of the gland compartment, which appears endoscopically as thick, enlarged gastric folds in the gastric body and fundus. Numerous cystically dilated gland structures (*arrow*), reminiscent of those seen in fundic gland polyps (*see* Chap. 23) are present

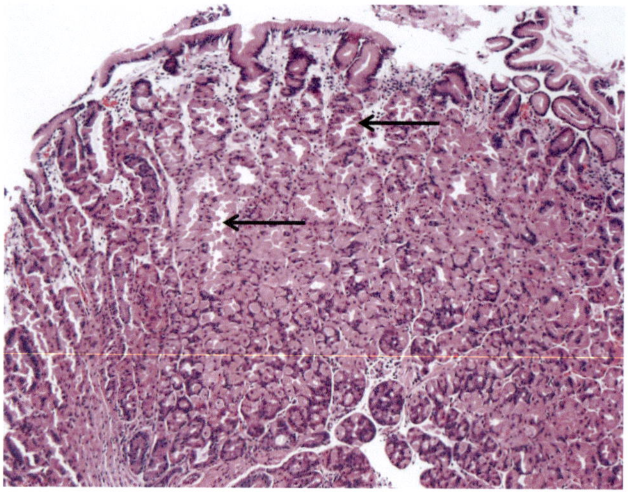

Fig. 20.26 At higher magnification, the hypertrophy of individual parietal cells is apparent, with apical cytoplasmic "snouts" extending from the surface of the parietal cells (*arrows*). This differs histologically from Ménétrier's disease (*see* Chap. 22), in which the hypertrophy of the mucosa is caused by foveolar (pit) hyperplasia associated with atrophy of the gland compartment

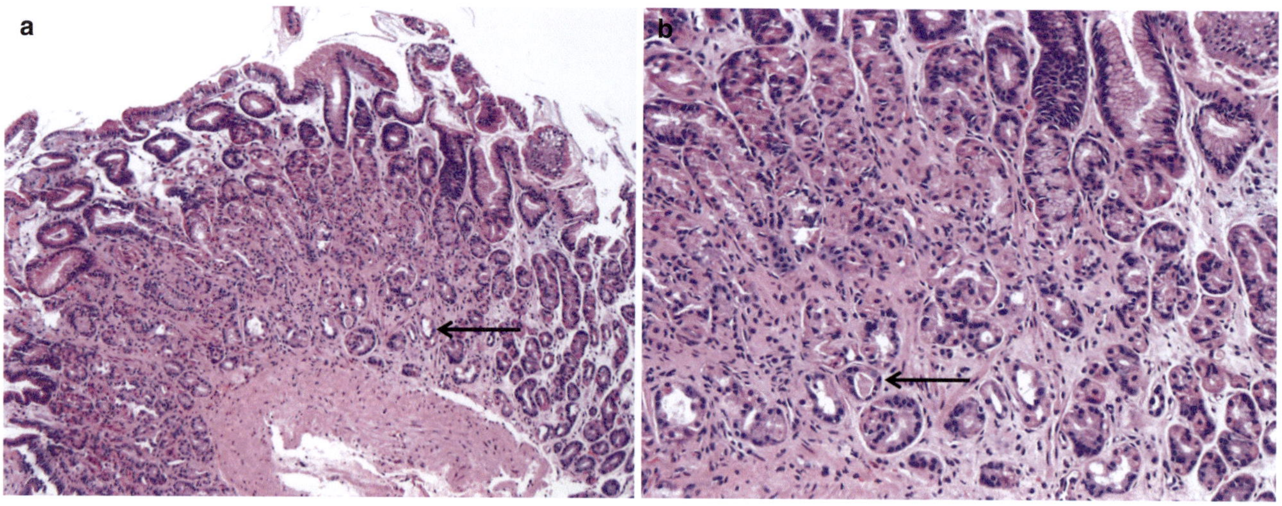

Fig. 20.27 Graft-vs.-host disease (GVHD) is an immune-mediated attack on recipient tissues by donor T lymphocytes after allogeneic transplants, most often of bone marrow. Clinically, involvement of the GI tract can lead to nausea, vomiting, diarrhea, abdominal pain, and bleeding, depending on the part of the gut that is involved. Histologically, the hallmark of GVHD is epithelial apoptosis, although this finding can be seen in a variety of other conditions, including infectious diseases that can also plague immunosuppressed patients after transplantation. (**a**) At low magnification, this patient's stomach is almost normal, but has some regenerative changes at the base of the mucosa (*arrow*). (**b**) At higher magnification, some of the basal glands (*arrow*) appear attenuated

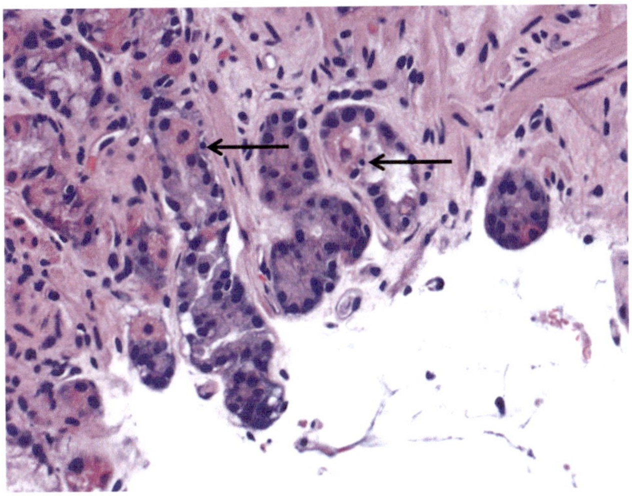

Fig. 20.28 At high magnification, the regenerative basal glands can be seen to contain rare apoptotic bodies (*arrows*). There has been controversy about how to report GVHD. A four-tier grading system has been used historically, where grade 1 = epithelial apoptosis only; grade 2 = injury and early loss of individual glands/crypts; grade 3 = loss of groups of glands/crypts; and grade 4 = necrosis and denudation of large areas of mucosa. This scheme does not always correlate with clinical severity, however, so more recent practice has centered on reporting whether GVHD is absent, possibly present, probably present, or unequivocally present. In our experience, the stomach is not affected as often or to the same degree as the small intestine and colon

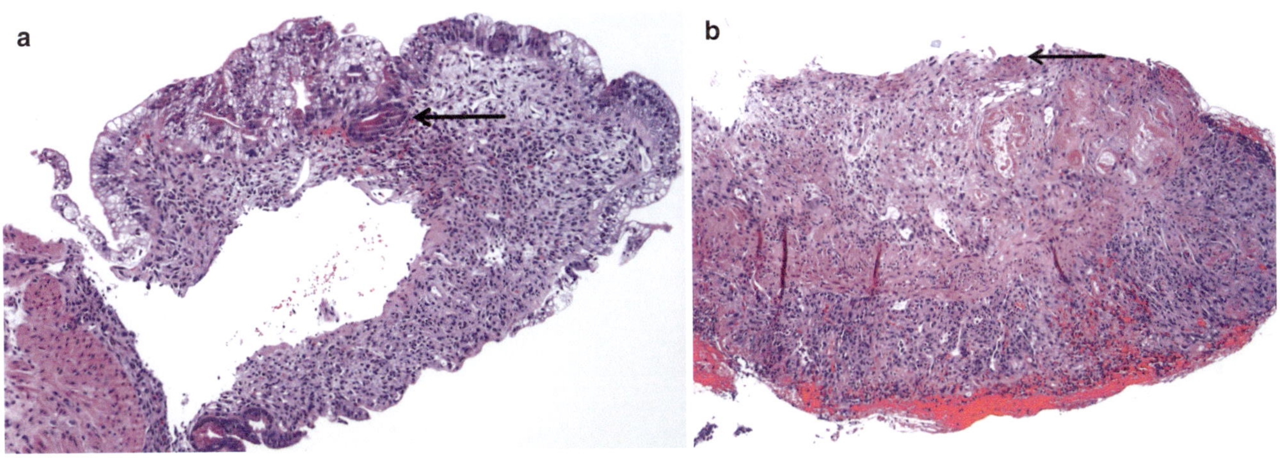

Fig. 20.29 (**a**) In this case of GVHD, there is nearly complete loss of the architecture of the mucosa, with only a few intensely regenerative epithelial structures remaining (*arrow*). (**b**) This case has led to complete mucosal necrosis and denudation, with a fibrinous exudate on the surface (*arrow*). As the mucosa regenerates after such an extensive injury, there can be architectural distortion reminiscent of that seen in inflammatory bowel disease

21 Infectious Diseases and Organisms

The discovery that most gastric ulcers and nearly all duodenal ulcers are related to an infectious disease revolutionized the treatment of peptic ulcer disease in the late 20th century. A significant part of our practice involves examining gastric biopsies accompanied by a clinical request to "rule out *Helicobacter pylori*," but this is not the only infectious disease that affects the stomach. It is, however, arguably the most important, because it can lead not only to gastric and duodenal ulcers but also to an increased risk for epithelial and lymphoid malignancy. Fortunately, *H. pylori* gastritis has a characteristic microscopic appearance that allows one to suspect it easily. Other infectious diseases, such as certain viral infections, require a higher index of suspicion and can be challenging to discriminate from other processes in the differential diagnosis.

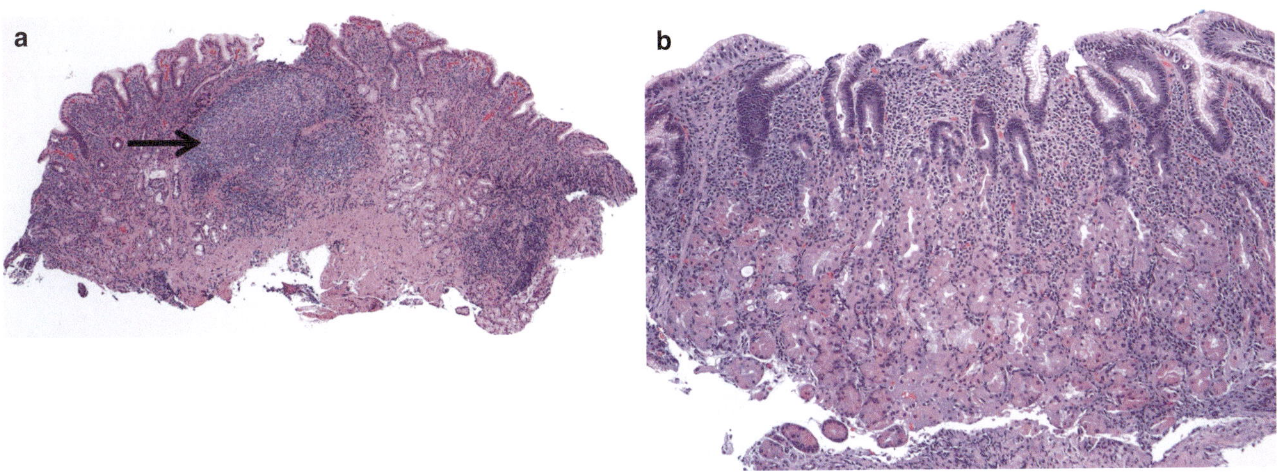

Fig. 21.1 At low magnification, gastritis caused by *H. pylori* consists of a band-like chronic inflammatory infiltrate in the superficial mucosa (in the pit and very superficial gland compartments). (**a**) Often, this inflammation is punctuated by lymphoid aggregates (or even germinal centers) in the deeper mucosa (*arrow*). Typically, the infection and associated gastritis are confined to the gastric antrum, but cases of *H. pylori* pangastritis with involvement of the body/fundus (**b**) and even the cardia can occur, particularly in patients who have received acid-suppression therapy with proton pump inhibitors

S.R. Owens, H.D. Appelman, *Atlas of Esophagus and Stomach Pathology*, Atlas of Anatomic Pathology,
DOI 10.1007/978-1-4614-8084-6_21, © Springer Science+Business Media New York 2014

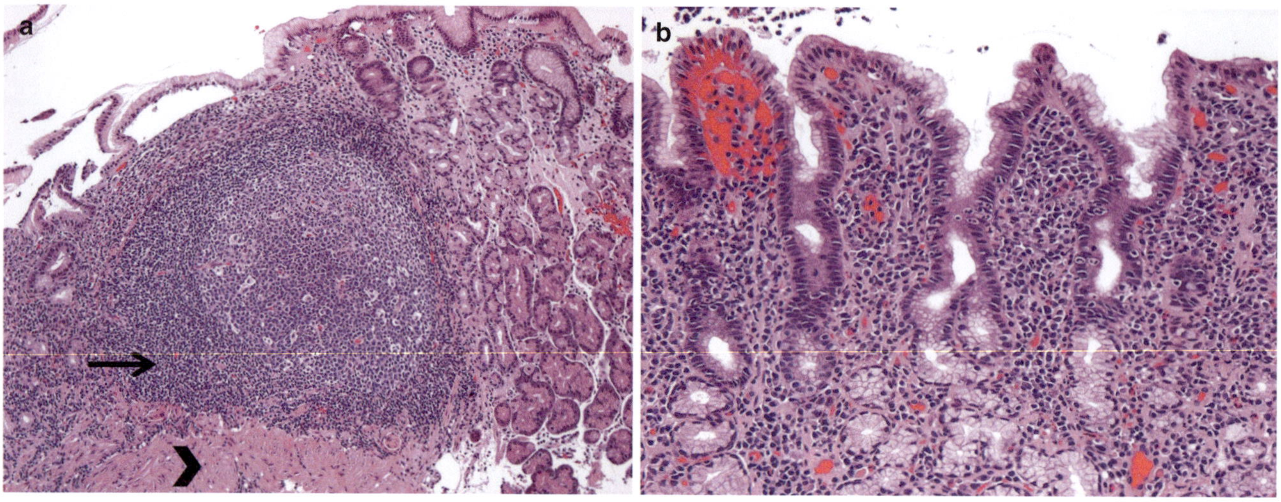

Fig. 21.2 (**a**) At higher magnification, a fully formed germinal center with a well-developed mantle zone (*arrow*) is visible, abutting the muscularis mucosae (*arrowhead*). (**b**) At this magnification, the prominent mononuclear inflammatory infiltrate in the lamina propria of the pit compartment is visible. At low and medium magnification, this moderate-to-severe band-like inflammatory infiltrate, imparting a very "blue" appearance to the mucosa, is highly characteristic of *H. pylori* gastritis and should prompt a search for the infectious organisms

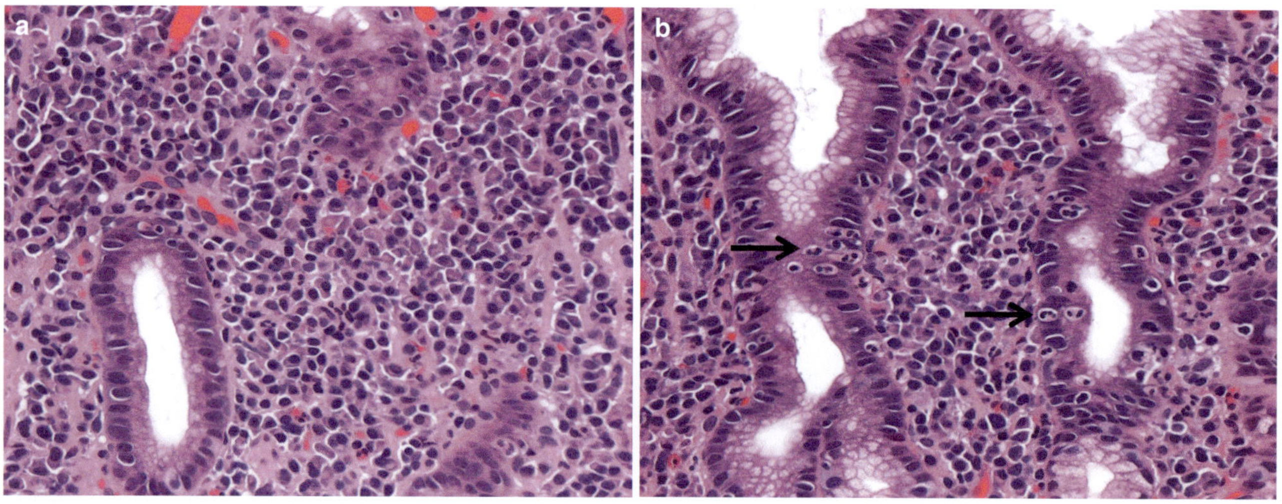

Fig. 21.3 (**a**) At high magnification, the inflammatory infiltrate in the superficial mucosa can be seen to contain a prominent population of plasma cells. (**b**) Active infection is often characterized by an infiltration of neutrophils (*arrows*) where the gastric pits join the superficial glands (the "mucous neck" region). The pits and mucosal surface in areas with this neutrophilic "activity" are the best place to begin a search for the infectious organisms, which will be found within the mucin. The combination of lymphoplasmacytic and neutrophilic inflammation leads to the characterization of *H. pylori* gastritis as "chronic active gastritis (CAG)"

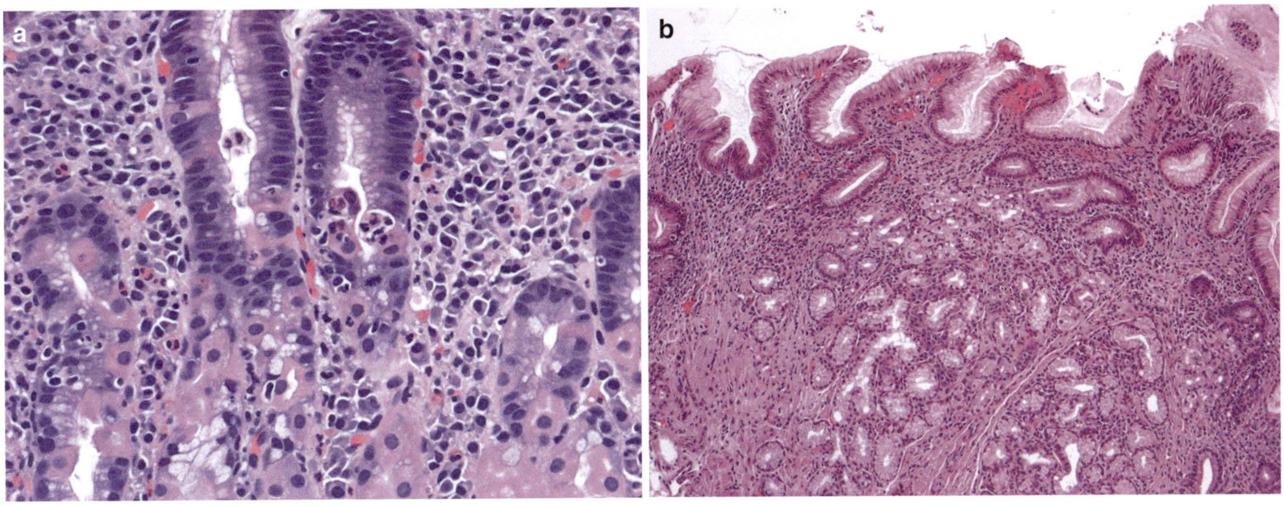

Fig. 21.4 As noted above, some patients with *H. pylori* infection develop pangastritis, with involvement of the body/fundus mucosa (**a**, with oxyntic glands visible at the bottom of the frame) and the gastric cardia (**b**). The gastric cardia is a frequent site of chronic inflammation (discussed in Chap. 16), so one must hold out for the band-like lymphoplasmacytic inflammatory infiltrate characteristic of *H. pylori* gastritis to make a fruitful search for the infectious organisms

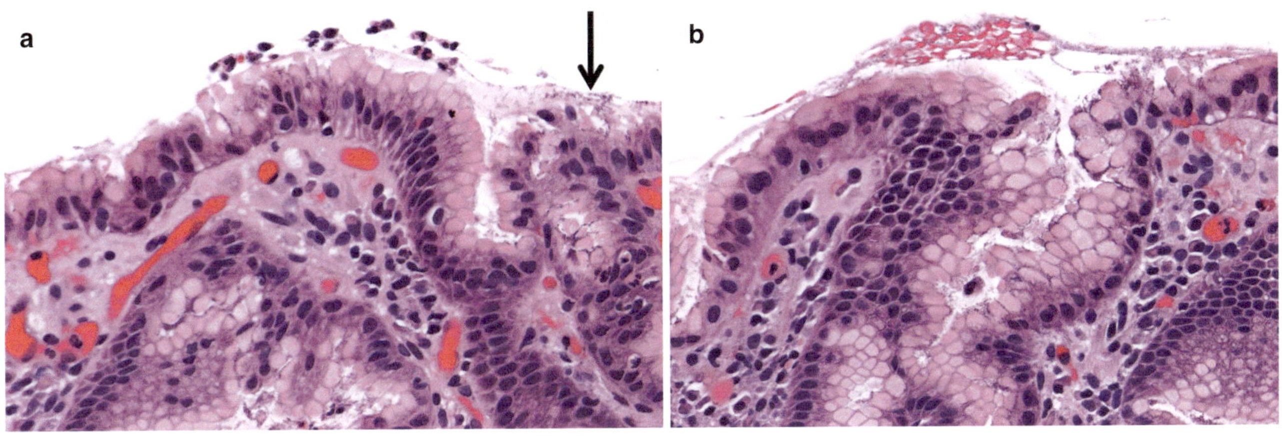

Fig. 21.5 *H. pylori* organisms can be found on routine hematoxylin and eosin (H&E)-stained sections. The organisms reside in the pit and surface mucin and appear as curvilinear, somewhat basophilic forms. (**a**) There are surface neutrophils and micro-erosions (*arrow*) of the surface epithelium. The *H. pylori* organisms tend to adhere to the apical surface of the epithelial cells. (**b**) Clusters of organisms are visible in the mucin of this pit, as well as on the epithelial surface. When surface and pit mucin is absent or difficult to find in the biopsy, it can be extremely difficult to find the organisms on H&E-stained sections. *H. pylori* gastritis is a common cause of gastric ulcer, and patients with this infection have approximately a four-fold increased risk of stomach ulcer compared with non-infected individuals

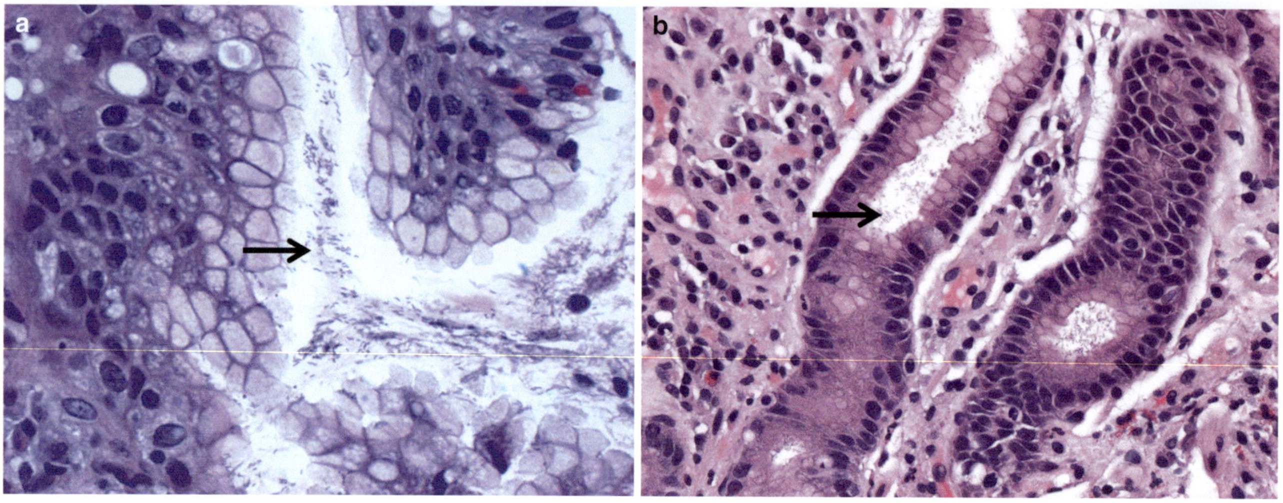

Fig. 21.6 At very high magnification, this heavily infested patient's stomach has clusters of organisms in the mucin of the gastric pits (**a** and **b**, *arrows*). With a careful search, organisms can almost always be located using routine H&E-stained sections

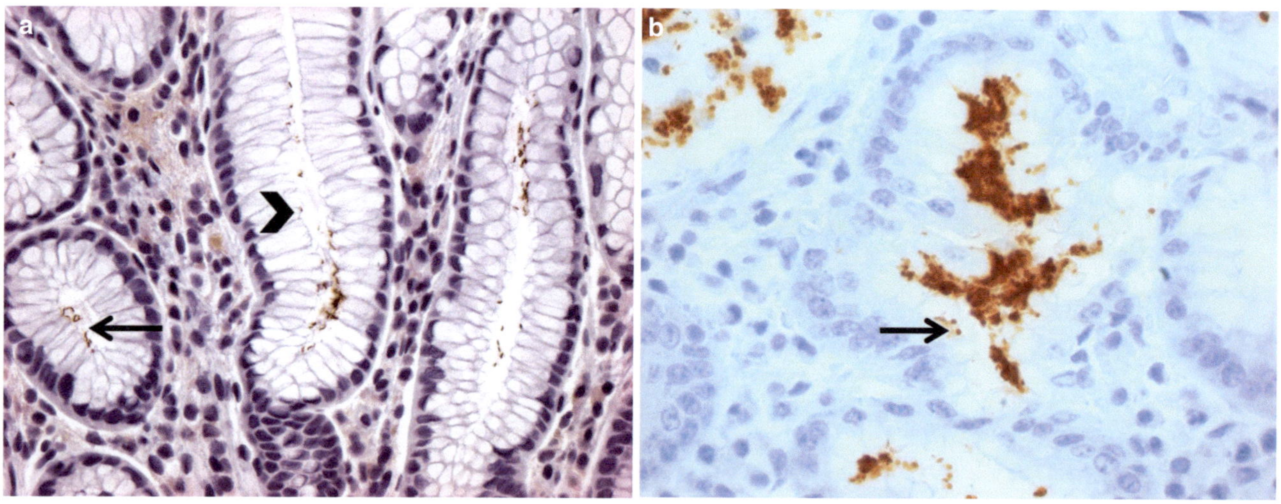

Fig. 21.7 A sensitive immunohistochemical (IHC) stain is available to aid in the diagnosis of *H. pylori* gastritis, and should be obtained, if available, when the characteristic gastritis is present in biopsies but the organisms cannot be located on H&E-stained tissue. The IHC highlights the curvilinear shape of the organisms ((**a**) *arrow*). In addition, a few of the bacteria have assumed a rounded, "coccoid" form (*arrowhead*), which is thought to be a response to stress such as hypoxia or partial eradication therapy. These coccoid *H. pylori* are indicative of true infection and should not be misinterpreted as nonspecific staining. (**b**) In some cases, particularly in resection specimens in our experience, clusters of coccoid bacteria can appear in the deep glands of the mucosa and conventional bacteria can be difficult or impossible to identify, even using the immunohistochemical stain. Again, such an appearance is truly indicative of *H. pylori* infection when accompanied by gastritis and should not be interpreted as nonspecific staining or debris. A few individual coccoid forms are visible (*arrow*)

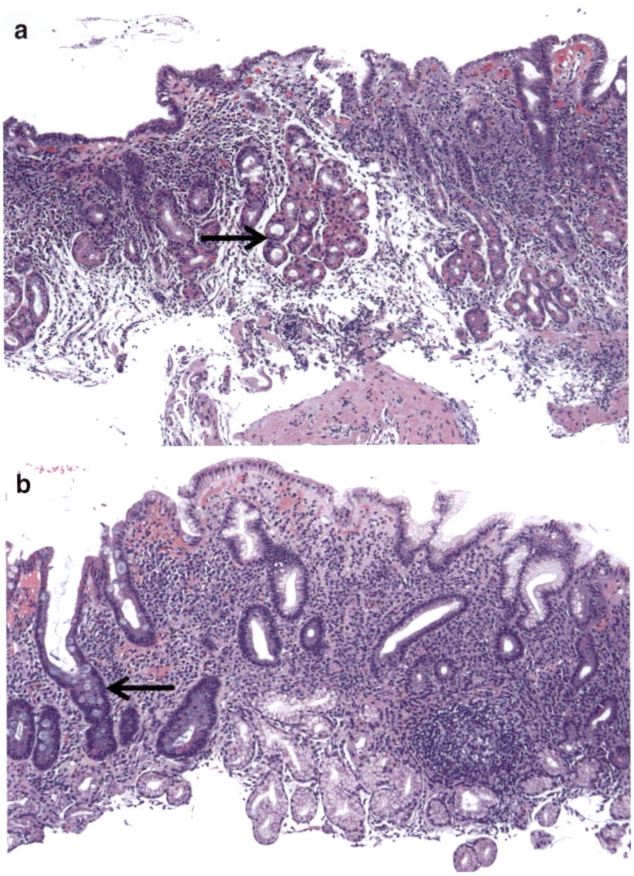

Fig. 21.8 Longstanding infection with *H. pylori* can result in mucosal atrophy, characterized by loss of gland mass and, often, intestinal metaplasia. (**a**) In this example, the glands are found in discrete lobules or "packets" (*arrow*) with intervening, inflamed lamina propria. The intense inflammation suggests that the causative organism is still present. (**b**) This case is also inflamed, and has a focus of intestinal metaplasia (*arrow*) as well as a deep lymphoid aggregate. The atrophy caused by longstanding *H. pylori* infection may be antral-predominant, or may occur more widely throughout the stomach (so-called "multifocal atrophic gastritis," discussed in Chap. 22) in patients with pangastric infection

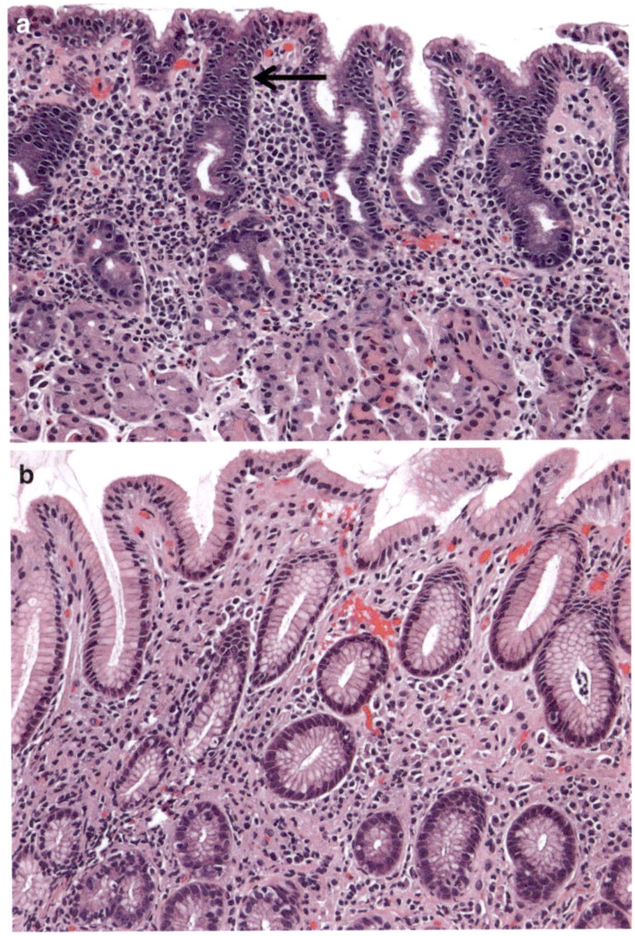

Fig. 21.9 (**a**) *H. pylori* gastritis is one condition associated with the histological appearance of "lymphocytic gastritis," in which prominent lymphocytes can be seen infiltrating the epithelium of the mucosal surface and the gastric pits (*arrow*), each surrounded by a non-staining "halo". The finding of intraepithelial lymphocytes is not specific to any one disease, however, and has also been reported in a number of conditions including celiac disease, inflammatory bowel disease, and others. It is discussed in greater detail in Chap. 20. Note the presence of the characteristic, band-like plasma cell infiltrate in the superficial lamina propria suggesting *H. pylori* infection. (**b**) In this case of treated *H. pylori* gastritis, the inflammatory infiltrate is less intense than in the cases seen previously, and an "active" (neutrophilic) component is missing. This finding can be seen in patients treated for *H. pylori* eradication, and the presence or absence of organisms (which are often difficult to locate, if present) depends on the time course of the therapy. If organisms are demonstrably absent, this type of finding can be diagnosed as "chronic gastritis resembling treated *H. pylori* gastritis"

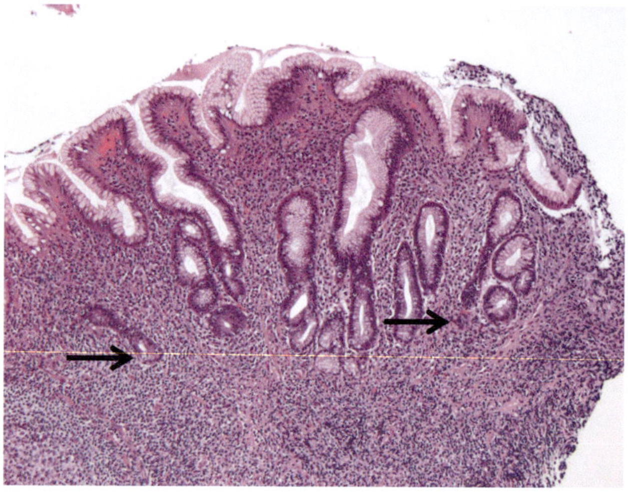

Fig. 21.10 Another potential outcome of persistent *H. pylori* gastritis is B cell lymphoma, most often extranodal marginal zone lymphoma of mucosa-associated lymphoid tissue (MALT lymphoma). Gastric lymphomas are addressed in detail in Chap. 28, but the diagnosis can be suggested when a diffuse infiltrate of lymphocytes markedly expands the lamina propria and leads to destruction of normal mucosal structures. In this case, the mucosal glands are being infiltrated and destroyed by lymphoma cells (*arrows*), producing so-called "lymphoepithelial lesions." Often, but not always, this is accompanied by macroscopic mucosal changes such as malignant-appearing ulcer and/or thickened mucosal folds. The lymphoma in this case spans the entire thickness of the mucosa, but the more superficial component is identical to *H. pylori* gastritis, and the causative organisms may be found on close inspection. With this etiologic association and the stepwise progression from inflammation to lymphoma, the distinction between severe *H. pylori* gastritis and incipient/early MALT lymphoma can be very difficult

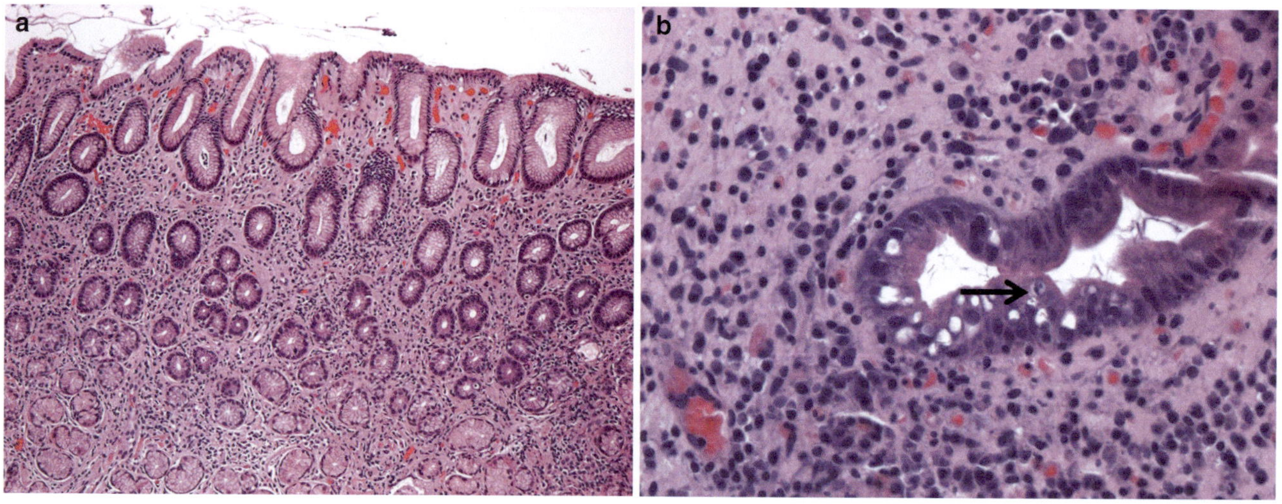

Fig. 21.11 Like *H. pylori*, *Helicobacter heilmannii* causes a chronic gastritis that can lead to upper gastrointestinal (GI) symptoms such as pain and dyspepsia. Unlike *H. pylori*, however, *H. heilmannii* is thought to be much less associated with gastric and duodenal ulcers, lymphoma, and gastric adenocarcinoma. (**a**) In addition, the chronic gastritis caused by *H. heilmannii* is usually less intense than that seen with *H. pylori*, meaning that a search for causative *Helicobacter* organisms should be undertaken even in cases of moderately severe gastritis such as this. (**b**) Furthermore, active neutrophilic inflammation is much less prominent in *H. heilmannii* gastritis, with only a rare neutrophil present in the mucous neck region in this case (*arrow*)

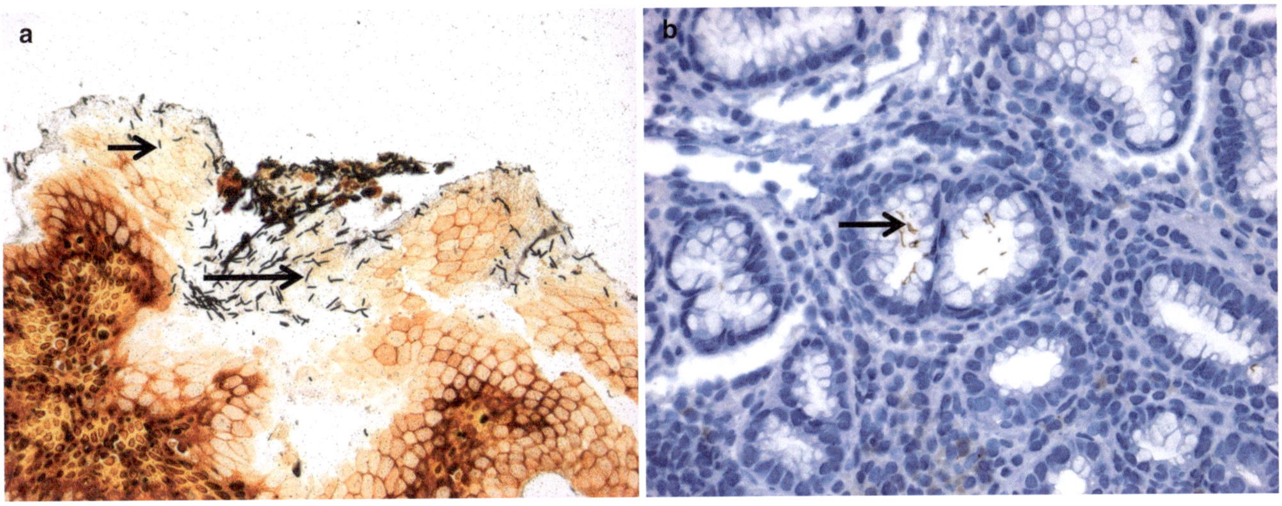

Fig. 21.12 (**a**) *H. heilmannii* can be highlighted with silver-based stains, as can *H. pylori*. The two organisms my coexist in a given case of gastritis, and recognizable *H. pylori* forms (*short arrow*) can be seen in this case alongside the larger, more tightly coiled *H. heilmannii* bacteria (*long arrow*). *H. heilmannii* infection is common in farm animals and domestic pets, and may be a zoonotic disease in humans. (**b**) Immunohistochemical stains directed at *H. pylori* cross-react with *H. heilmannii*, so the latter may be revealed on these stains as well (*arrow*). They tend to be found "floating free" in the pit or gland lumens or in the surface mucin, and do not adhere to the apical surface of the epithelial cells in the same way that *H. pylori* organisms do

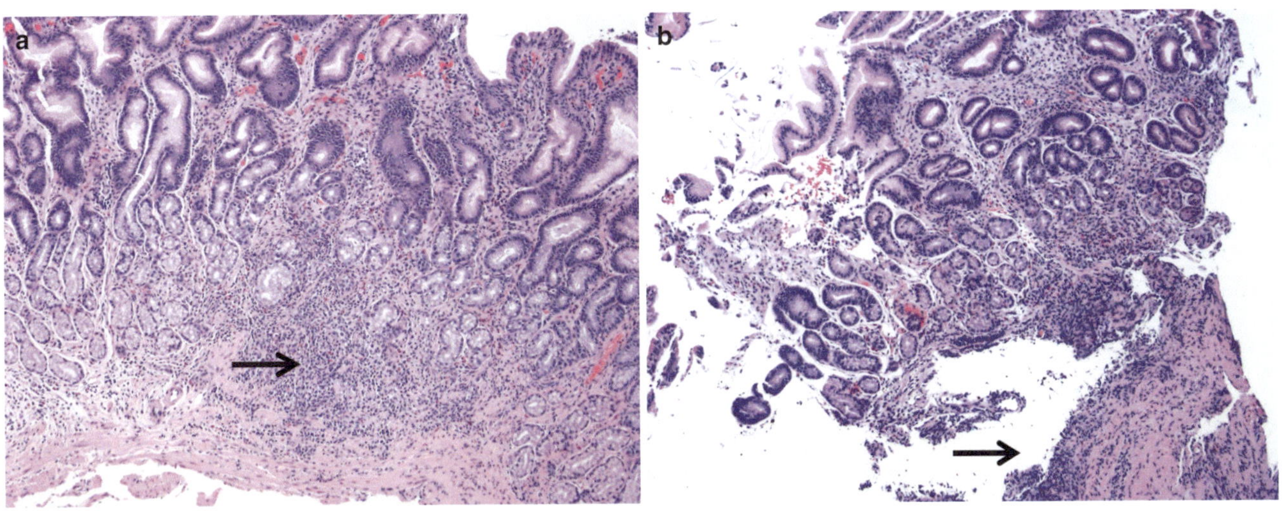

Fig. 21.13 Most commonly found in immunocompromised patients, cytomegalovirus (CMV) gastritis can cause upper gastrointestinal symptoms, and may often be found in other sites throughout the GI tract. (**a**) This gastric biopsy contains a dense, mixed inflammatory infiltrate (*arrow*) localized around a cluster of gastric glands. (**b**) Frequently, the inflammation caused by CMV will be accompanied by an ulcer (*arrow*)

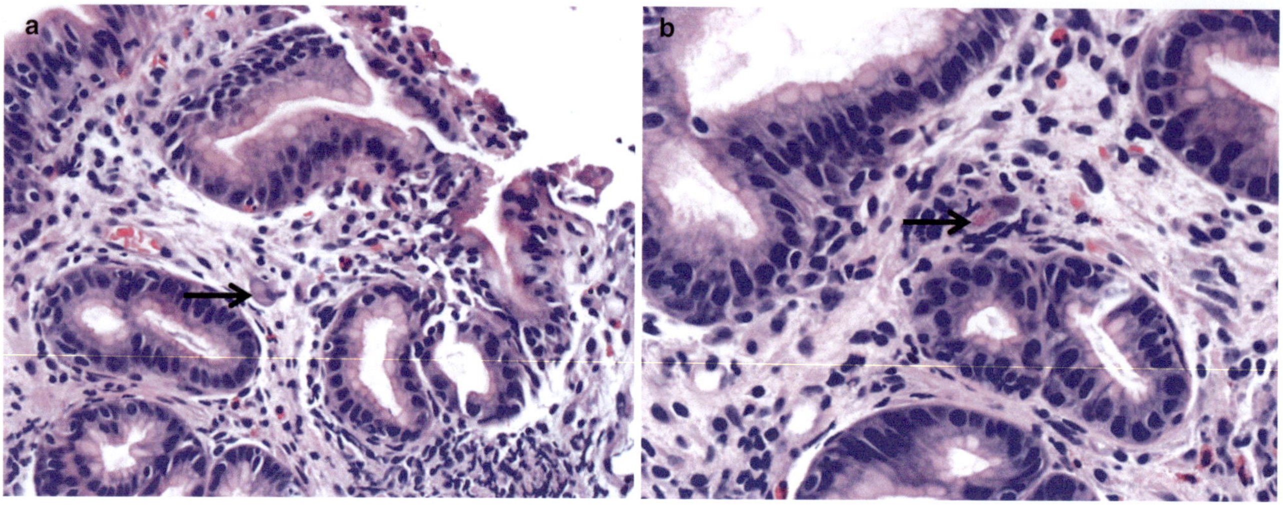

Fig. 21.14 At high magnification, the mixed inflammatory infiltrate is visible, containing lymphocytes, plasma cells, neutrophils, and eosinophils. Two cells with characteristic nuclear and cytoplasmic inclusions are visible (**a** and **b**, *arrows*). The "virocytes" are often endothelial cells, but infection of other cell types such as fibroblasts and macrophages is possible. Apoptotic bodies may be found among epithelial cells in CMV infection and this can lead to confusion, as prominent epithelial apoptosis is a feature of graft-versus-host disease (discussed in Chap. 20), which affects a similar, immunosuppressed patient population

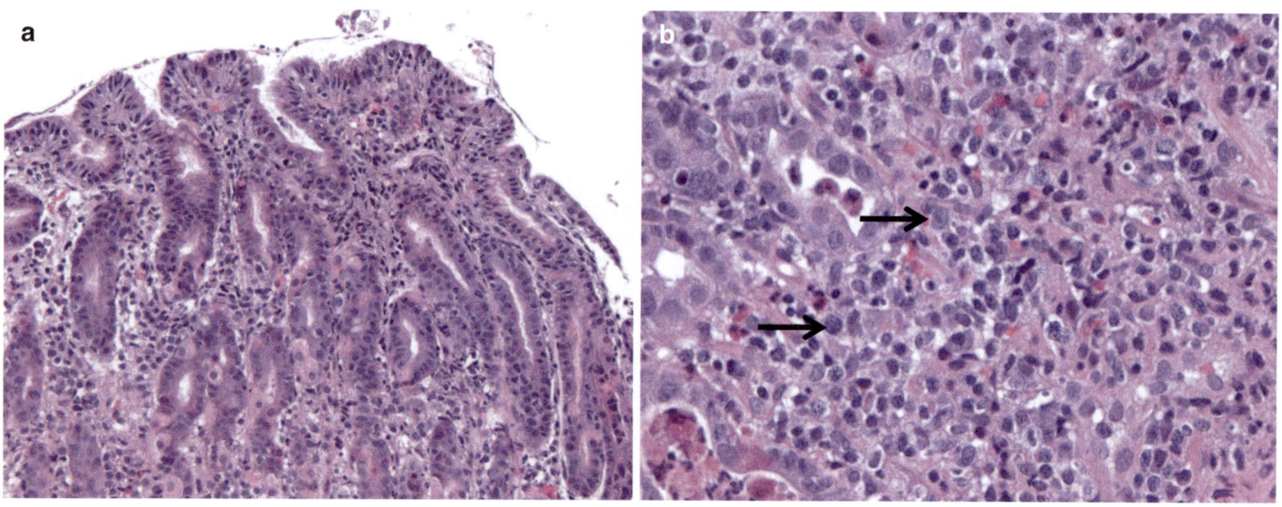

Fig. 21.15 Gastritis associated with Epstein-Barr virus (EBV) infection has been rarely reported, including in patients with a viral syndrome attributable to infection. The main importance in recognizing this entity is to differentiate it from a malignant hematolymphoid process, as it can mimic gastric large cell lymphoma (having been termed "pseudolymphoma" by some observers). (**a**) At low magnification, this gastric biopsy from a symptomatic 18 year old contains a diffuse lamina propria infiltrate of atypical lymphoid-appearing cells. (**b**) At high magnification, these cells are large and atypical-appearing (*arrows*), but can also be seen to mix with other inflammatory cells such as neutrophils and eosinophils. Many of the large cells are CD20-positive B cells, which can lead to a misdiagnosis as large B-cell lymphoma

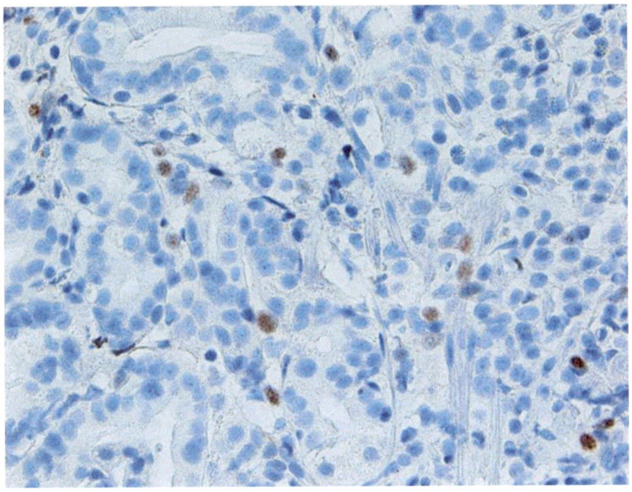

Fig. 21.16 Scattered nuclei in the large, atypical B cells in a case of EBV gastritis are positive for EBV RNA on in situ hybridization (brown staining, in this instance)

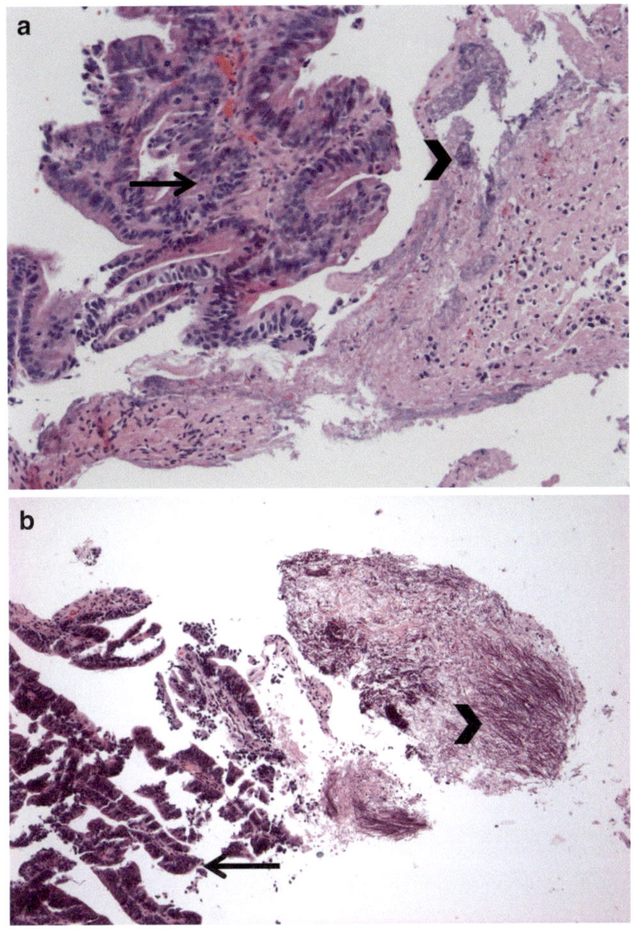

Fig. 21.17 Gastric neoplasia will be discussed in detail elsewhere but one useful microbial clue to the diagnosis of malignancy bears mentioning in this chapter. We have noticed the presence of clouds of filamentous organisms, for which we currently have no name, in association with ulcers in the stomach and esophagus. While some older reports have associated similar organisms with ulcers of any cause, we have found them to nearly always colonize malignant ulcers due to carcinomas or lymphomas. These panels illustrate two gastric adenocarcinomas (*arrows*) that were associated with such organisms. (**a**) The organisms in this case were mixed with copious ulcer exudate (*arrowhead*), and appear as small collections of basophilic material. (**b**) In this case, the organisms (*arrowhead*) were more easily seen at low magnification, and their filamentous nature is apparent

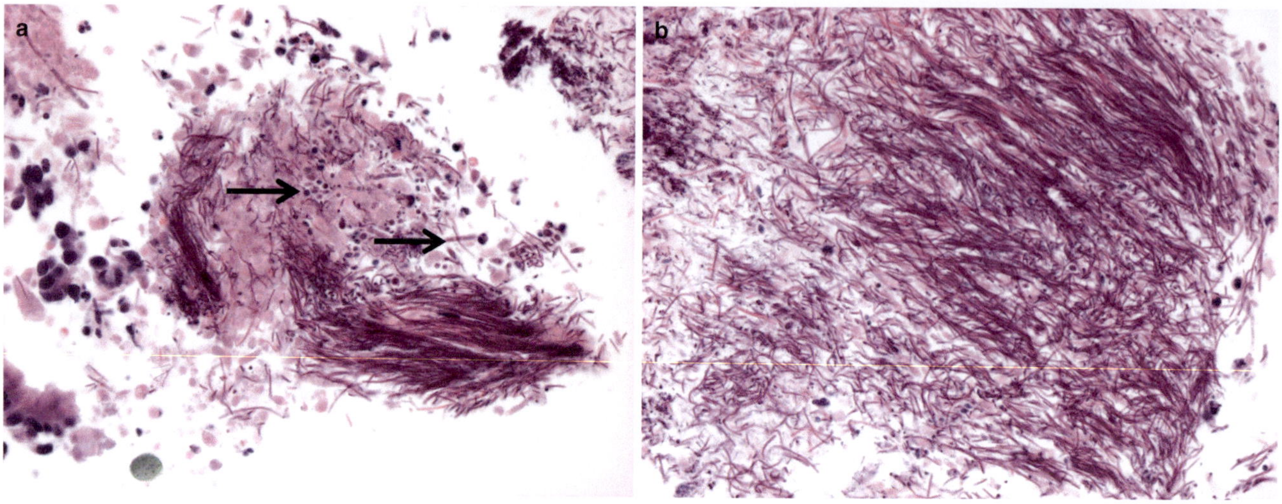

Fig. 21.18 At high magnification, the organisms have a filamentous appearance, with individual filaments that are thicker than actinomycetes, but thinner than *Candida* pseudohyphae. In this particular case, the organisms were admixed with *Candida* yeasts and pseudohyphae (**a** *arrows*) but were easily discerned (**b**)

22 Hyperplastic/Metaplastic Conditions

A few conditions can cause alterations in the gastric mucosa that are characterized by either an increase in mucosal mass (hyperplasia) or a loss of mucosal mass (atrophy). Focal mucosal hyperplasia can take the form of mucosal polyps, which are commonly encountered and discussed in Chap. 23, but in this chapter we will address more widespread mucosal hyperplasia, which is rare. We much more commonly encounter mucosal atrophy, especially in the setting of long-standing infection by *Helicobacter pylori*. It is important to find and mention atrophy in mucosal biopsies because it is accompanied by intestinal metaplasia, which is a risk factor for gastric adenocarcinoma. Finally, a (typically incidental) collection of foamy, lipid-laden macrophages (xanthelasma) is addressed, predominantly because it should be recognized as benign and not mistaken for other more serious diseases.

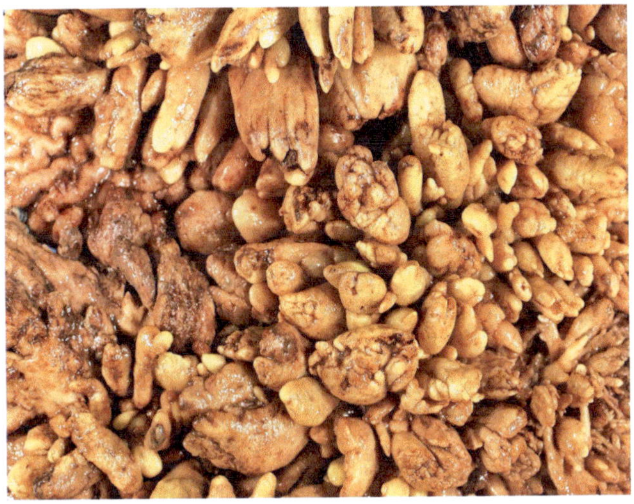

Fig. 22.1 Grossly, Ménétrier disease is characterized by giant, complex gastric folds that are restricted to the mucosa of the gastric body and fundus, with sparing of the antrum. The disease occurs in middle-aged patients, with a male predominance, and is associated with weight loss, hypoproteinemia, and decreased gastric acid production (hypochlorhydria)

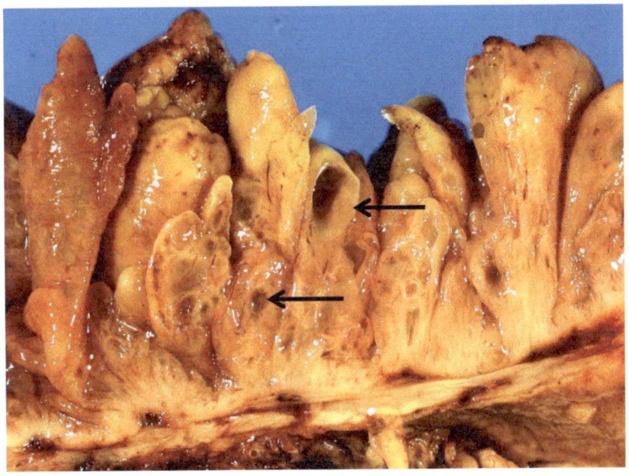

Fig. 22.2 The cut surfaces of the giant gastric folds in Ménétrier disease often have cystically dilated gastric glands (*arrows*). The etiology of the disease is unknown but may be related to changes in mucosal homeostasis, and possibly overexpression of transforming growth factor-α (TGF-α). Each of these giant polyp/fold structures resembles a gastric hyperplastic polyp, but the mucosal surface is carpeted with such structures in Ménétrier disease

S.R. Owens, H.D. Appelman, *Atlas of Esophagus and Stomach Pathology*, Atlas of Anatomic Pathology,
DOI 10.1007/978-1-4614-8084-6_22,

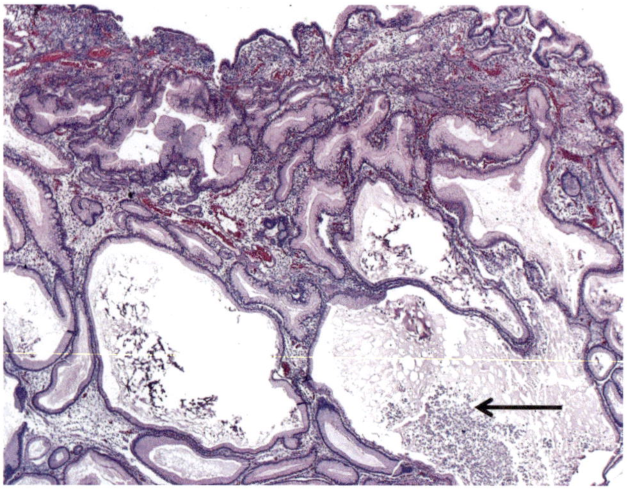

Fig. 22.3 The enlarged gastric folds in Ménétrier disease are characterized by dilated gastric pit and gland structures, corresponding to the cystic spaces seen grossly (*arrow*). There is extensive foveolar hyperplasia, and the lamina propria contains a mixture of inflammatory cells that vary in number. In isolation, the histological features are indistinguishable from a gastric hyperplastic polyp (see Chap. 23)

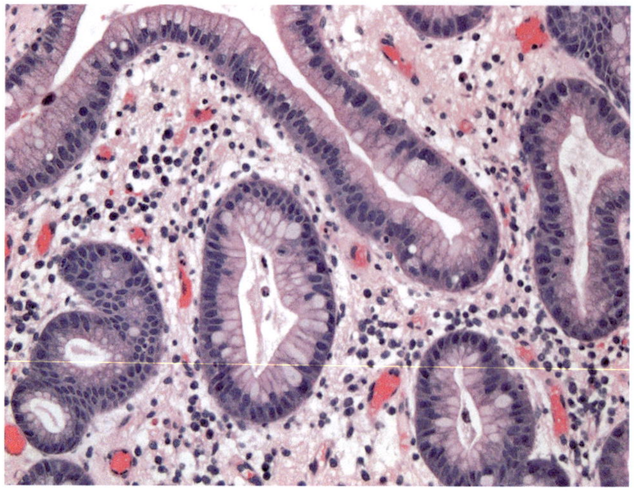

Fig. 22.4 At high magnification, the hyperplastic gastric pits are surrounded by edematous lamina propria that contains inflammatory cells. Because these features are identical to those seen in a hyperplastic polyp, correlation with the clinical features of hypoproteinemia and diffuse giant folds restricted to the gastric body/fundus on endoscopic examination is essential in making the diagnosis

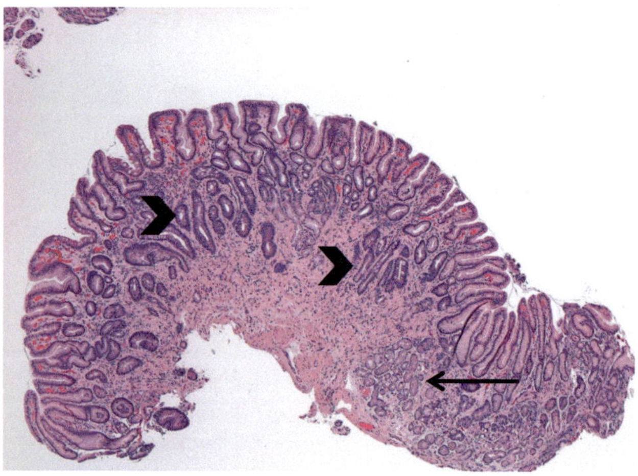

Fig. 22.5 Multifocal atrophic gastritis (MAG) is most often caused by longstanding *H. pylori* infection, typically in patients with early acquisition of the infection in endemic areas. It is characterized by loss of mucosal gland mass throughout the gastric mucosa. At low magnification, this is reflected in small clusters or "packets" of residual glands (*arrow*) surrounded by an expanded lamina propria. In addition, there is multifocal intestinal metaplasia, which is seen at low power as collections of darkly staining tubules (*arrowheads*)

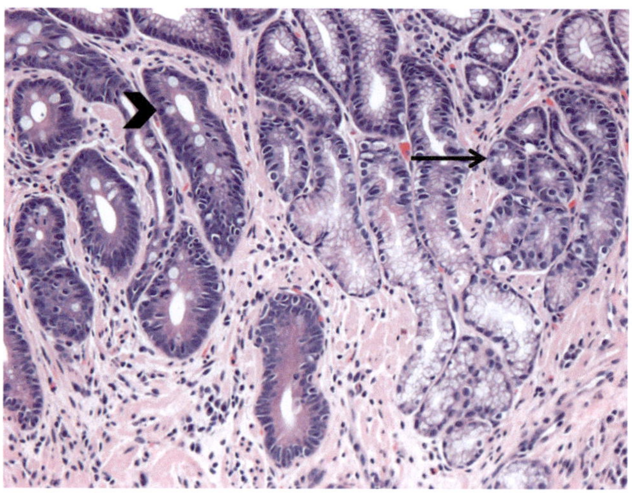

Fig. 22.6 At higher magnification, this antral biopsy contains residual antral glands with G cells (*arrow*), as well as tubules lined by metaplastic intestinal-type epithelium containing goblet cells (*arrowhead*). A true loss of gland mass (as opposed to simple expansion of the lamina propria by inflammation, which does not constitute atrophy) is apparent. The intestinal metaplasia puts MAG patients at increased risk for the development of epithelial dysplasia and adenocarcinoma

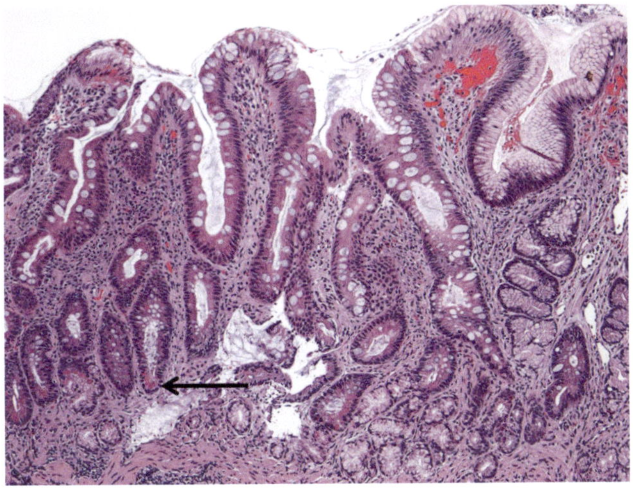

Fig. 22.7 This antral biopsy from a patient with MAG has extensive intestinal metaplasia, including Paneth cells (*arrow*). Some cases, such as this, have relatively abundant background inflammation in the lamina propria, potentially reflecting the genesis of the condition in *H. pylori* gastritis. Sometimes, the infection and early MAG coexist; patients with such findings should be treated for *H. pylori* eradication. Often, however, the change in mucosal microenvironment, with decreased acid and alteration in mucus chemistry, leads to an absence of the organisms

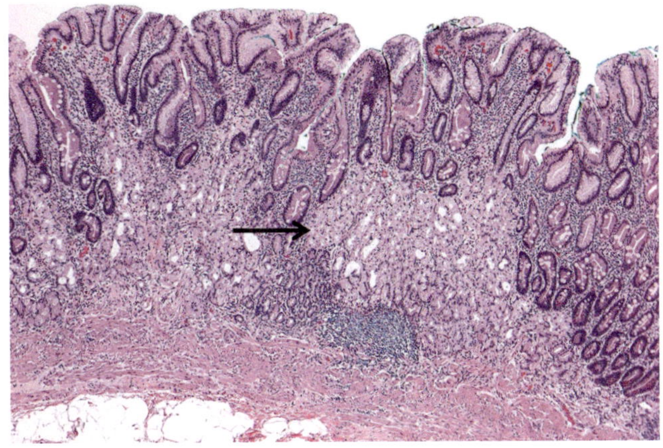

Fig. 22.8 As suggested by the name, MAG occurs in both oxyntic and antral mucosa, as opposed to antral-predominant mucosal atrophy, which may also follow *H. pylori* infection. Here, residual clusters of oxyntic glands (*arrow*) are separated by intestinal metaplasia. In addition, there is a basal lymphoid aggregate. MAG can be separate from autoimmune-type atrophic gastritis (see Chap. 20) by the distribution of the process, and the lack of enterochromaffin-like (ECL) cell hyperplasia in MAG

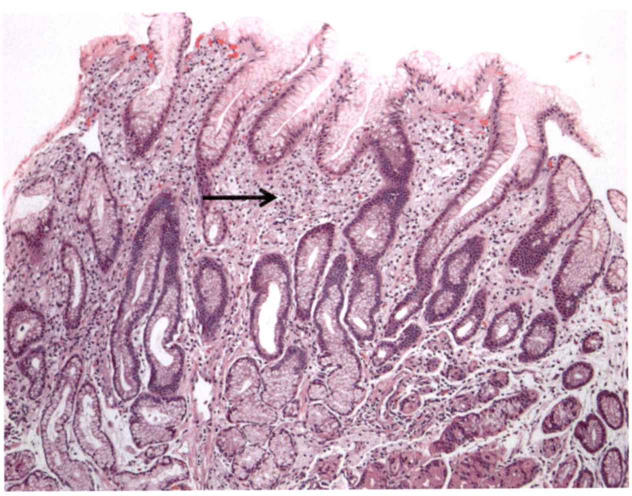

Fig. 22.9 Gastric xanthelasma (sometimes termed "xanthoma") appears as a yellow plaque or nodule on the mucosal surface, often on the lesser curvature. At low magnification, an expansion of the lamina propria by pale-appearing cells (*arrow*) is apparent

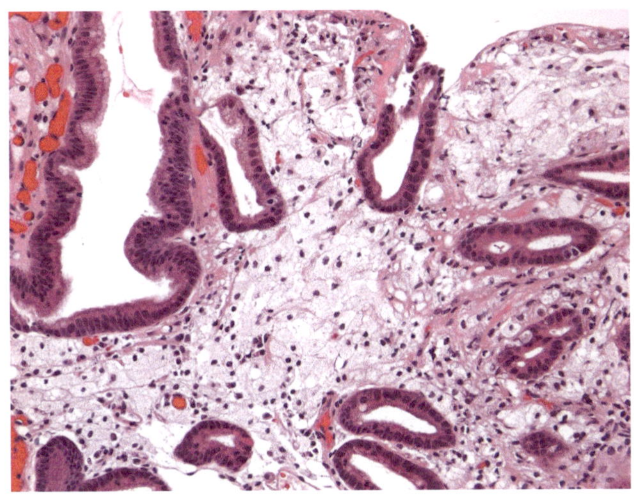

Fig. 22.10 The pale cells in the expanded lamina propria are foamy histiocytes, and they can be highlighted immunohistochemically using macrophage markers such as CD68. The cause of most xanthelasmas is unknown and they are usually found incidentally. They are more frequently seen, however, in patients who have undergone gastric surgery, such as Billroth II gastrojejunostomy. Xanthelasmas can also be found in patients with *H. pylori* infection and hypercholesterolemia

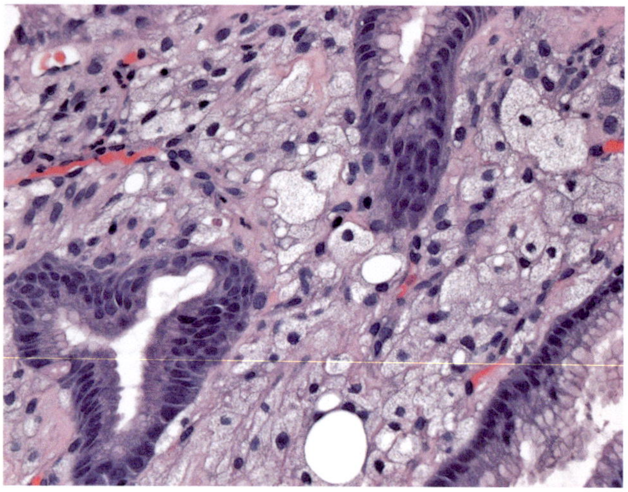

Fig. 22.11 At high magnification, the bland appearance of the foamy histiocytes is apparent. This innocuous histology, along with the endoscopic appearance, helps to separate an incidental xanthelasma from other entities in the differential diagnosis, including signet-ring cell carcinoma and metastatic clear cell carcinoma. In the appropriate clinical setting, one must also consider infectious processes such as mycobacterial infection (especially *M. avium-intracellulare*) and Whipple disease

23 Benign Tumors and Polyps

Only a few types of benign polyps occur in the stomach. The main polyps encountered routinely in gastric biopsies are the fundic gland polyp and the hyperplastic polyp, which are composed mainly of oxyntic glands and elongated foveolae/pits, respectively. These polyps rarely harbor epithelial dysplasia and, even when they do, the connection of such dysplasia with gastric cancer is controversial. Some gastric polyps are associated with underlying polyposis syndromes. These include fundic gland polyps with a higher frequency of dysplasia, which occur in the setting of familial adenomatous polyposis. Most other syndromic gastric polyps strongly resemble (and can be indistinguishable from) gastric hyperplastic polyps, including those occurring in Peutz–Jeghers syndrome, juvenile polyposis, and others. Thus, it is important to keep these syndromes in the differential diagnosis when encountering numerous or recurrent benign gastric polyps in any given patient. Lastly, the "inflammatory fibroid polyp" (IFP), actually a submucosal fibroinflammatory proliferation, can appear like a polyp endoscopically and may make an appearance in gastric biopsies.

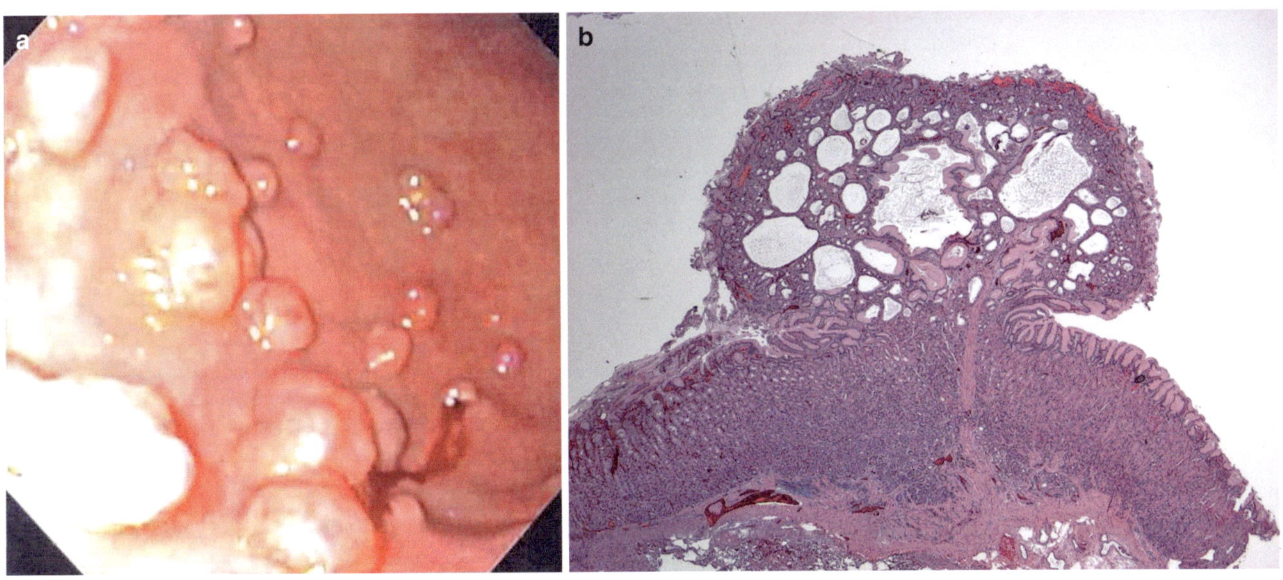

Fig. 23.1 Fundic gland polyps (FGP) are a very common finding on upper endoscopy, and may be solitary or multiple. Most are small (<2 mm), but they can be larger. (**a**) Endoscopically, FGP appear as sessile polyps in the gastric body and/or fundus (*ie*, in oxyntic mucosa). Typically, they are the same color (pale pink) as the surrounding mucosa, and have a smooth surface. (**b**) In this example, seen at extremely low magnification, an FGP appears "stuck on" the surrounding oxyntic mucosa with a broad base. Even at this low magnification, the characteristic morphology, with cystically dilated gland-like structures, is apparent

S.R. Owens, H.D. Appelman, *Atlas of Esophagus and Stomach Pathology*, Atlas of Anatomic Pathology,
DOI 10.1007/978-1-4614-8084-6_23, © Springer Science+Business Media New York 2014

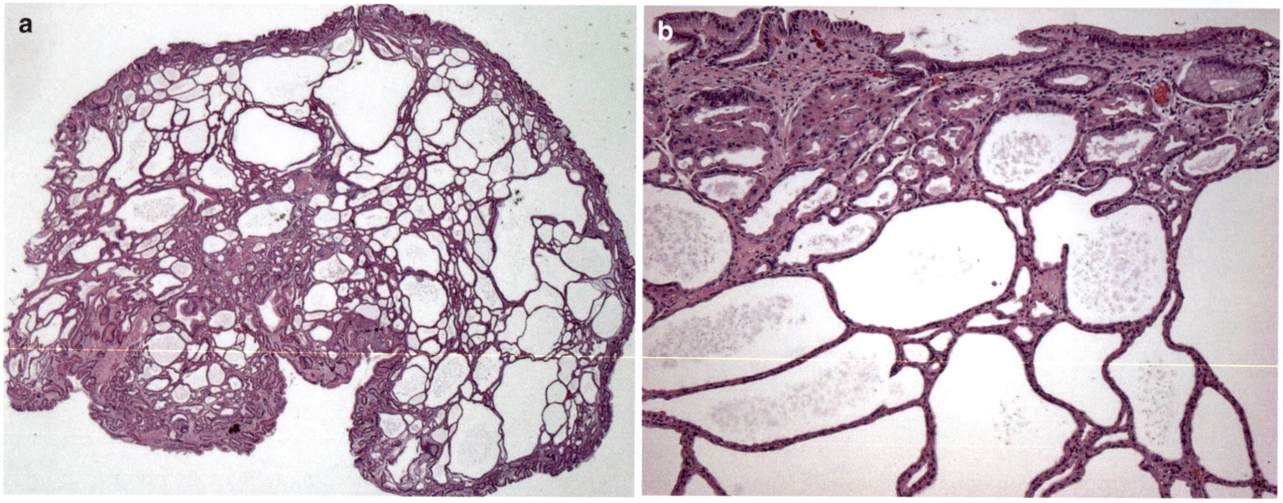

Fig. 23.2 The characteristic feature of FGPs is their composition by *glands*. The pit/foveolar compartment is attenuated and the oxyntic glands occupy almost the entire thickness of the polypoid mucosa. (**a**) In this example, the cystic dilation of the glands is very prominent, although this is not always the case. At the surface of the polyp, the near absence of the pit compartment is apparent, even at this low magnification. (**b**) The glands (cystically dilated or not) always have at least a component of parietal cells lining them, whether or not there are foveolar and/or chief cells

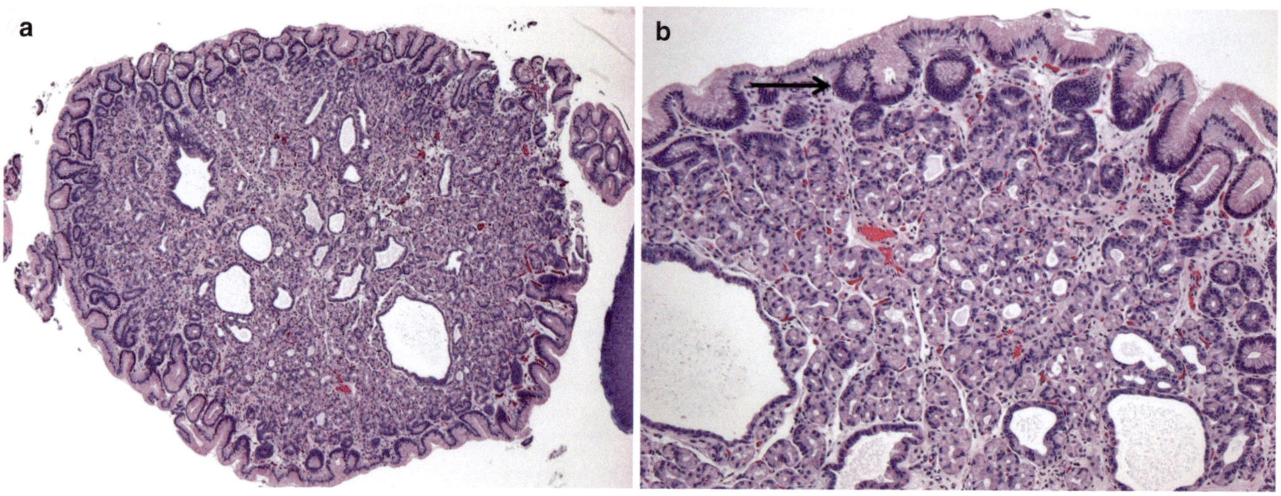

Fig. 23.3 (**a**) This classic-appearing FGP has a mixture of small oxyntic-type glands as well as a few cystically dilated examples, particularly in the deeper reaches of the polyp. (**b**) At higher magnification, the attenuation of the pit compartment is apparent (*arrow*). The background lamina propria often appears edematous. FGP occur sporadically, but they are also associated with familial adenomatous polyposis (FAP) syndrome. Syndromic examples tend to be found in younger patients (third vs. fifth to sixth decades) but are otherwise morphologically indistinguishable

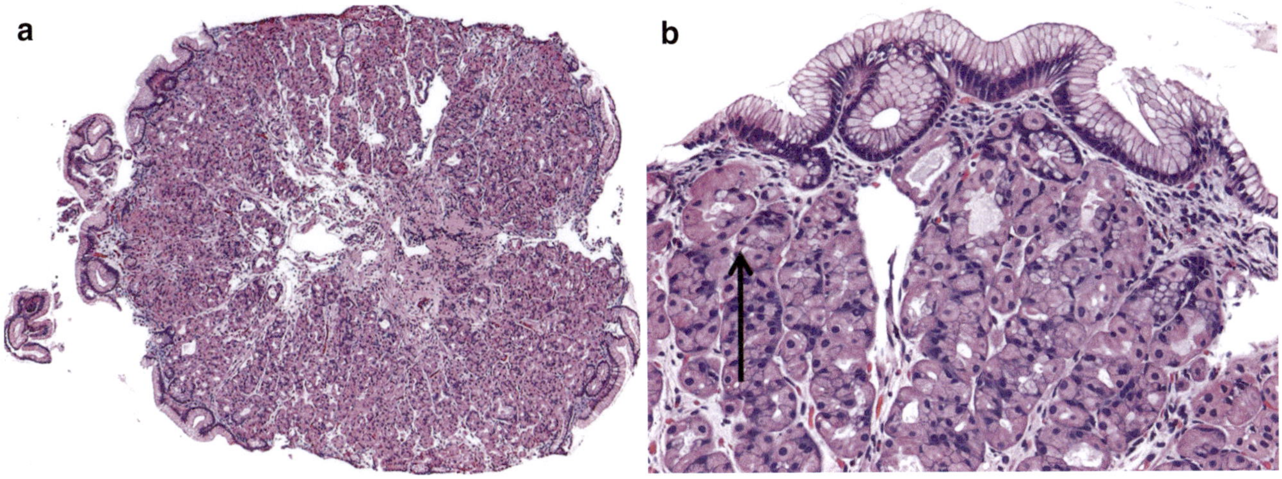

Fig. 23.4 (**a**) This particular FGP has almost no cystically dilated glands. It is recognizable at low magnification, nonetheless, because of the predominance of glands and the almost-nonexistent pit compartment. (**b**) At higher magnification, the tendency of the oxyntic glands to sit immediately beneath the surface epithelium (*arrow*) is apparent. This feature alone is sufficient to make the diagnosis, even without the dilated glands, when a polyp is seen endoscopically in the body/fundus. In addition, note the prominence of the parietal cells in many of the glands. One of the putative etiologies of FGP (or at least a contributing factor) is thought to be proton pump inhibitor (PPI) therapy. The apical "snouts" seen in many of these glands are suggestive of PPI therapy

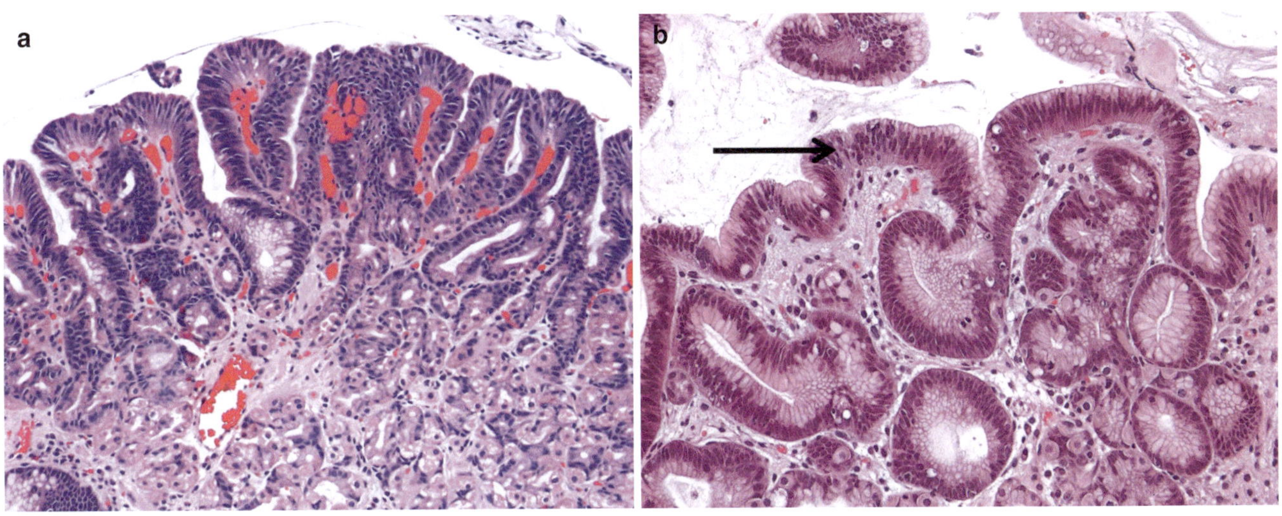

Fig. 23.5 FGP may harbor epithelial dysplasia. This is most common in syndromic examples (associated with FAP), but also can occur in sporadic examples. The combination of FGP and epithelial dysplasia should prompt the observer to at least give thought to the possibility of FAP. (**a**) This patch of low-grade foveolar-type dysplasia, predominantly in the surface/pit epithelium, was found in an FGP in an FAP patient. Although not always true, the dysplasia in FGP tends to favor the superficial epithelium. Occasionally, it will appear in the dilated gland structures. (**b**) Even in the setting of FAP, the dysplasia is morphologically identical to that seen in nonsyndromic polyps, and is characterized by enlarged and hyperchromatic nuclei (*arrow*). For FAP patients, the risk of dysplasia is associated with the number of polyps. The occurrence of high-grade dysplasia is rare, even in syndromic examples. The risk of progression to invasive adenocarcinoma is controversial, and seems to occur extremely rarely, if at all

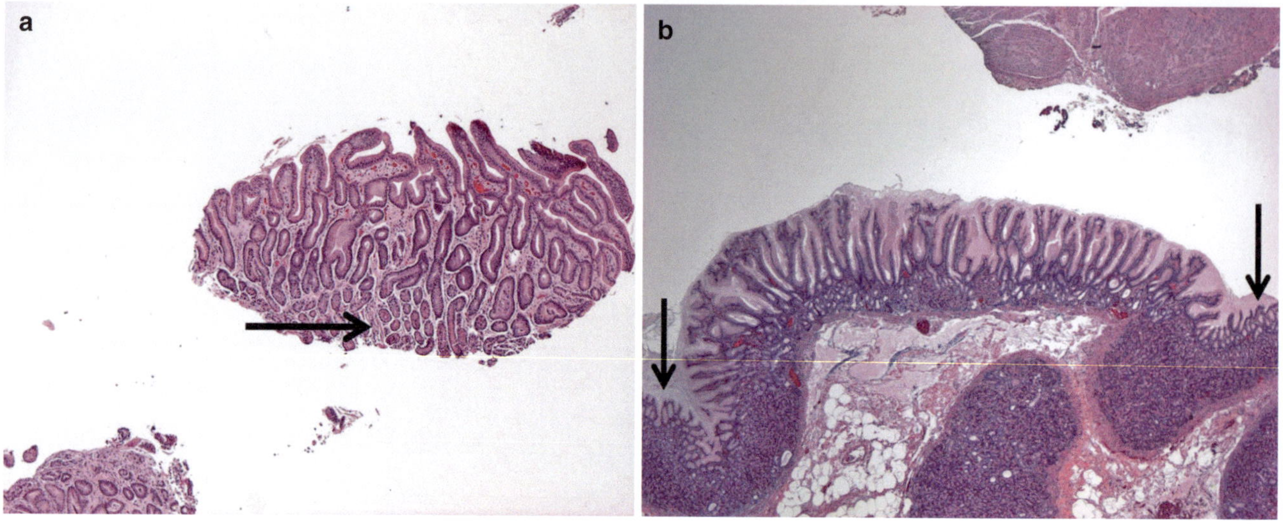

Fig. 23.6 Focal (or "polypoid") foveolar hyperplasia (FFH) can produce endoscopically visible protrusions on the mucosa. Really, this is on a spectrum with gastric hyperplastic polyps (discussed in the next section), and FFH tends to appear more polypoid by endoscopy than it does by histology. (**a**) In contrast to FGP, FFH is an expansion of the pit/foveolar compartment. In this biopsy, essentially no gland compartment is present at the base of the biopsy (*arrow*). (**b**) This is very apparent in this excision specimen, where a distinct patch of foveolar hyperplasia is apparent at the center of the figure, surrounded by more normal-appearing mucosa (*arrows*). The distinction between a large focus of FFH and a small hyperplastic polyp is difficult, and likely varies from observer to observer. Some observers use a size criterion of 1 cm for the distinction (<1 cm = FFH; >1 cm = hyperplastic polyp)

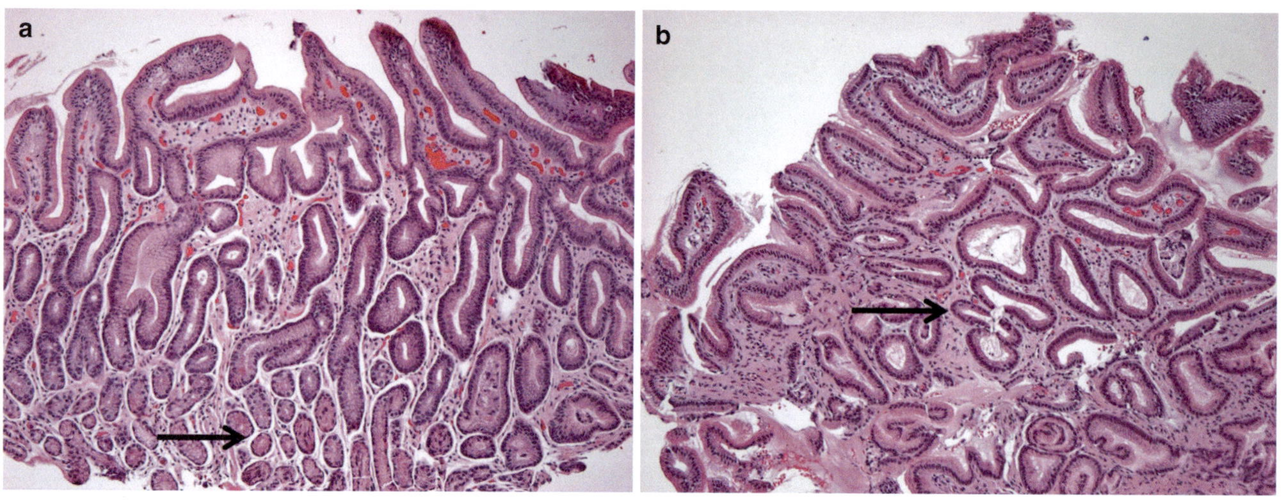

Fig. 23.7 (**a**) At higher magnification, the "pit-heavy" composition of this biopsy is visible. Only a few glands are seen at the very bottom of the image (*arrow*). (**b**) This biopsy of FFH has no glands at all, and only consists of irregularly shaped pit/foveolar structures (*arrow*). Sometimes, these can become dilated, mimicking the dilated glands seen in FGP. The low-power impression of "all pits" versus "all glands" is helpful in such situations, as is the presence of at least some parietal cells in the dilated gland of FGP

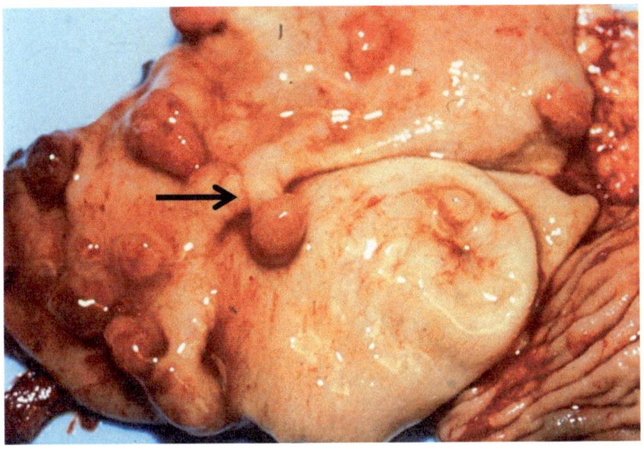

Fig. 23.8 Gastric hyperplastic polyps (GHP) are thought to be associated with mucosal injury and regeneration. In contrast to FGP, GHP often have a broad stalk or pedicle (*arrow*), and can have a red-appearing, eroded surface on endoscopic examination

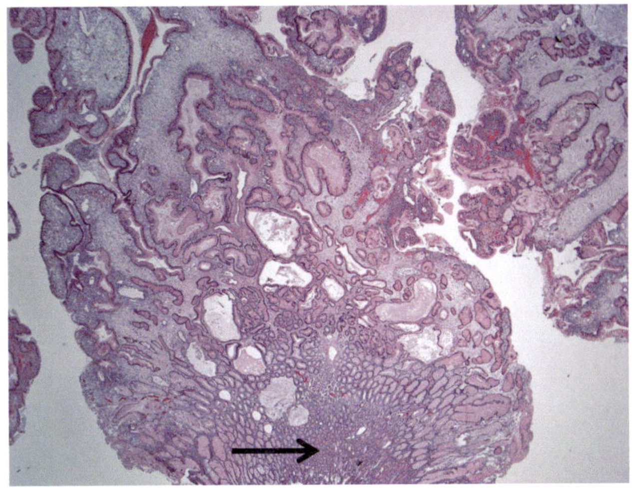

Fig. 23.9 While the constitutive feature of FGP is *glands*, GHP are composed of a hyperplasia of the *pit* compartment ("it's the pits!"). GHP can become quite large, and can occur in the setting of chronic mucosal injury caused by *H. pylori*, bile reflux, autoimmune gastritis, and near gastroenterostomies, as well as other settings. In this example, the gland compartment is at the bottom of the image (*arrow*) and the markedly expanded foveolar compartment occupies most of the polyp

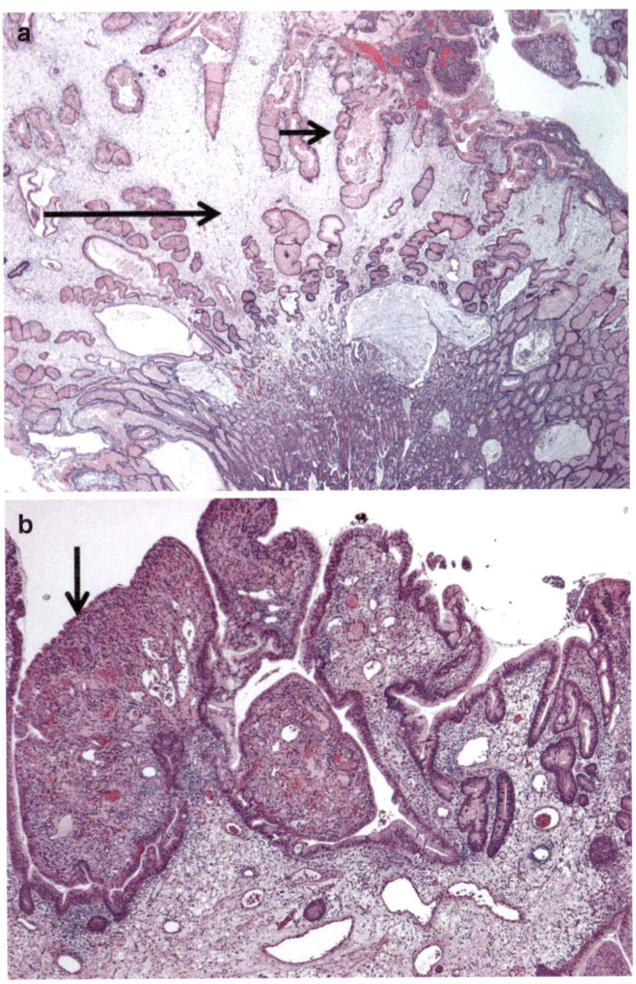

Fig. 23.10 (**a**) At higher magnification, the foveolar mucin of the expanded pit compartment is visible (*short arrow*). The lamina propria between the pits (*long arrow*) is edematous and often contains a mixture of inflammatory cells. (**b**) Many GHP have erosions of the surface epithelium (*arrow*), and the adjacent intact epithelium can appear reactive and hyperchromatic, mimicking dysplasia

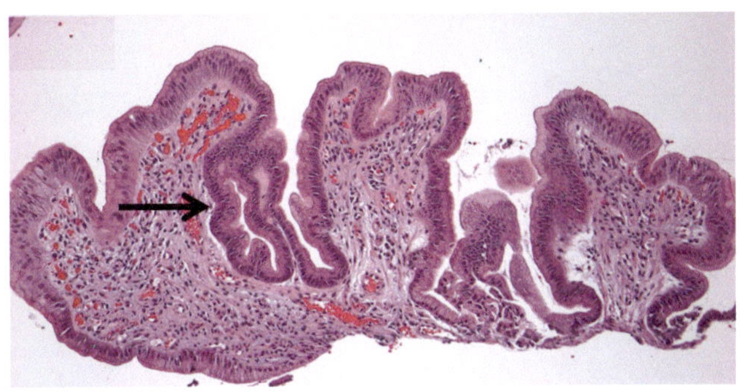

Fig. 23.11 This superficial biopsy of a GHP has edematous and inflamed lamina propria, prominent capillaries, and reactive atypia of the epithelium (*arrow*), all reflecting the background of mucosal injury that is thought to underlie these polyps. Although hyperchromatic, the epithelium maintains the basal location of its nuclei and some mucin production, including at the mucosal surface

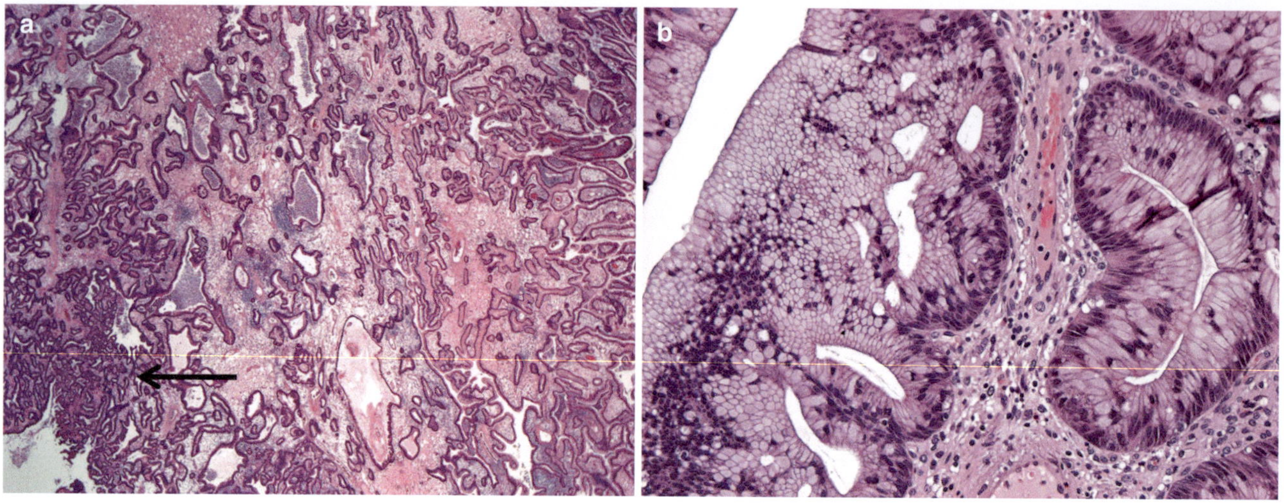

Fig. 23.12 Rarely, GHP may harbor dysplasia, as in this case. (**a**) At extremely low magnification, the composition of this polyp by expanded foveolae is apparent (essentially no glands are present) and, in the left part of the image (*arrow*), the epithelium is very hyperchromatic. (**b**) At high magnification, the epithelium can be seen to be truly dysplastic, with stratified and irregular nuclei and mitotic activity, despite the abundance of mucin production in this case

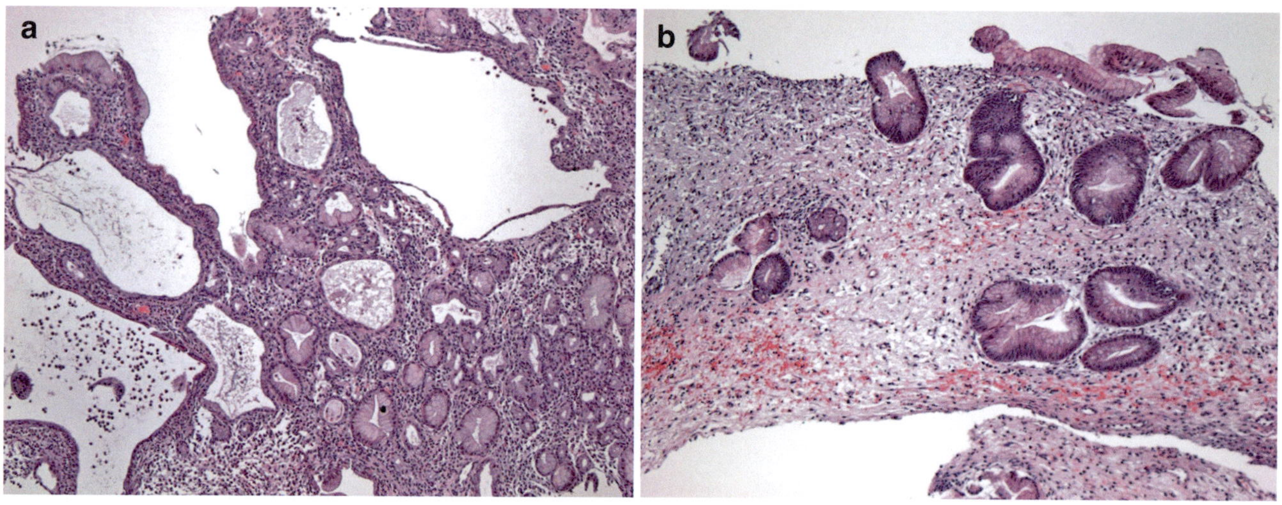

Fig. 23.13 While many of the inherited polyposis syndromes have their most characteristic expression outside the stomach, syndromic hamartomatous polyps occur in the stomach as well. Unfortunately, most such polyps strongly resemble GHPs and can easily be mistaken for them without a clue from the clinical history and an index of suspicion. (**a**) This example of a gastric polyp in a patient with Cronkhite–Canada syndrome (CCS) has expanded, dilated, and irregularly-shaped pits with numerous inflammatory cells in the lamina propria. (**b**) In other areas, polyps from the same patient had a more fibrotic-appearing lamina propria, but were still primarily composed of pit/foveolar structures. CCS patients also have ectodermal features such as skin and nail abnormalities

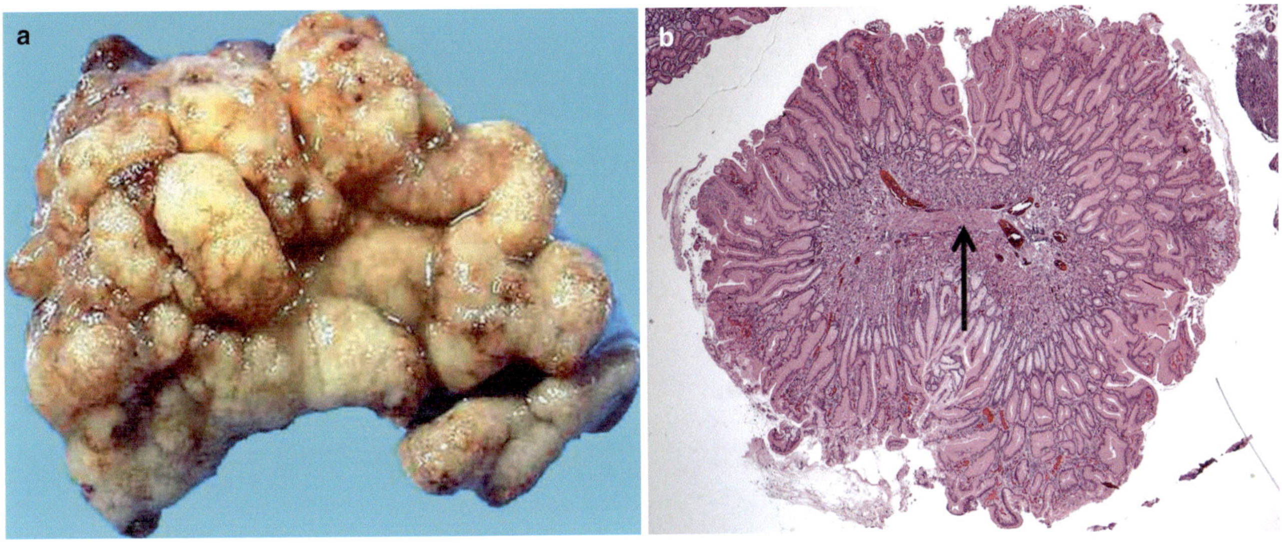

Fig. 23.14 This gastric polyp is from a patient with Peutz-Jeghers syndrome (PJS). (**a**) Grossly, it has a lobulated appearance. (**b**) This polyp, too, is mostly composed of expanded pits reminiscent of a GHP, which can be appreciated at low magnification. The hamartomatous polyps of PJS have their most characteristic expression in the small intestine, where they have prominent, arborizing smooth muscle bundles that are decorated with disorganized-appearing mucosa. In the very center of this polyp (*arrow*), there is a subtle collection of smooth muscle fibers

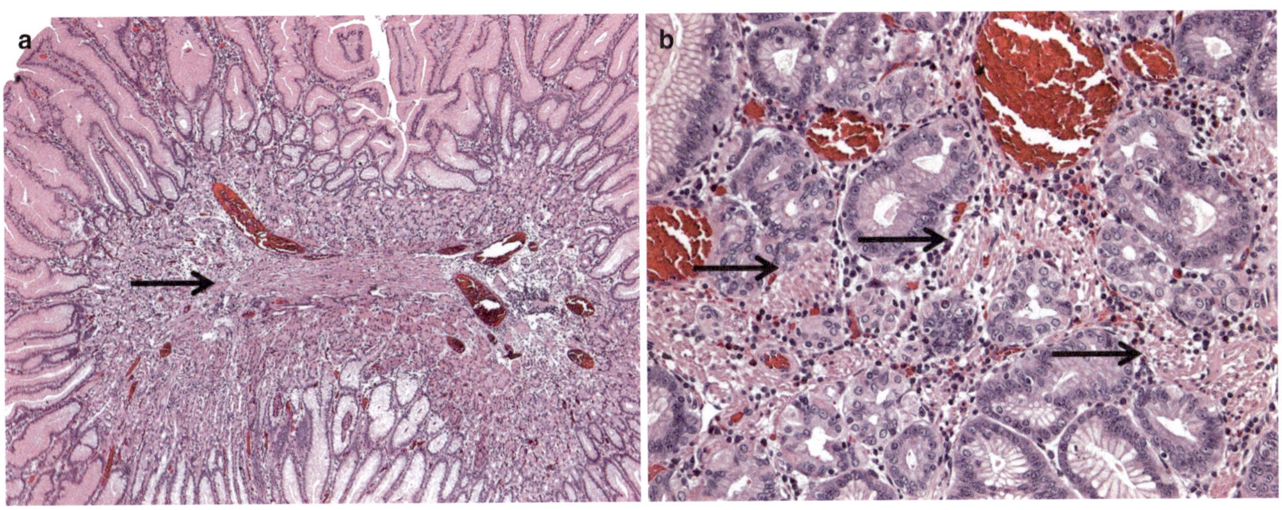

Fig. 23.15 (**a**) At higher magnification, the muscle bundle (*arrow*) in this PJS polyp is more visible, as is the expansion and irregularity of the pit compartment. (**b**) At very high magnification, some subtle bundles of smooth muscle can be seen traversing the mucosa (*arrows*)

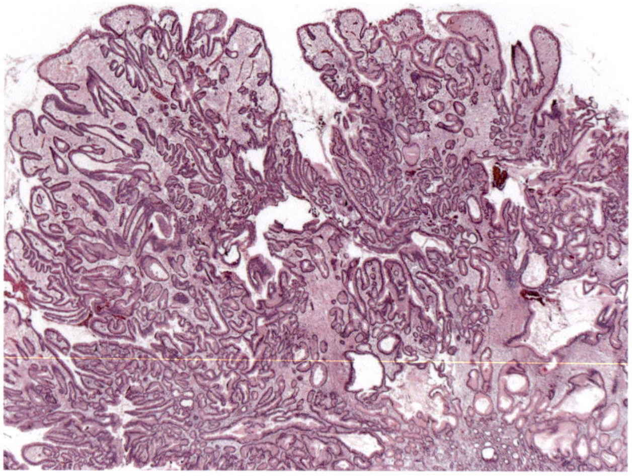

Fig. 23.16 This polyp is from a patient with juvenile polyposis syndrome (JPS). This syndrome is associated with germline mutations in two genes, *SMAD4* and *BMPR1A*. Patients who have *SMAD4* mutations have the highest risk of gastric polyposis and gastric cancer. Once again, however, the polyps are strongly suggestive of GHP, and this particular example has an abundance of dilated, elongated, and irregular foveolar structures

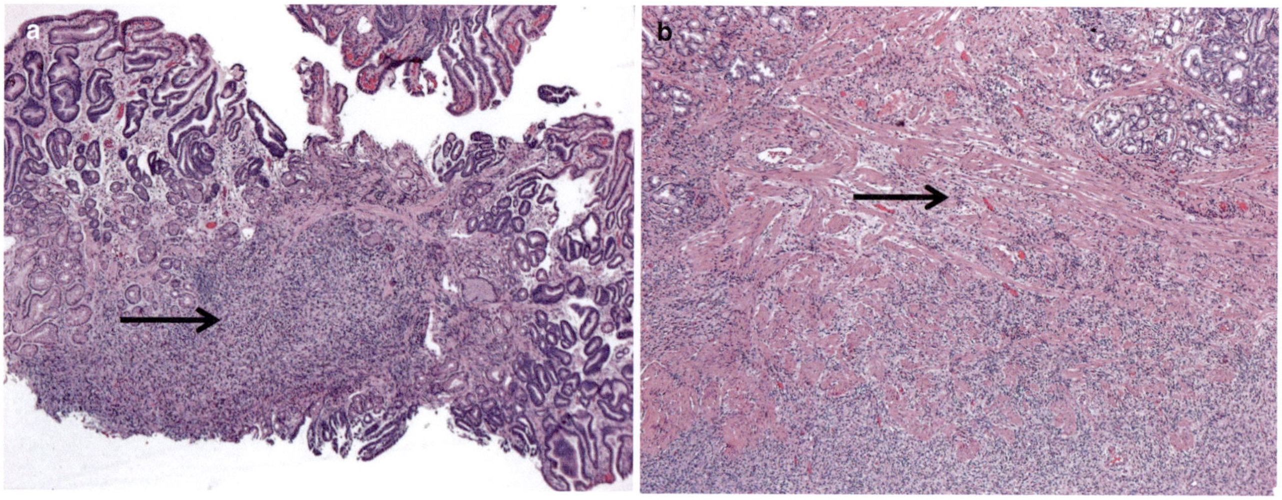

Fig. 23.17 IFP may occur throughout the gastrointestinal tract, but the gastric antrum is the most common site of involvement. These rare lesions contain a proliferation of fibrous tissue with an eosinophil-rich inflammatory infiltrate and a prominent vascular component. (**a**) At low magnification, they are centered in the submucosa (*arrow*) and extend into the deep mucosa, which may have reactive changes as in this example. In the gastric antrum, IFP may lead to gastric outlet obstruction, and biopsies of the process may not sample much submucosa. (**b**) IFP tend to disrupt the fibers of the muscularis mucosae (*arrow*) as they extend into the deep mucosa

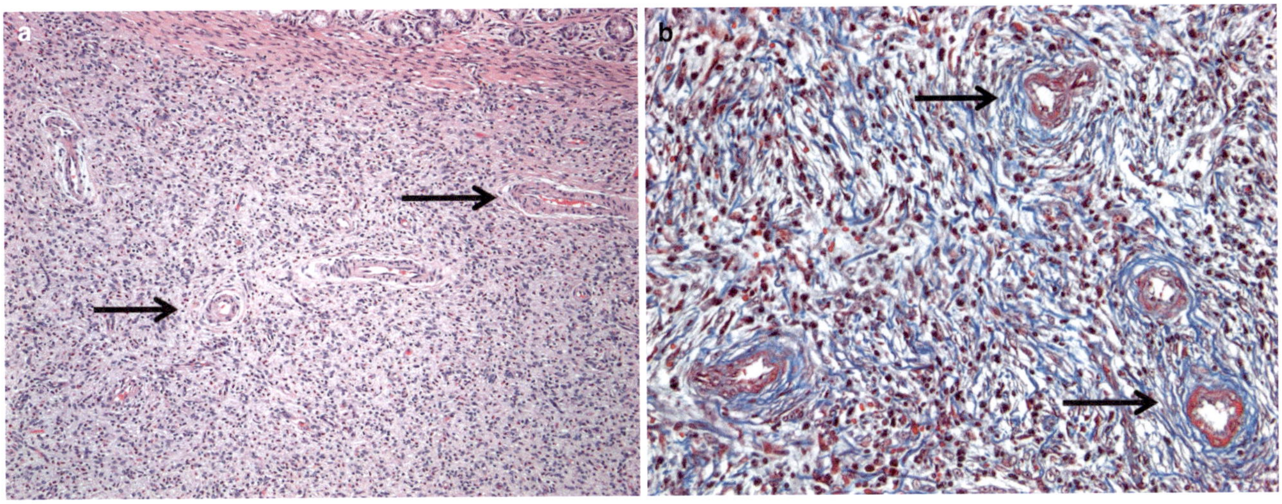

Fig. 23.18 (**a**) The main part of an IFP contains an infiltrate of bland spindle cells that spread out diffusely. In gastric IFP, there is a characteristic condensation around blood vessels (*arrows*), giving an "onion-skin" appearance. These cells are admixed with inflammatory cells, with a prominent population of eosinophils, which can just be discerned as red spots at this magnification. (**b**) The "onion-skin" pattern is especially visible around the vessels (*arrows*) on this trichrome stain, which highlights the strands of collagen in the lesion. IFP are usually positive for CD34 on immunohistochemistry, and are negative for CD117 (c-kit), which helps to separate them from gastric stromal tumors (GISTs)

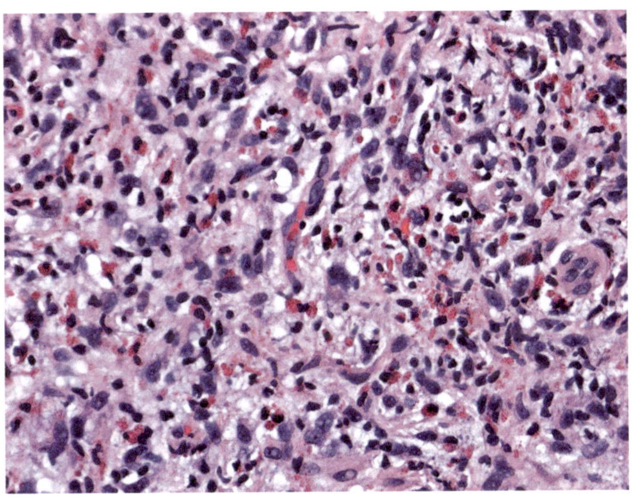

Fig. 23.19 At high magnification, the bland, spindle-shaped lesional cells are visible, as are the prominent eosinophils. Neutrophils are not a prominent feature the inflammatory infiltrate. Recent evidence has connected mutations in the *PDGFRA* gene to the pathogenesis of IFP. Exon 18 mutations are found in gastric examples

24 Epithelial Dysplasia and Adenomas

In the stomach, the term "adenoma" is used to describe polypoid dysplasia that does not fit into one of the other named polyp categories (*ie*, a recognizable fundic gland polyp with superimposed dysplasia would not technically be deemed an adenoma). In places where gastric cancer is common (such as East Asia), gastric adenomas are common as well. Here in the United States, we rarely encounter adenomas in biopsies from the stomach. By definition, an adenoma should appear as a polyp or nodule endoscopically. Most adenomas that we do encounter contain dysplastic intestinal-type epithelium. Rarer subtypes harbor dysplastic foveolar-type epithelium (so-called "type II" dysplasia) or are composed of pyloric gland-like structures. These polyps can contain low-grade or high-grade dysplasia, and must be carefully searched for evidence of an early adenocarcinoma invading the lamina propria ("intramucosal adenocarcinoma;" see Chap. 25). In the West, we use a two-tiered grading system for dysplasia that utilizes cytological and architectural features, and we require unequivocal evidence of invasion to diagnose adenocarcinoma. In Asia, more emphasis is placed on cytological features in making a carcinoma diagnosis. While this chapter focuses on polypoid gastric dysplasias, the approach to diagnosis and grading is similar for flat dysplasias in the stomach.

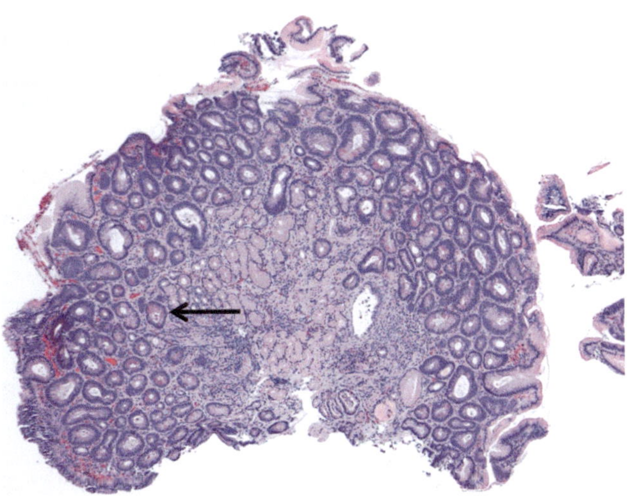

Fig. 24.1 In the United States, adenomas in the stomach are rare. When they occur, they are most commonly composed of intestinal-type epithelium, and are thought to arise in the background of intestinal metaplasia, such as that seen in the mucosal atrophy that follows long-standing *Helicobacter pylori* infection (Chaps. 21 and 22). The dysplastic epithelium in the superficial part of the polyp is crowded and hyperchromatic, and these changes extend to the mucosal surface. Even at this low magnification, some evidence of mucosal atrophy and background intestinal metaplasia is evident in this polypoid collection of dysplastic tubules. Note the cluster of tubules containing eosinophilic Paneth cells (*arrow*)

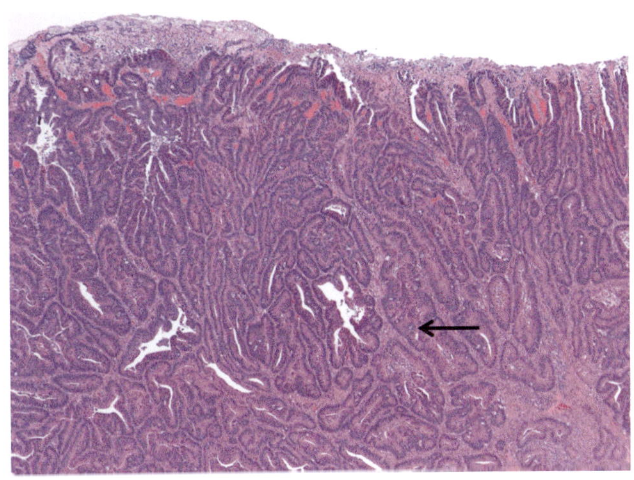

Fig. 24.2 At slightly higher magnification, this adenoma contains crowded tubules lined by epithelium with hyperchromatic, but basally oriented, nuclei indicative of low-grade dysplasia. The epithelium in intestinal-type adenomas parallels that seen in colonic adenomas. At this power, the lack of foveolar mucin is apparent, and a few goblet cells can be seen in the tubules (*arrow*)

S.R. Owens, H.D. Appelman, *Atlas of Esophagus and Stomach Pathology*, Atlas of Anatomic Pathology,
DOI 10.1007/978-1-4614-8084-6_24,

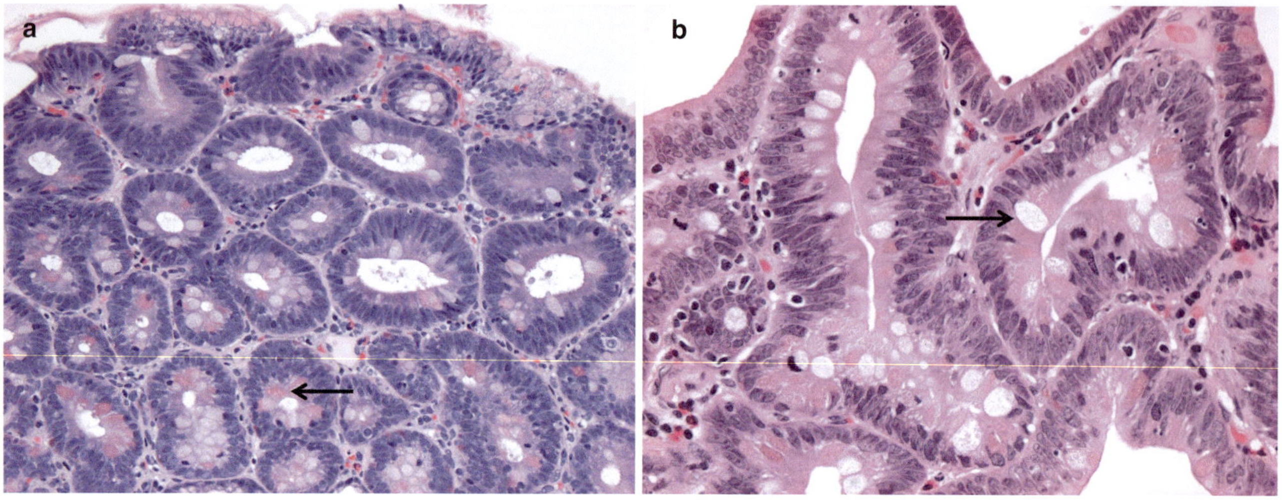

Fig. 24.3 At high magnification, the characteristic features of low-grade intestinal-type dysplasia are evident. The nuclei are crowded, dark, elongated, and, in areas, pseudostratified. They are, however, basally oriented, with some remaining mucin production in the apical cytoplasm of the cells. (**a**) This adenoma is relatively rich in Paneth cells (*arrow*). (**b**) This example contains numerous goblet cells (*arrow*). Intestinal-type gastric dysplasia is characterized by MUC2 expression, which can be demonstrated using immunohistochemistry

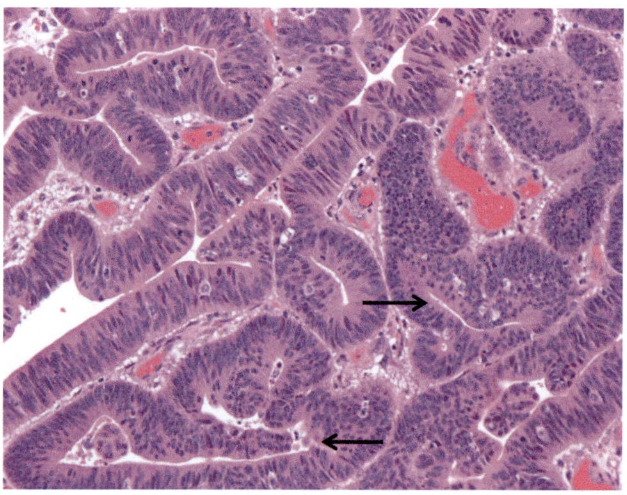

Fig. 24.4 High-grade dysplasia has more complex architecture as well as more striking cytological changes. In this intestinal-type adenoma, some of the tubules have a complex branching appearance (*arrows*). The epithelium also exhibits full-thickness nuclear stratification, abundant mitotic activity and apoptotic debris, and almost no mucin production

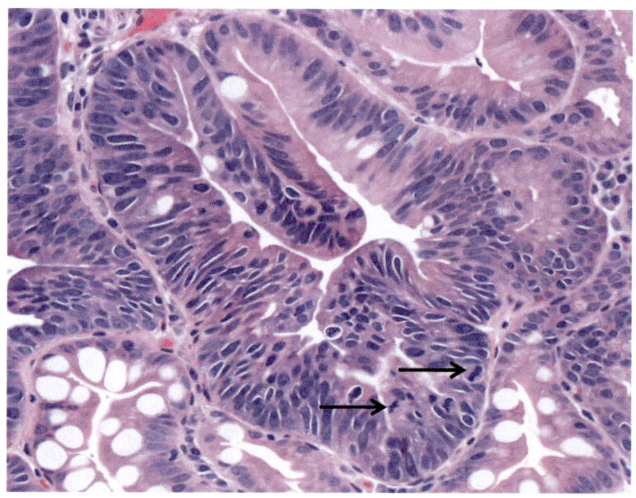

Fig. 24.5 This example of high-grade dysplasia arising in the background of mucosal atrophy with intestinal metaplasia has both very complex architecture and striking cytological atypia. This tubule has a cribriform architecture. Almost no mucin is apparent in the apical cytoplasm of the most atypical epithelium, and numerous mitotic figures (*arrows*) are visible. At the bottom left and right, two nondysplastic tubules with goblet cells reflect the background intestinal metaplasia

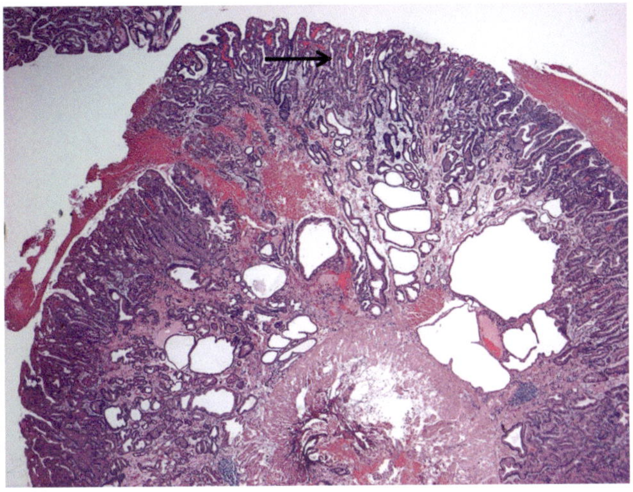

Fig. 24.6 In contrast to the more common intestinal-type, gastric adenomas with foveolar-type dysplasia are reminiscent of hyperplastic polyps at low magnification. They tend to have more abundant, frothy, apical mucin in the epithelium. The same pattern of crowded and hyperchromatic superficial tubules (*arrow*) is present, however

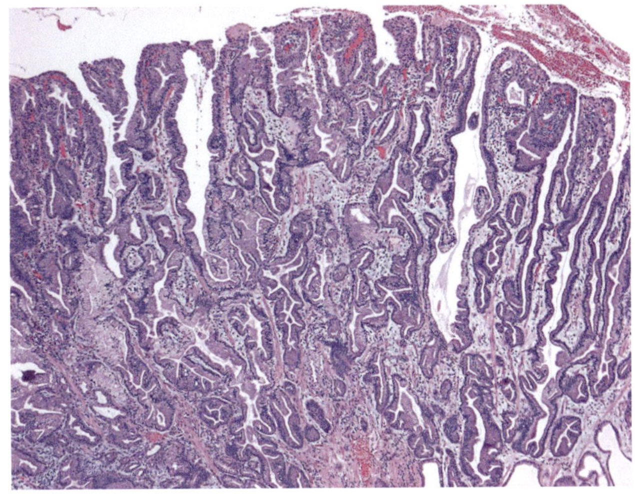

Fig. 24.7 At higher magnification, the "pit-predominant" nature of this gastric foveolar adenoma is apparent. The foveolae are markedly elongated and irregular, and are lined by epithelium with crowded and hyperchromatic, but basally oriented, nuclei. The "serrated" architecture of many of the dysplastic foveolae is a common feature

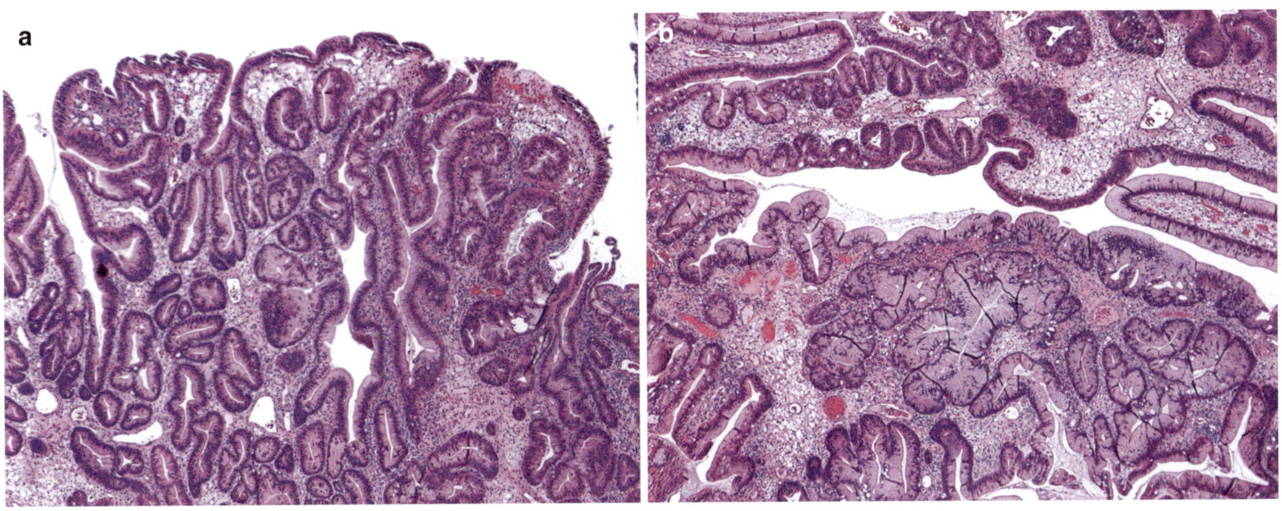

Fig. 24.8 (**a**, **b**) The architectural component of dysplasia is more difficult to assess in foveolar-type gastric adenomas, due to the common finding of serrated or irregular foveolar structures. True budding or cribriform architecture, however, is typical of the architectural atypia of high-grade dysplasia. In this example, note the abundant foveolar-type mucin (which is immunohistochemically positive for MUC5AC) superimposed on the hyperchromatic and crowded nuclei

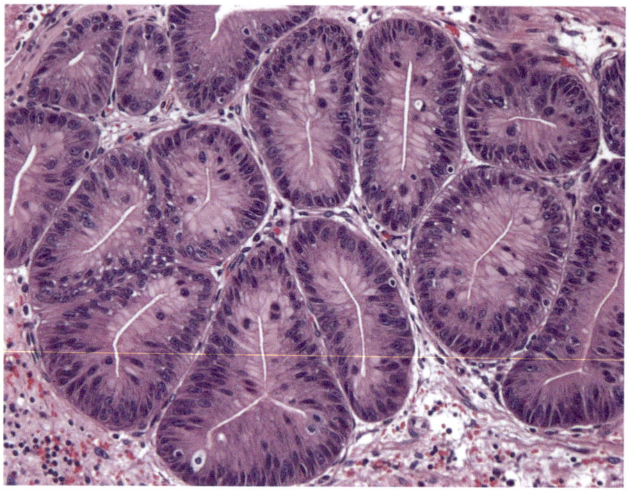

Fig. 24.9 At high magnification, the abundant apical mucin is apparent in this foveolar-type adenoma. In this example, the epithelial atypia is more pronounced, with nuclei that are more pseudostratified and more frequent mitotic figures. The architecture, however, remains simple

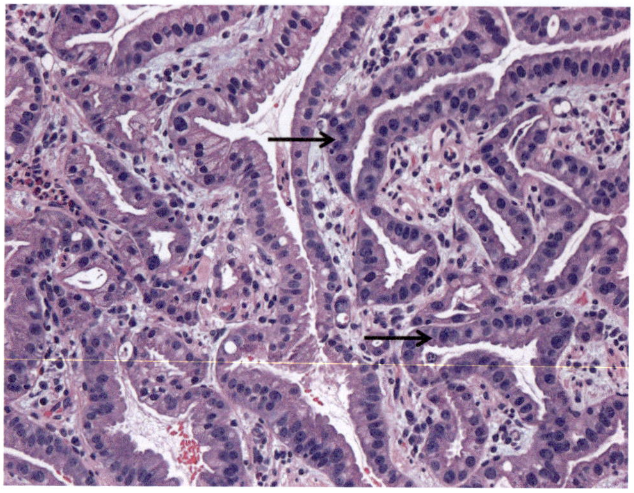

Fig. 24.10 In this foveolar-type adenoma, there is a mixture of low-grade and high-grade dysplasia. The tubules are more complex and closely packed than those seen in the earlier examples. In addition, several (*arrows*) are lined by epithelium that produces almost no mucin and has rounded, hyperchromatic, and pleomorphic nuclei, diagnostic of high-grade dysplasia

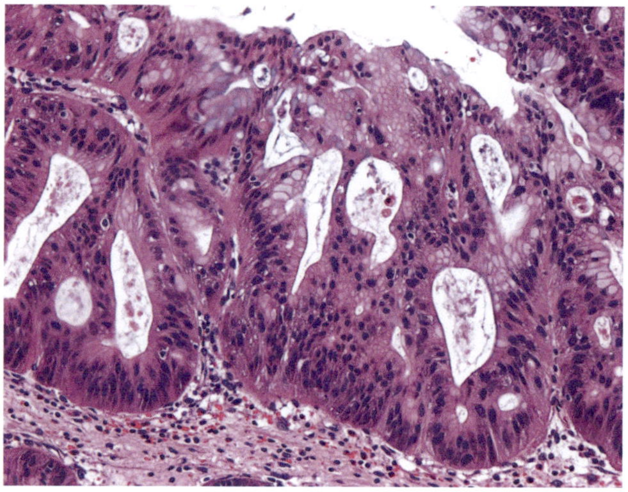

Fig. 24.11 This foveolar-type adenoma has both architectural and cytological features indicative of high grade dysplasia. The tubules have a cribriform architecture with numerous lumens, and the epithelial cells have stratified and pleomorphic nuclei. When such architectural changes are extensive, one must begin to contemplate the diagnosis of "intramucosal adenocarcinoma" (*ie*, carcinoma invading the lamina propria). In Japan, this focus would likely receive an outright diagnosis of carcinoma

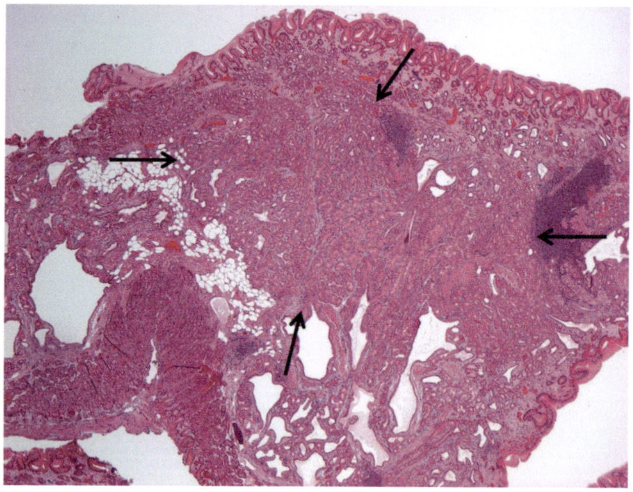

Fig. 24.12 Pyloric gland adenoma (PGA) is a rare (or at least rarely diagnosed) epithelial proliferation that can occur in several different parts of the gastrointestinal tract, including the stomach. These neoplasms seem to have a propensity to affect the stomach of women with autoimmune gastritis, and are associated with background intestinal metaplasia. In this example, there is a dense, discrete collection of bland-appearing gland-like structures in the deep mucosa (*arrows*)

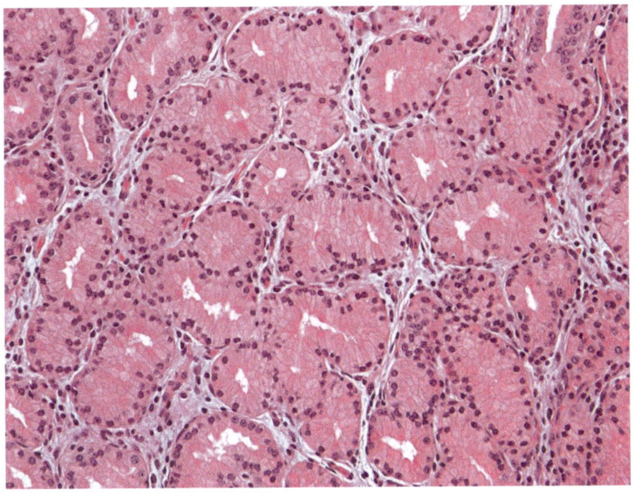

Fig. 24.13 At higher magnification, the composition of this polyp by bland-appearing glands/tubules with abundant, frothy cytoplasm is apparent. The nuclei are round and basally oriented, and the structures are essentially identical to pyloric-type glands in the distal stomach. This example is not dysplastic

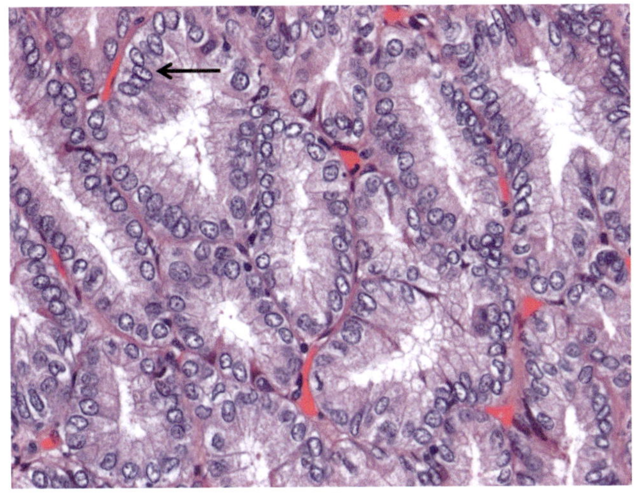

Fig. 24.14 At high magnification, the frothy (or "ground-glass") apical cytoplasm is visible, as are the relatively bland-appearing, round nuclei with inconspicuous nucleoli. Assessment of dysplasia is similar to that in other gastric adenomas, although the different appearance of the cells from intestinal-type adenomas and the relative rarity of this type of polyp can make grading somewhat more difficult. This example has low-grade dysplasia, with slightly larger and more crowded nuclei that have subtle stratification in areas (*arrow*). In addition, the tubules are a bit more irregular than the example in Fig. 24.13

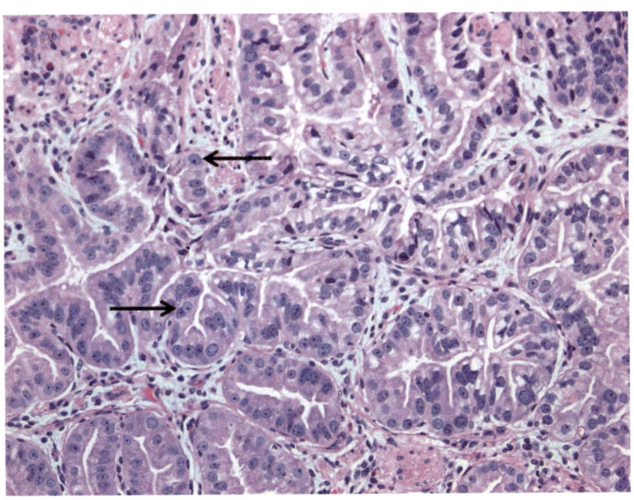

Fig. 24.15 This PGA contains high-grade dysplasia, characterized by more irregular architecture, more pleomorphic nuclei that lack basal polarity, and a few conspicuous nucleoli (*arrows*)

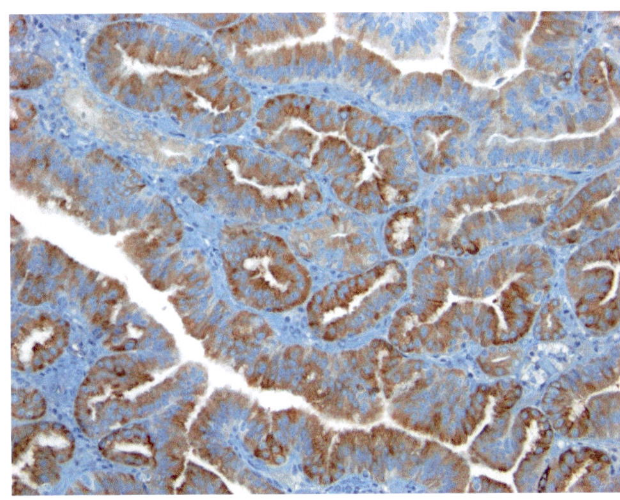

Fig. 24.16 PGAs express pyloric-type mucin, as evidenced by this positive MUC6 immunohistochemical stain

25 Carcinoma of the Stomach

We do not see very much gastric cancer in the United States, compared to our colleagues in the Far East and, to some extent, Eastern Europe, Central America, and South America. As a result, we in the United States are not nearly as adept at diagnosis and classification of this disease and have not studied it as comprehensively as, in particular, the Japanese. Cancer in the proximal stomach (in and around the gastroesophageal junction) is dealt with in association with Barrett's mucosa in the esophagus section of this text. Most of the remaining adenocarcinomas affecting the stomach occur in the distal organ (antrum and pylorus) and the most important etiology/risk factor seems to be infection with *Helicobacter pylori*, although smoking, certain dietary intake (smoked and salt-preserved foods), and bile reflux have also been implicated. Traditionally, gastric adenocarcinoma has been divided by the Laurén classification into "intestinal type" (*ie*, cancers that make tubules and/or papillary structures) and "diffuse type" (composed of dyscohesive cells that may have a signet-ring appearance). Using this scheme, a small number of cases have overlap between the patterns, precluding definitive classification. The World Health Organization (WHO) has recognized five major types of carcinoma (tubular, papillary, mucinous, "poorly cohesive," and mixed) and there are several other variants that do not fit into either of these classification schemes and which are really rare. Grossly, gastric cancers may appear polypoid, fungating, ulcerating, or infiltrative. Classically, the diffuse type spreads throughout the gastric wall, causing diffuse desmoplasia and giving the stomach a semi-rigid "linitis plastica" (or "leather bottle") character. This chapter will basically follow the Laurén classification, with an emphasis on biopsy diagnosis and an occasional nod to some of the rare variants.

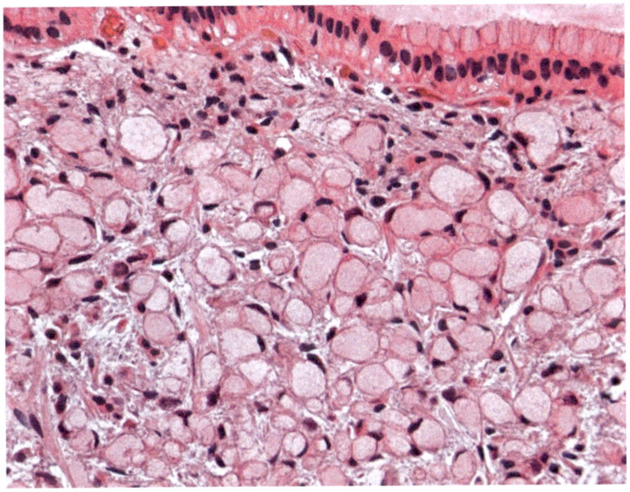

Fig. 25.1 The diffuse type of gastric adenocarcinoma is characterized by the infiltration of the lamina propria (and, often, the gastric wall) by dyscohesive cells with eccentric nuclei and abundant cytoplasm. Often, they will contain a discrete mucin vacuole that pushes the nucleus to the edge of the cell, imparting a so-called "signet-ring cell (SRC)" appearance

S.R. Owens, H.D. Appelman, *Atlas of Esophagus and Stomach Pathology*, Atlas of Anatomic Pathology, DOI 10.1007/978-1-4614-8084-6_25,

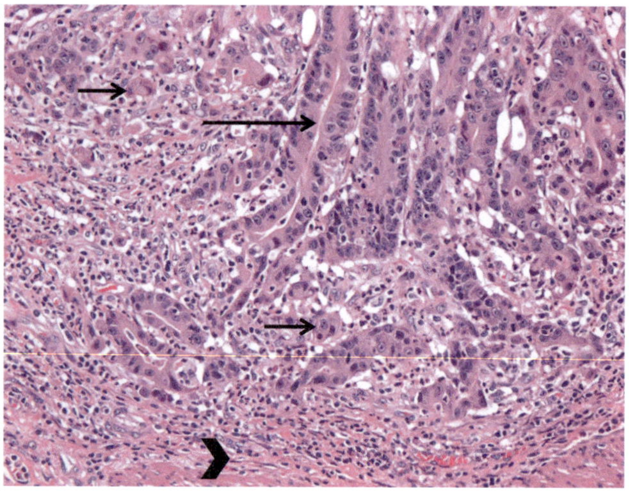

Fig. 25.2 In contrast, the intestinal type of gastric adenocarcinoma makes tubular or papillary structures. One of the risks of longstanding *H. pylori* infection is atrophic gastritis with intestinal metaplasia, which can precede intestinal type carcinoma. So-called "incomplete" intestinal metaplasia (that with a mixture of gastric- and intestinal-type mucin profiles) has been found in some studies to be particularly associated with cancer risk. In this case of superficially invasive cancer, which was restricted to the gastric mucosa, the muscularis mucosae can be seen at the bottom of the field (*arrowhead*). There are several recognizable tubular structures (*long arrow*), but in other areas, individual cells and small clusters infiltrate the lamina propria (*short arrows*). This so-called "early gastric cancer," limited by definition to the mucosa and submucosa (*ie*, pT1 in the TNM staging scheme), has been very well studied in the Japanese literature, because it is found in that country by endoscopic screening programs

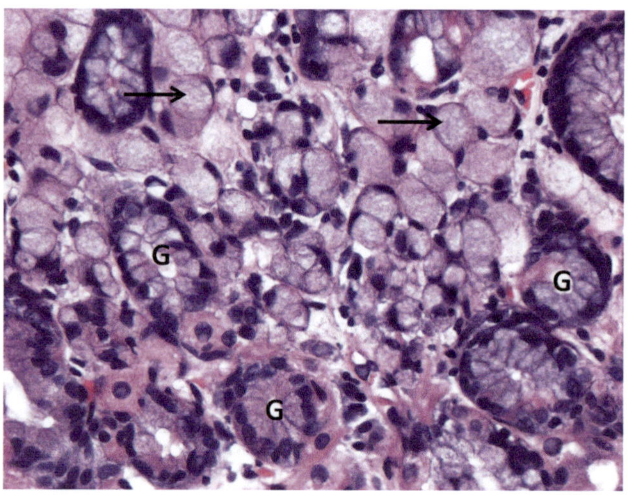

Fig. 25.4 At high magnification, this diffuse gastric adenocarcinoma is composed of SRC with a globoid vacuole of amphophilic or slightly basophilic mucin (*arrows*). These malignant cells insinuate between the normal gastric glands (*G*)

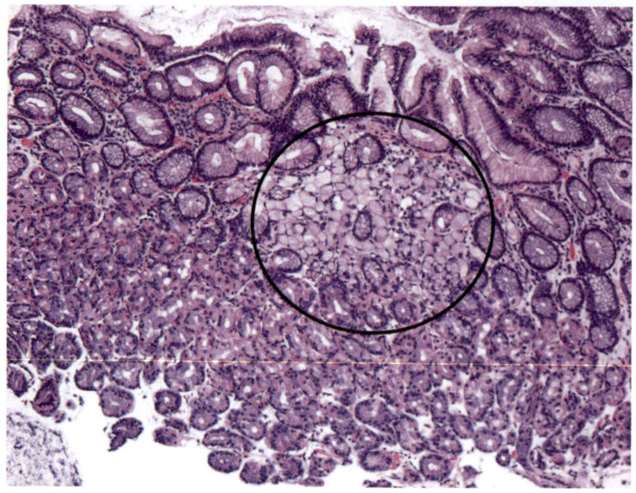

Fig. 25.3 This gastric biopsy contains a microscopic focus of SRC (diffuse) carcinoma involving only the mucosa (*inside circle*). While this focus creates a distinct collection of cells that stand out from the normal mucosa, this type of carcinoma can be very subtle and difficult to recognize when the cells infiltrate individually between the normal mucosal structures

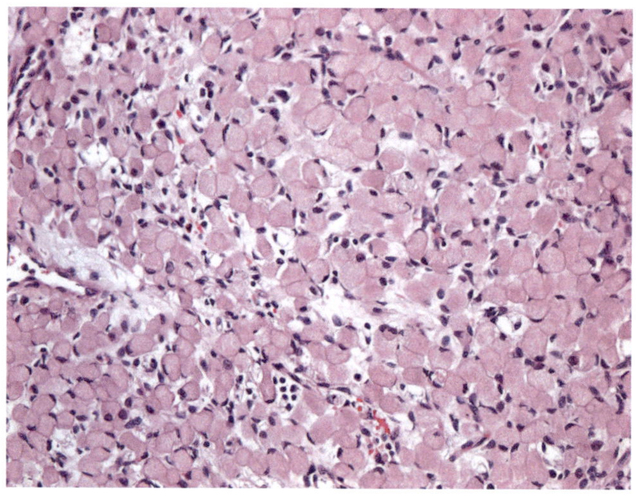

Fig. 25.5 This diffuse gastric adenocarcinoma has sheets of SRC with more eosinophilic cytoplasm. No normal mucosal structures are visible. In some cases of diffuse gastric carcinoma, the individual SRC will float in pools of mucin

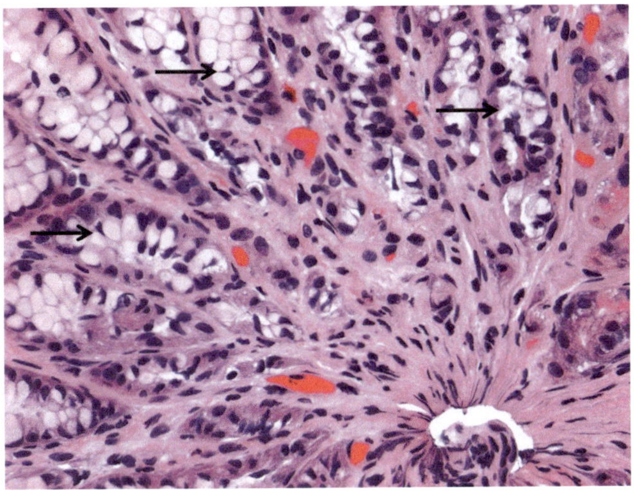

Fig. 25.6 Some patients inherit an autosomal dominant cancer susceptibility syndrome termed "hereditary diffuse gastric cancer," resulting from a germline mutation in the E-cadherin (*CDH1*) gene. This leads to an increased risk of diffuse gastric cancer and lobular breast carcinoma and these patients can develop multifocal SRC carcinomas in their gastric mucosa. A preinvasive lesion is called "signet-ring cell carcinoma in situ" and is characterized by a disorganized, "depolarized" appearance to the mucin cells in the gastric pits (*arrows*). These are, essentially, malignant SRC that still reside within the basement membrane. Unfortunately, this appearance can be mimicked by other nonneoplastic processes such as early degeneration of the epithelium when it is marginally preserved. True carcinoma in situ, however, is characterized by a decreased or absent expression of E-cadherin by immunohistochemistry, analogous to that found in lobular breast carcinoma

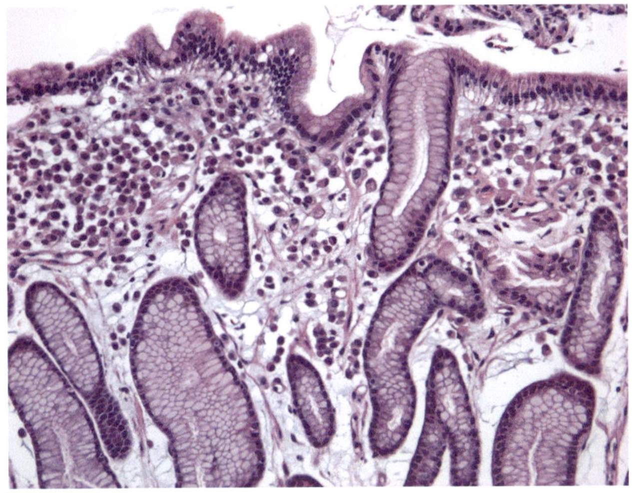

Fig. 25.7 In this case of diffuse gastric carcinoma, the cells that fill the lamina propria have a less conspicuous signet-ring appearance and instead mimic plasma cells or histiocytes. A cytokeratin immunohistochemical stain can help to confirm their epithelial nature. Compare the normal gastric pit cells here to those in the previous figure

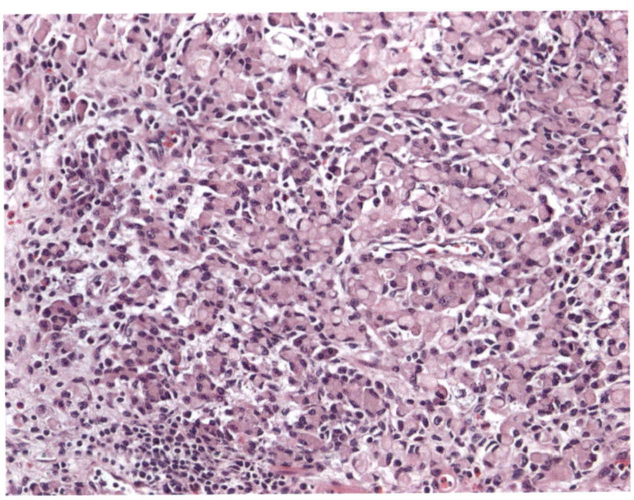

Fig. 25.8 Here, the SRC collect in clusters and cord-like structures. In our experience, this pattern can mimic the normal gastric gland structure of the mucosa at low magnification, yet another potential pitfall in the diagnosis of diffuse gastric adenocarcinoma

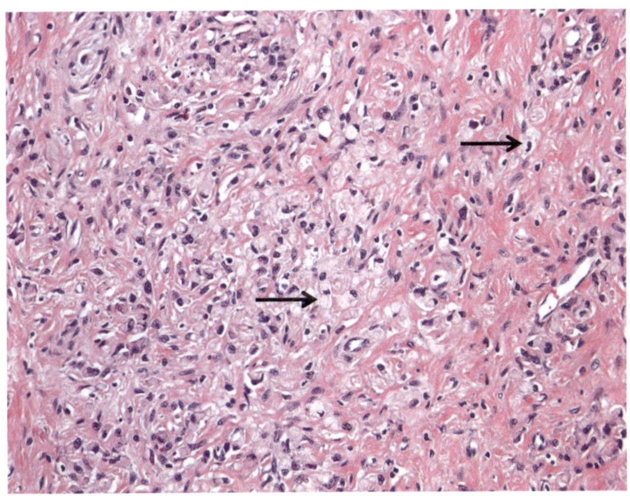

Fig. 25.9 Here, a diffuse gastric adenocarcinoma infiltrates the submucosa and leads to a dense desmoplastic stromal response. The carcinoma cells (*arrows*) have a foamy appearance and many are surrounded by eosinophilic collagen bundles. This type of stromal reaction throughout the gastric wall in a widely infiltrating diffuse cancer leads to the "linitis plastica" phenotype when it involves most or all of the stomach

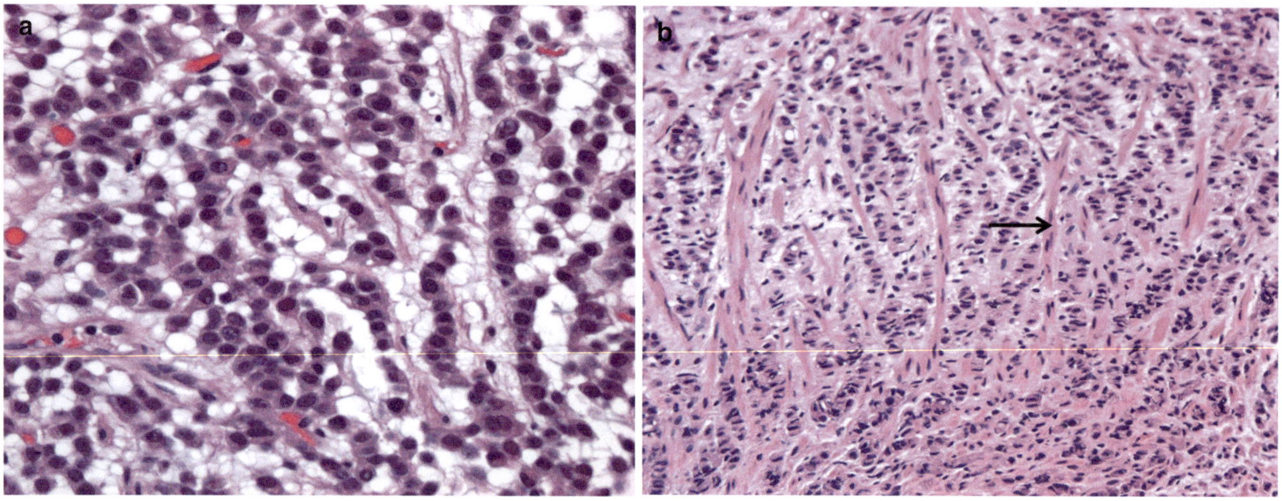

Fig. 25.10 This diffuse gastric adenocarcinoma consists of undifferentiated carcinoma cells that infiltrate the mucosa (**a**) and fibers of the muscularis mucosae (**b** *arrow*) in single-file cords reminiscent of lobular breast carcinoma. Indeed, the stomach is a favorite site of involvement by truly metastatic lobular carcinoma (Chap. 29), and care should be taken not to overlook the possibility of a primary breast tumor

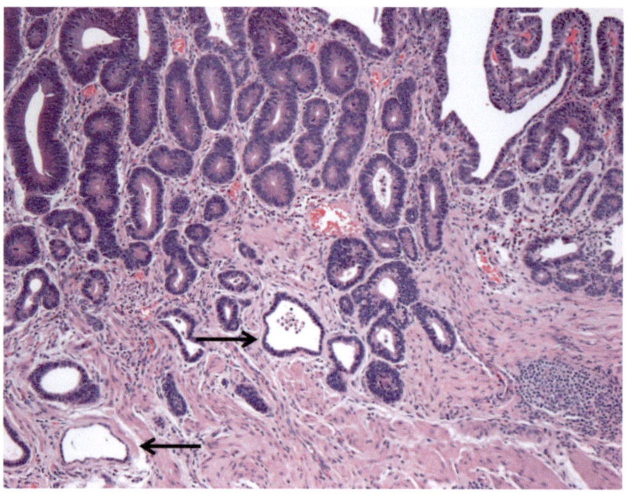

Fig. 25.11 Intestinal-type gastric adenocarcinoma is composed of tubular structures. In this case, a superficially invasive adenocarcinoma (*arrows*) arises at the base of a patch of intestinal-type dysplasia which, in turn, arose in the setting of intestinal metaplasia. The carcinoma is infiltrating fibers of the muscularis mucosae at the bottom of the field

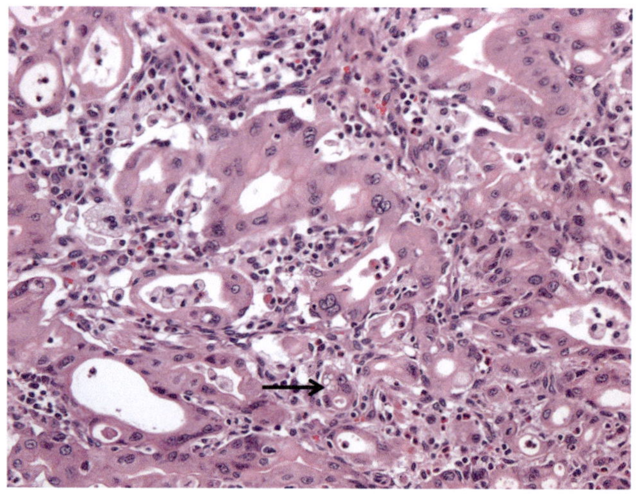

Fig. 25.12 This gastric adenocarcinoma is composed of irregular, poorly formed, and interconnecting tubular structures lined by pleomorphic cells with abundant eosinophilic cytoplasm. Small collections of cells bud from the larger tubules and infiltrate the lamina propria (*arrow*)

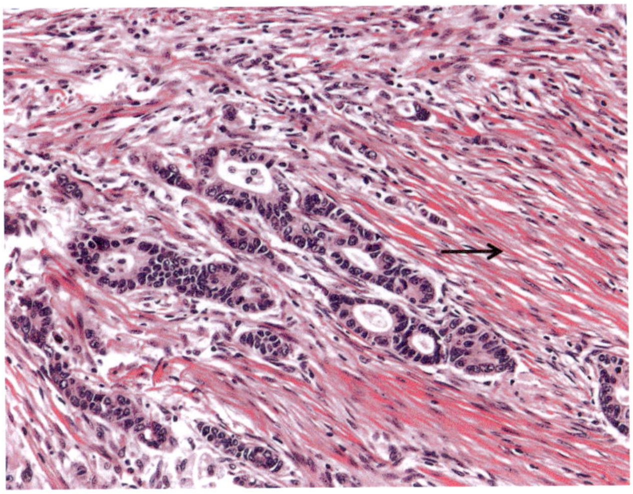

Fig. 25.13 Infiltrating intestinal type gastric cancers also elicit a desmoplastic stromal response, although they are not typically associated with the linitis plastica phenotype as they are more localized. Here, the neoplastic tubules infiltrate fibers of the muscularis propria (*arrow*)

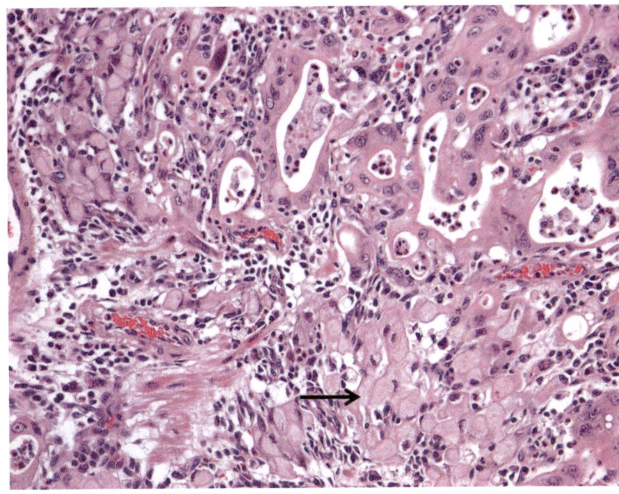

Fig. 25.14 This is an example of a "mixed type" gastric adenocarcinoma that contains a combination of malignant tubules and clusters of SRC (*arrow*), defying the Laurén classification. This particular tumor also has a rather prominent lymphoid infiltrate surrounding the malignant cells. One unusual variant of gastric carcinoma has a very striking lymphoid stroma in which it can be difficult to recognize the epithelial cells, imparting an appearance of so-called "medullary" carcinoma. Such "lymphoepithelioma-like" carcinomas are frequently associated with Epstein–Barr virus (EBV) infection

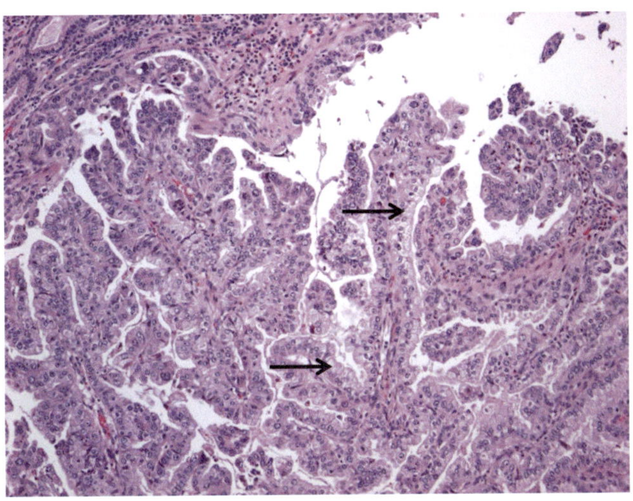

Fig. 25.15 This well-differentiated gastric carcinoma has a papillary appearance, with structures lined by malignant cells with abundant foveolar-type apical mucin (*arrows*). Included in intestinal type carcinoma in the Laurén classification, it rates its own category according to the WHO

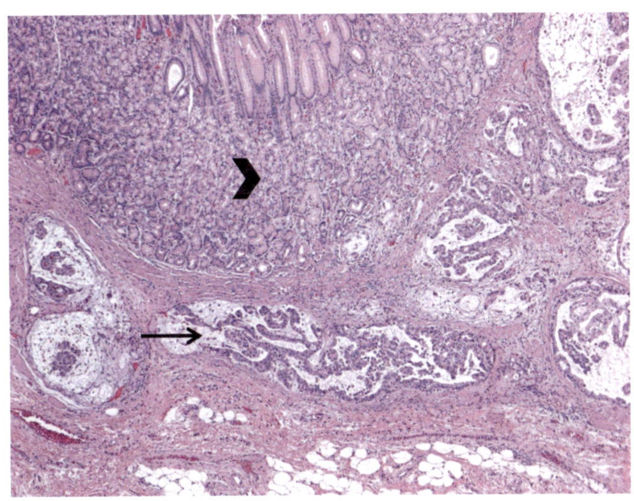

Fig. 25.16 This invasive papillary type gastric cancer contains large collections of carcinoma cells floating in pools of mucin (*arrow*). The cells are arranged in papillary structures and infiltrate beneath the overlying mucosa (*arrowhead*)

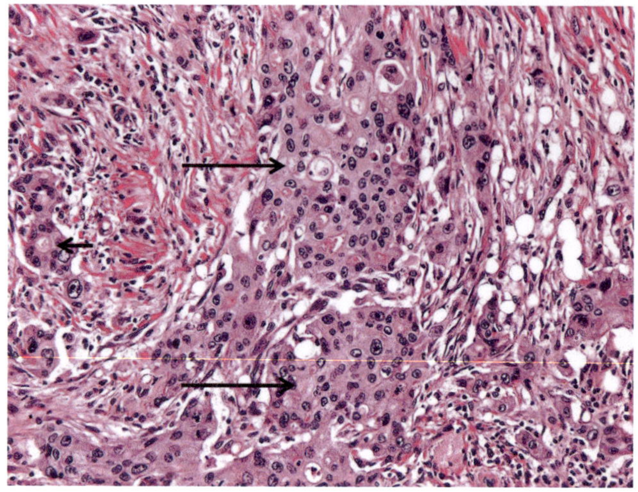

Fig. 25.17 This poorly differentiated adenocarcinoma has a few recognizable tubules (*short arrow*) but also contains sheets of polygonal carcinoma cells with abundant eosinophilic or occasionally cleared cytoplasm (*long arrow*). These cells are reminiscent of hepatocellular carcinoma cells, and another rare variant of gastric carcinoma is the so-called "hepatoid" type. Tumors with this pattern can express α-fetoprotein and even make bile

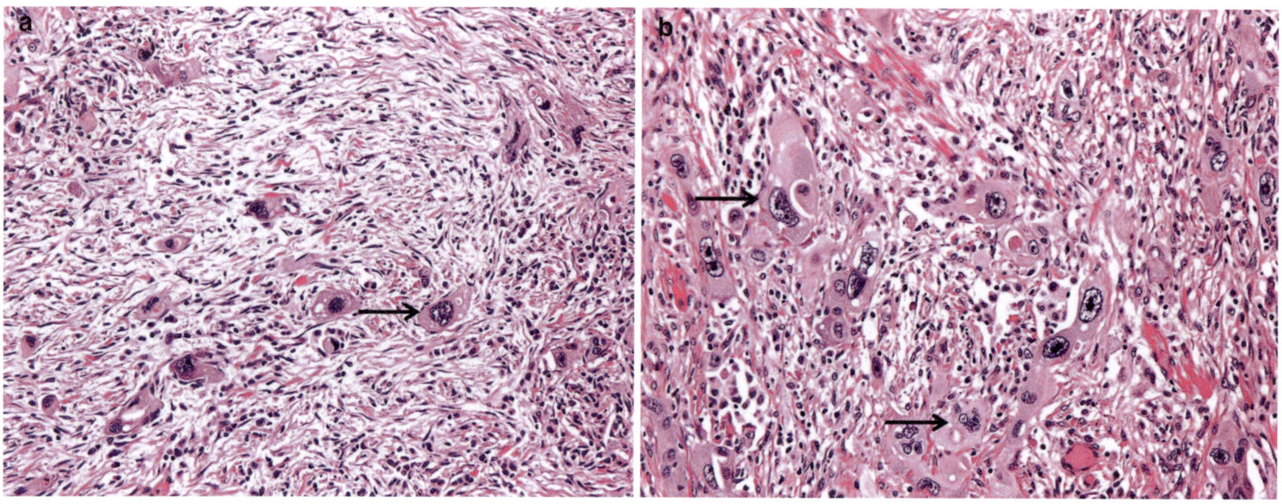

Fig. 25.18 (**a**) This tumor consists of individually infiltrating anaplastic cells (*arrow*) surrounded by an abundant desmoplastic stroma. (**b**) In a few places the cells have a fused or syncytial appearance (*arrows*). Another rare gastric carcinoma variant is gastric choriocarcinoma, in which cytotrophoblastic and syncytiotrophoblastic cells are admixed with traditional adenocarcinoma. β-HCG production can be demonstrated in this variant by immunohistochemistry

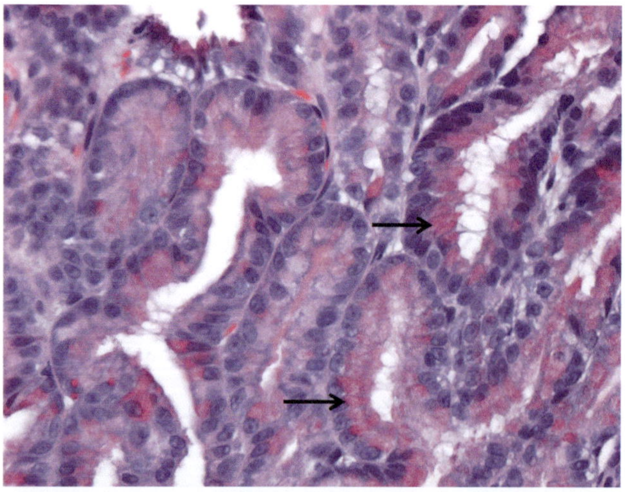

Fig. 25.19 Some gastric cancers have a parietal cell phenotype or differentiation, at least in areas. This is characterized by the production of abundant eosinophilic granules (*arrows*)

26 Carcinoid Tumor of the Stomach

Gastric carcinoid tumors (in fact, carcinoid tumors of the gastrointestinal [GI] tract in general) have undergone a dizzying array of name changes over the years, reflecting their ability to behave aggressively while appearing rather banal. Thus, a tumor with bland morphology can invade vascular structures and metastasize to lymph nodes or liver. While generally categorized as "neuroendocrine" tumors (NET), they have been classified by some observers as "well-differentiated neuroendocrine tumors," "well-differentiated neuroendocrine carcinomas," and so on. Bona fide small-cell carcinomas and large-cell neuroendocrine carcinomas can occur in the stomach, but they are rare. Thus, we will concentrate on the most frequently encountered entities here, which—even after all of the arguing about nomenclature—are still commonly called gastric "carcinoids." Most such tumors in the stomach consist of enterochromaffin-like (ECL) cells that have been induced to undergo hyperplasia/proliferation by a hypergastrinemic state. To sort out the variety of situations in which these tumors occur, they have been categorized into several types. "Type 1" tumors arise in the setting of ECL cell hyperplasia brought on by autoimmune atrophic gastritis (AAG; see Chap. 20) and account for the vast majority of gastric carcinoids. "Type 2" tumors arise in the setting of Zollinger-Ellison syndrome (ZES; also in Chap. 20), and usually occur when this condition is associated with multiple endocrine neoplasia type 1 (MEN-1). "Type 3" ("sporadic") gastric carcinoids are thought to arise from true enterochromaffin cells (ECC) and are often larger and more aggressive than the ECL cell-derived tumors. Finally, some patients with defective parietal cell acid-secreting machinery unrelated to AAG or ZES have hypergastrinemia and can develop ECL cell-derived carcinoid tumors designated "Type 4." Types 1, 2, and 4 (the ECL cell tumors) arise in the gastric body/fundus, whereas type 3 tumors can arise anywhere in the stomach. The ECL cell-derived tumors also have a good prognosis, compared to type 3 tumors.

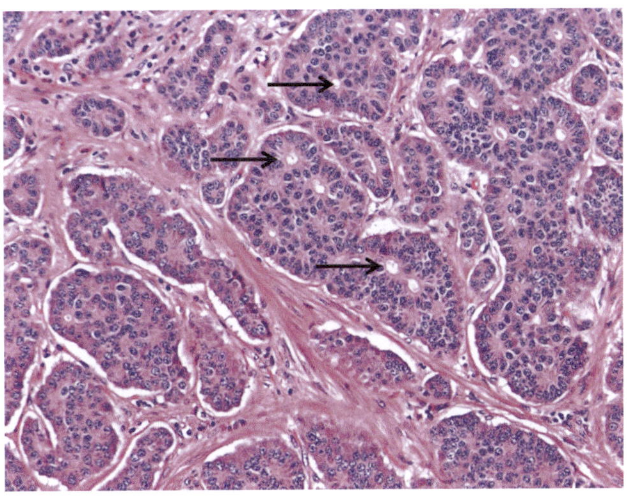

Fig. 26.1 Carcinoid tumors in the stomach are basically identical to those elsewhere. That is, they consist of nests and cords of cells with finely stippled chromatin that may occasionally form tubules (*arrows*)

S.R. Owens, H.D. Appelman, *Atlas of Esophagus and Stomach Pathology*, Atlas of Anatomic Pathology,
DOI 10.1007/978-1-4614-8084-6_26,

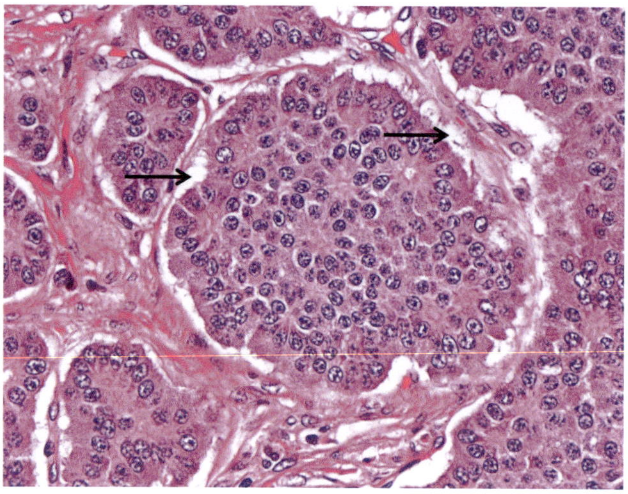

Fig. 26.2 At high magnification, the characteristic neuroendocrine "salt-and-pepper" nuclear chromatin is visible in this nest of cells from a carcinoid tumor. Commonly, there is retraction artifact (*arrows*) around the nests of tumor cells that may mimic angiolymphatic invasion. In most carcinoids, mitotic activity is sparse. Sporadic carcinoids are now graded based on mitotic activity and/or proliferation index as determined by Ki-67 immunohistochemistry. In this scheme, grade 1 tumors have fewer than two mitotic figures/10 high-power fields (HPF) or less than 2 % Ki-67 index, grade 2 tumors have 2–20 mitotic figures/10 HPF or 3–20 % Ki-67 index, and grade 3 tumors more than 20 mitotic figures/10 HPF or more than 20 % Ki-67 index. In the stomach, this grading system applies only to sporadic (type 3) tumors

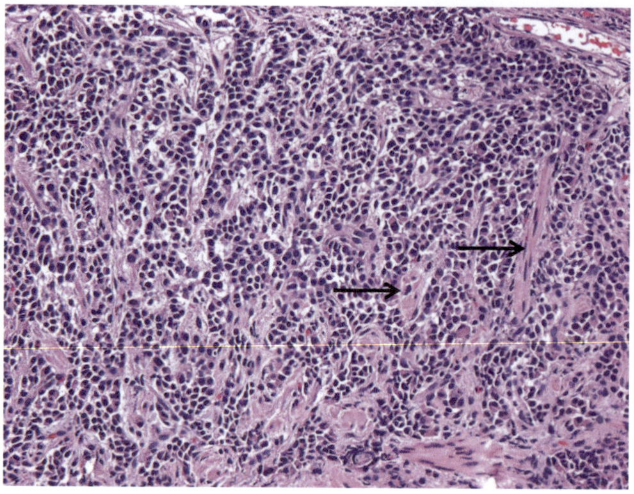

Fig. 26.3 This gastric carcinoid that arose in the setting of AAG has a ribbon-like arrangement of cells that infiltrate fibers of the muscularis mucosae (*arrows*). The cells are monotonous and relatively uniform

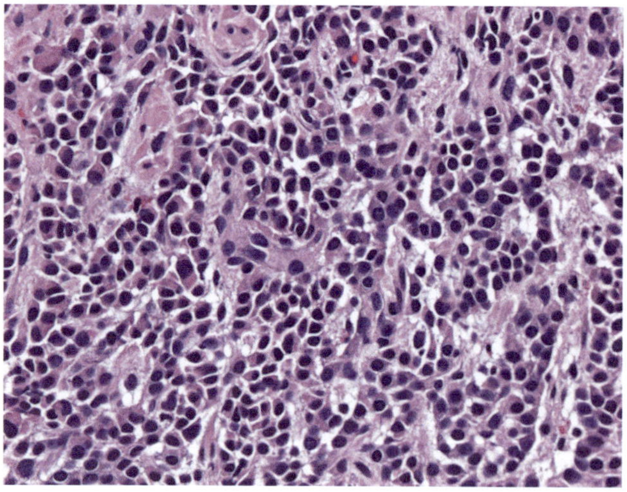

Fig. 26.4 At high magnification, the finely stippled chromatin is visible. Strictly, ECL cell proliferations are divided into three classes: *hyperplasia* (linear or nodular collections of ECL cells that form "chains" along gastric glands or nodules measuring <150 μm); *dysplasia* (nodules 150–500 μm, fused nodules, or proliferations filling the lamina propria); and *microcarcinoid tumors* (nodules >500 μm). In practice, however, we do not take such measurements. Usually, we either see biopsies of the background AAG with ECL cell hyperplasia, or true carcinoid tumors that appear as nodules endoscopically, prompting their sampling

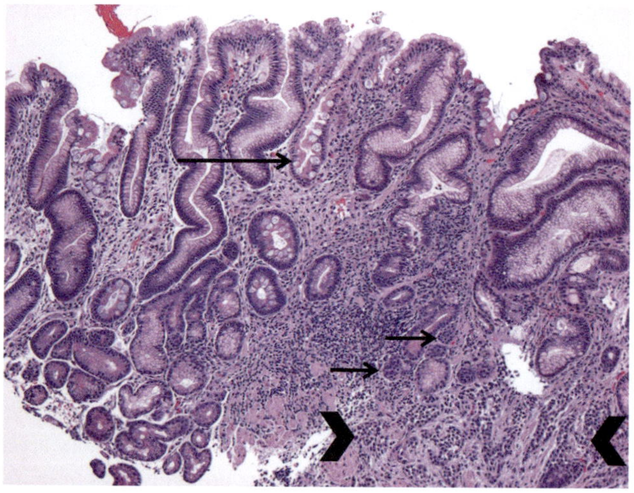

Fig. 26.5 As noted above, the large majority of gastric carcinoid tumors arise in the setting of autoimmune gastritis. At low magnification, this case of AAG contains intestinal metaplasia (*long arrow*), nodules of hyperplastic ECL cells (*short arrows*), and the edge of an infiltrating carcinoid tumor (*arrowheads*). This biopsy is from the gastric body, but there are no longer any intact oxyntic glands. Tumors arising the setting of ZES have a background of elongated and hypertrophic oxyntic glands (see Chap. 20)

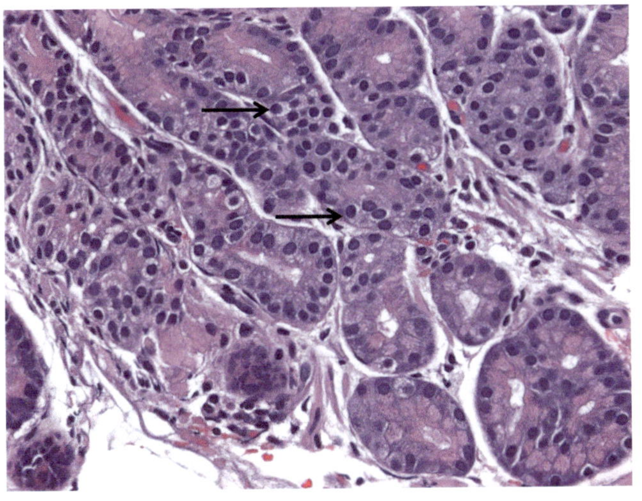

Fig. 26.6 This case of AAG has chains and clusters of hyperplastic ECL cells (*arrows*). When they do not make nodules, these cells can be difficult to appreciate on H&E-stained sections

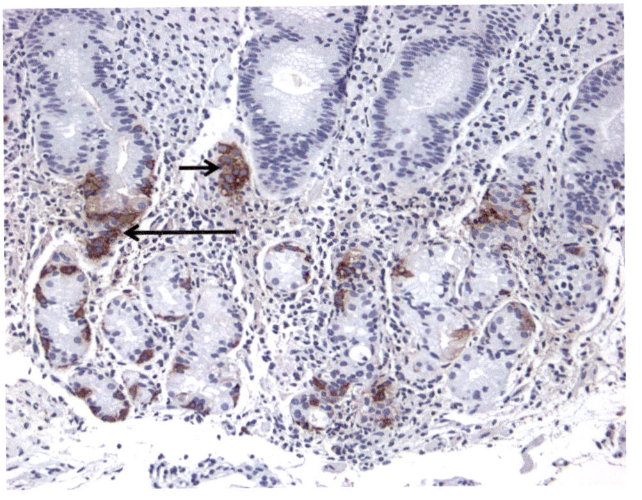

Fig. 26.7 Using immunohistochemistry for a neuroendocrine marker such as chromogranin, the chains (*long arrow*) and nodules (*short arrow*) of ECL cells are easily visible

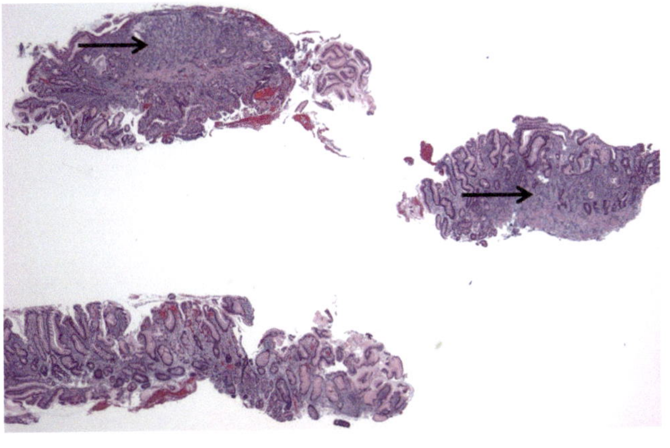

Fig. 26.8 This is a typical low-magnification view of a set of biopsies from a patient with AAG who was found to have two mucosal nodules on endoscopic examination. The piece at the bottom has mucosal atrophy and chronic inflammation reflecting the background atrophic gastritis, while the two other pieces contain nodular proliferations of ECL cells (*ie*, microcarcinoid tumors; *arrows*)

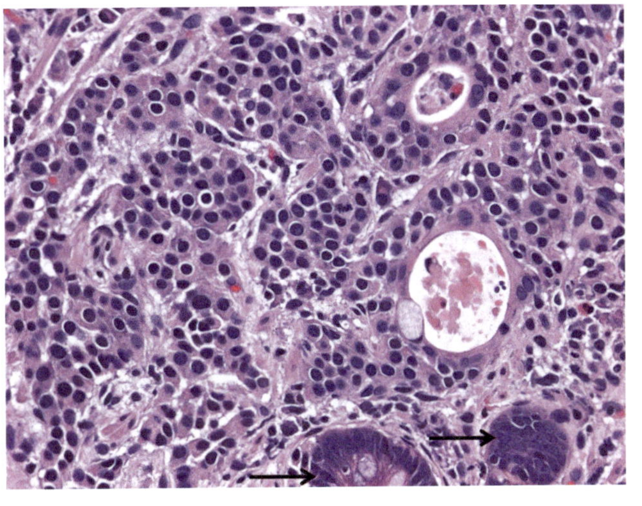

Fig. 26.9 At high magnification, one of the tumors from this patient is composed predominantly of small nests and anastomosing cords of monotonous cells. Occasionally, there are some tubular structures, which may be part of the tumor itself, of residual glandular structures being overgrown by the hyperplastic ECL cells. At the bottom (*arrow*), there are some tubules that are part of the background intestinal metaplasia

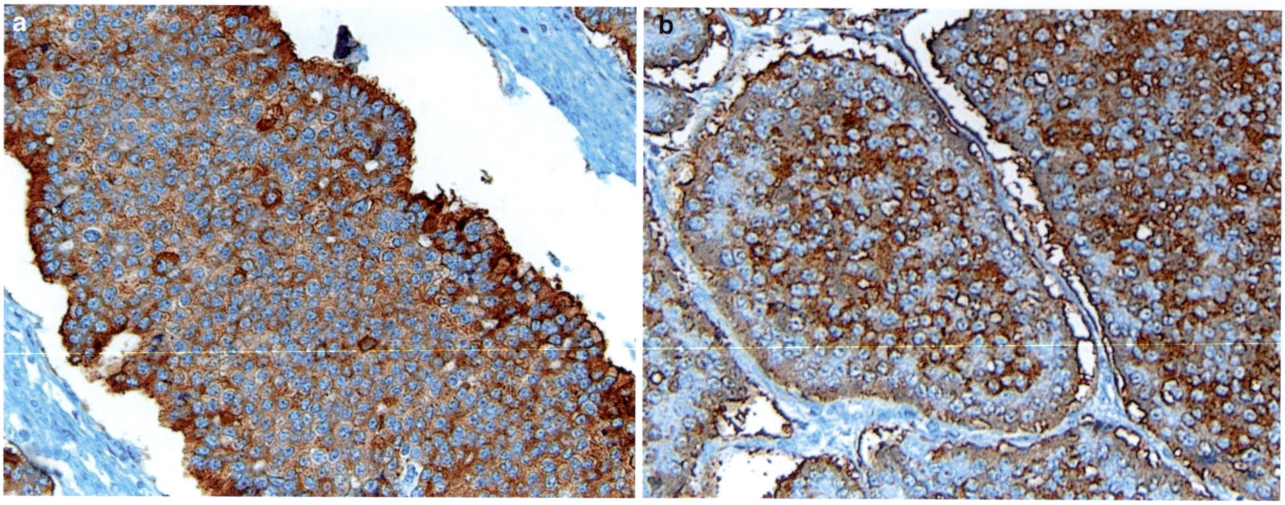

Fig. 26.10 Immunohistochemistry for synaptophysin (**a**) and/or chromogranin (**b**) is helpful in highlighting the neuroendocrine nature of gastric carcinoid tumors, regardless of their subtype

27 Mesenchymal Neoplasms

Mesenchymal or stromal tumors are not very common in the stomach, in comparison to other conditions discussed in this text. Because most are centered in the wall of the stomach, they are uncommonly encountered in endoscopically obtained gastric biopsies. Nonetheless, we occasionally see the superficial aspects of these tumors in biopsy specimens, and we can also encounter certain tell-tale signs in biopsies that suggest the presence of a mesenchymal tumor in the deeper gastric wall. Several different mesenchymal tumors can affect the stomach, but only the most frequently encountered of these uncommon lesions are discussed here. All can be treated by excision/resection.

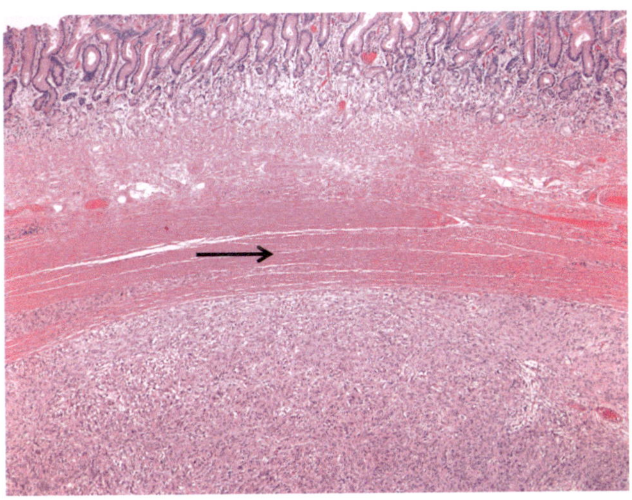

Fig. 27.1 Of the mesenchymal tumors affecting the stomach, the most common is the "gastrointestinal stromal tumor" (commonly referred to throughout the gastrointestinal tract as *GIST*). The stomach is the most common site for GISTs to occur. As in this case, most such tumors are centered in the muscularis propria, and so are not usually sampled in mucosal biopsies. Some expand into the submucosa or mucosa, however, so they may be encountered occasionally. In this low-magnification photomicrograph, a nodular proliferation of spindle cells is seen at the bottom of the field, with overlying fibers of the muscularis propria (*arrow*) and the gastric mucosa at the top of the field

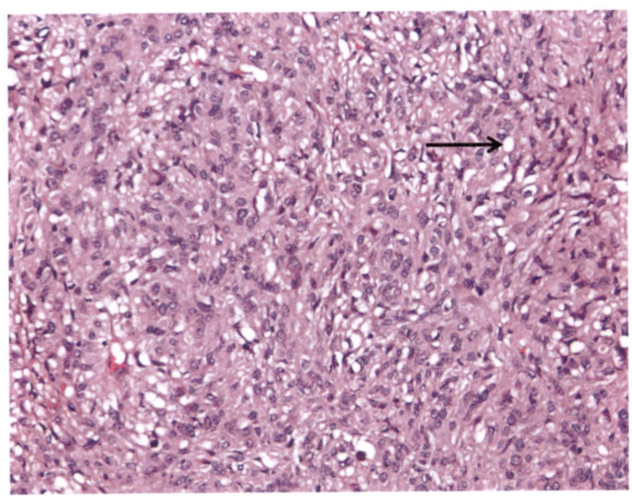

Fig. 27.2 At higher magnification, the composition of this GIST by predominantly spindled cells is apparent. In most tumors, the population is rather monotonous and bland appearing. The "empty" spaces (*arrow*) are cytoplasmic (often perinuclear) vacuoles, a common feature of GISTs. These tumors usually occur in middle-aged or older adults and are most often sporadic. The majority are the result of mutations in the *KIT* gene, which encodes a receptor tyrosine kinase. Non-sporadic tumors may be seen in families harboring a germline *KIT* mutation. Also, patients with type 1 neurofibromatosis (NF1) can develop GISTs, although most commonly in the small intestine

S.R. Owens, H.D. Appelman, *Atlas of Esophagus and Stomach Pathology*, Atlas of Anatomic Pathology,
DOI 10.1007/978-1-4614-8084-6_27, © Springer Science+Business Media New York 2014

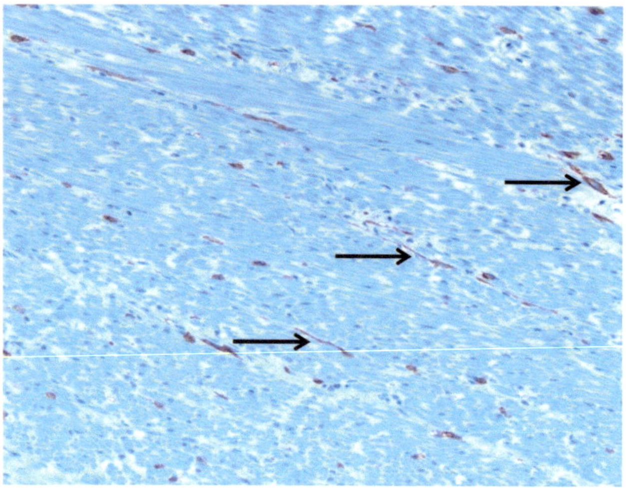

Fig. 27.3 The putative cell of origin for GIST is the interstitial cell of Cajal, a normal cell type that serves as an intermediary between the autonomic nervous system and the gastrointestinal musculature. In this c-kit immunohistochemical stain, the Cajal cells appear as elongated spindle cells (*arrows*). The smaller, ovoid cells expressing c-kit are individually scattered mast cells

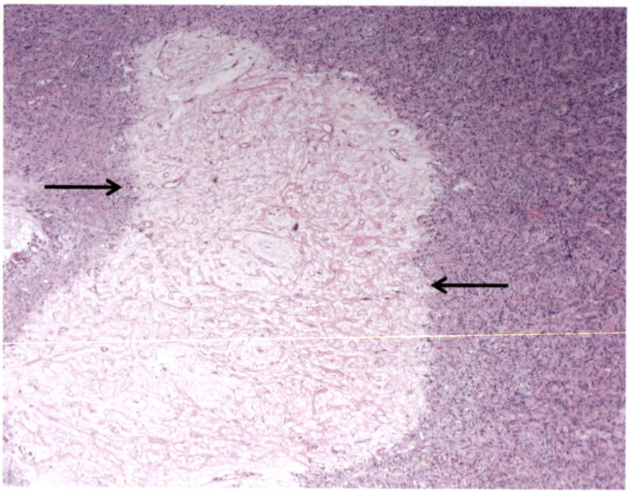

Fig. 27.4 In this GIST, there is an area of hyaline-type degeneration (*arrows*). This appearance is not uncommon and may progress to an empty, cystic appearance. Also common are hypocellular areas with a myxoid or "chondroid" appearance. True coagulative tumor necrosis is uncommon, and portends more aggressive behavior (*see below*)

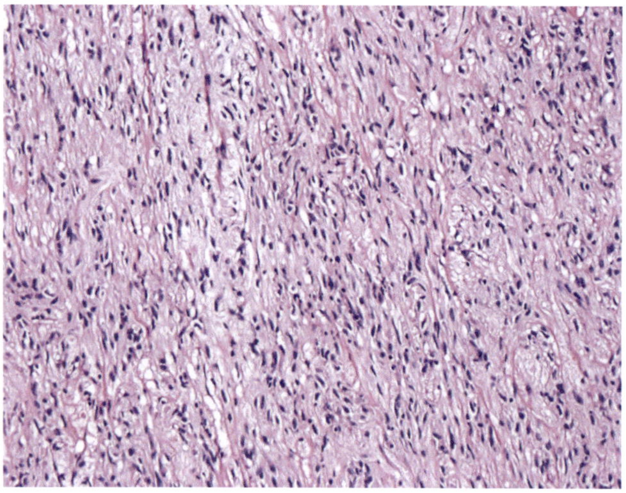

Fig. 27.5 This gastric stromal tumor has a similar appearance to the tumor above, but was associated with a different type of genetic mutation, this time in the *PDGFRA* gene. A minority of GISTs harbors this type of mutation, and a very small number are *KIT* and *PDGFRA* wild-type. Examples with *PDGFRA* mutations may have epithelioid cell morphology. Another potential abnormality in these tumors is a mutation in one of the succinate dehydrogenase (*SDH*) genes or a deficiency in the SDHB subunit. Tumors with these abnormalities have an epithelioid morphology and are associated with the Carney triad (SDHB-deficient; includes epithelioid GIST, pulmonary chondroma and extra-adrenal paraganglioma) or the Carney-Stratakis syndrome (*SDH* mutated, includes familial epithelioid GIST and paragangliomas)

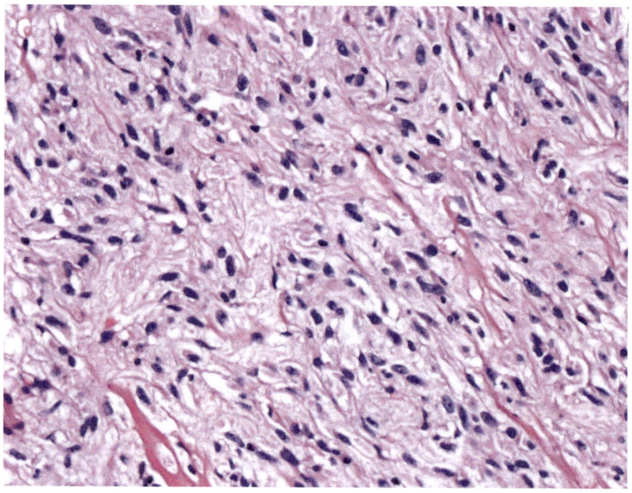

Fig. 27.6 At this high magnification, the cytoplasmic vacuoles in this GIST are easily seen. Note the uniformity of the cells and their overall tendency to stand apart from each other, imparting an impression of relatively sparse cellularity. These features are typical of tumors with a favorable clinical prognosis

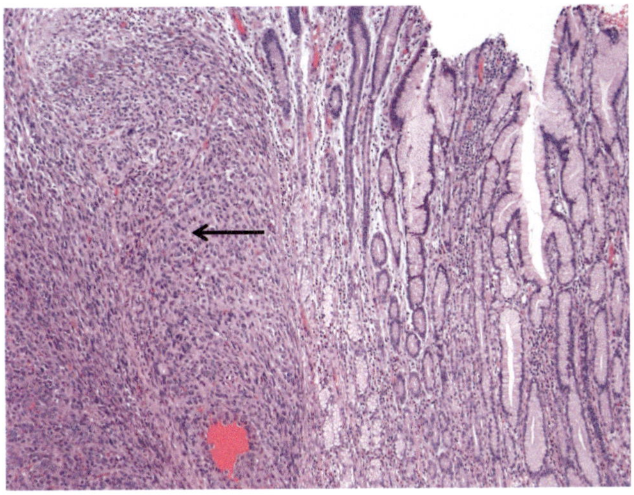

Fig. 27.7 In contrast to the previous examples, this gastric stromal tumor (*arrow*) is much more cellular. In addition, it invades the overlying mucosa, and causes an ulcer. Both aggressive and indolent GISTs can lead to mucosal ulcers. Aggressive examples can truly invade the mucosa (an unfavorable prognostic feature), whereas those with a favorable prognosis may expand and cause a mechanical ulcer as they compress the overlying mucosa. Because of this, overt or occult GI blood loss is a frequent presenting feature of these tumors. Invasion and/or ulceration of the mucosa can result in this normally mural tumor being sampled by an endoscopic biopsy

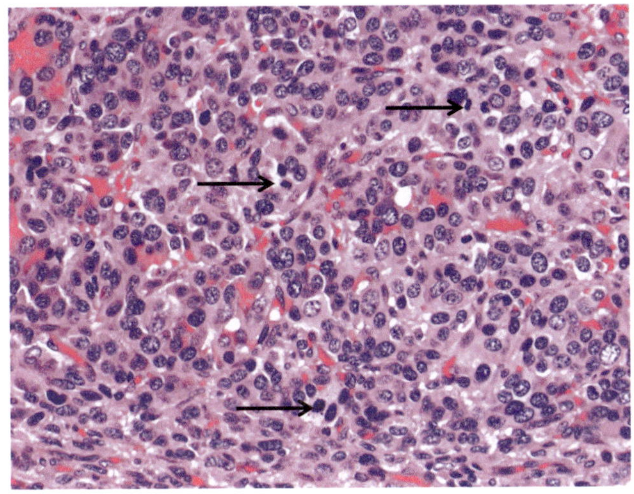

Fig. 27.8 The cells in this gastric GIST are epithelioid and densely packed together. Furthermore, the cells are pleomorphic and there are numerous mitotic figures (*arrows*) visible in this single field. All of these features portend an aggressive clinical behavior for this tumor. Most observers do not use a "benign vs. malignant" categorization for GISTs, but rather use a combination of site of origin, tumor size, and mitotic activity to generate a risk stratification for these tumors based on consensus criteria. Overall, gastric GISTs tend to have a better prognosis than those occurring in the small intestine

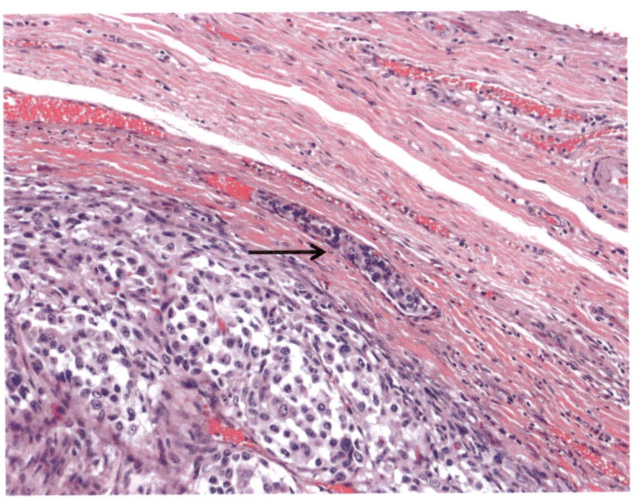

Fig. 27.9 In this field from the same tumor seen in Fig. 27.8, there is a clear focus of angiolymphatic invasion (*arrow*). This is unequivocal evidence of malignancy, and this particular tumor had already metastasized to the patient's liver

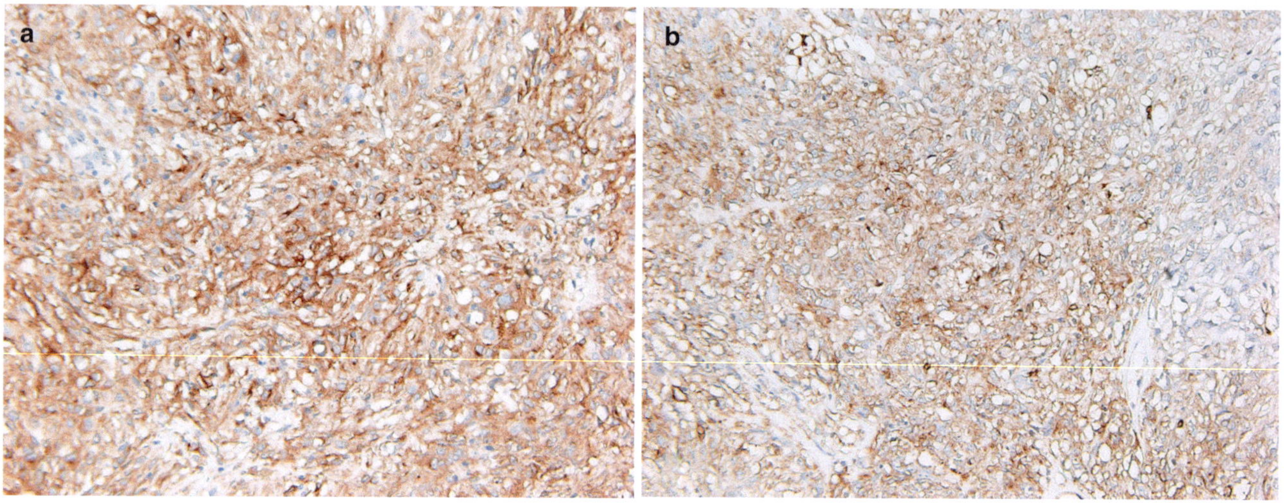

Fig. 27.10 Immunohistochemical stains are useful in the diagnosis of GIST. (**a**) Most examples are positive for c-kit, and even a small number of tumors with *PDGFRA* mutations express this marker. Care must be taken not to overinterpret staining of normal mast cells, which can be surprisingly abundant in other types of soft tissue tumors. The vast majority of GISTs (including most tumors with *PDGFRA* mutations) express another marker, DOG1 that will also highlight normal Cajal cells. (**b**) Around two-thirds of GISTs also express CD34

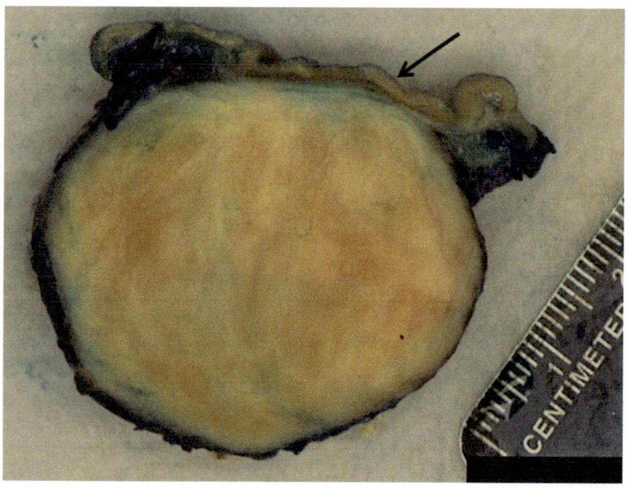

Fig. 27.11 Another mesenchymal tumor sometimes encountered in the stomach is a schwannoma. Like GISTs, schwannomas are usually based in the gastric wall (or sometimes the submucosa), but they can occasionally make an appearance in endoscopic biopsies when found on upper endoscopy. This example has a vaguely whorled, tan cut surface. The mucosa is draped over the top of the nodule (*arrow*)

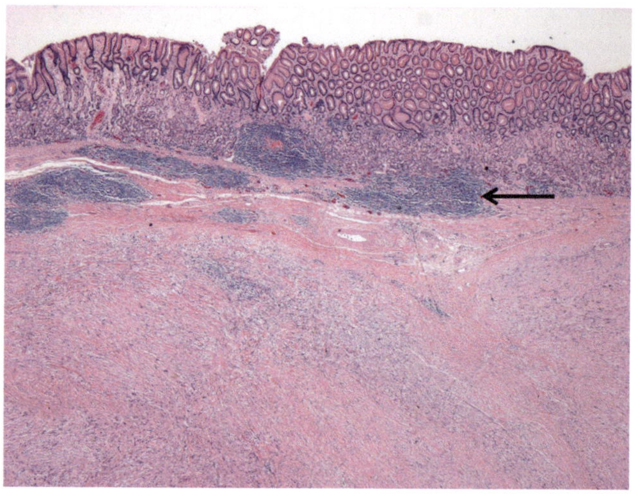

Fig. 27.12 One characteristic feature of schwannomas is their tendency to be surrounded by a "cuff" of lymphoid tissue (*arrow*). This can vary from relatively sparse to very dense, and may be more likely to appear in endoscopic biopsies than the cells of the schwannoma itself. We have seen occasional examples of gastric masses in which the lymphoid cuff surrounding a schwannoma was seen on biopsies, mistaken for a lymphoma, and extensively worked up with immunohistochemical stains before a rebiopsy finally revealed the underlying mesenchymal tumor

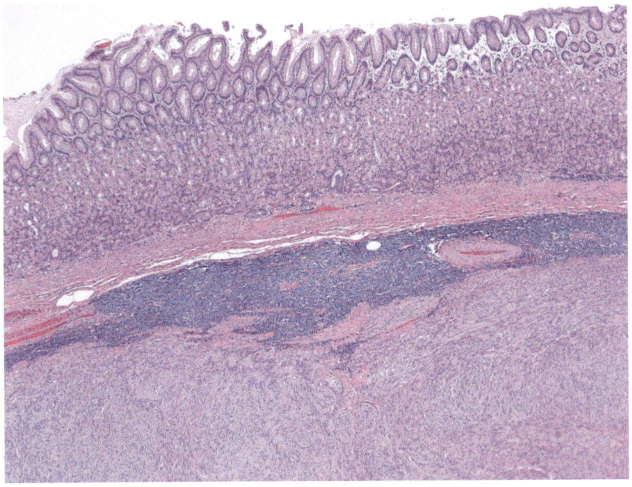

Fig. 27.13 Unfortunately, while characteristic and suggestive of an underlying schwannoma, the lymphoid cuff is not specific, as evidenced by this GIST with a similar-appearing ring of lymphoid tissue. This tumor was strongly positive for c-kit

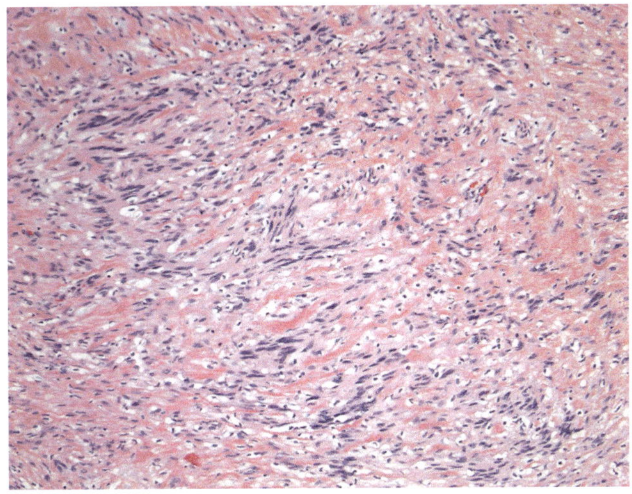

Fig. 27.14 At higher magnification, this gastric schwannoma has alternating areas of dense and sparse cellularity. Gastrointestinal schwannomas differ somewhat from their counterparts elsewhere in the soft tissue in that they lack abnormalities in the *NF2* gene (found in many conventional examples) and usually do not have the prominent, hyalinized blood vessels seen in other schwannomas

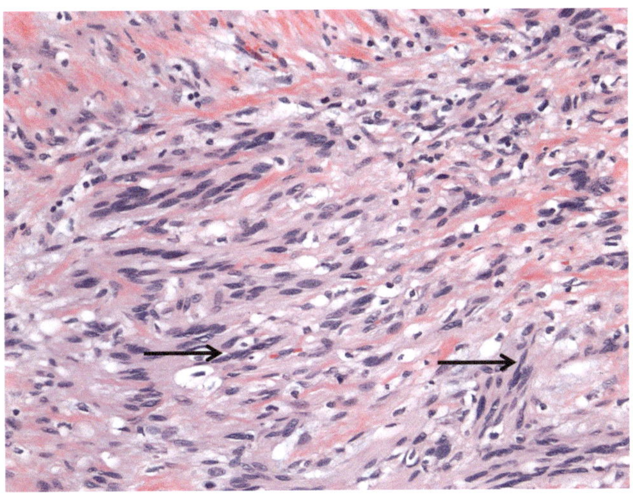

Fig. 27.15 At high magnification, the characteristic "wavy" Schwann cell nuclei (*arrows*) are apparent. A few dense, eosinophilic collagen bands are interspersed

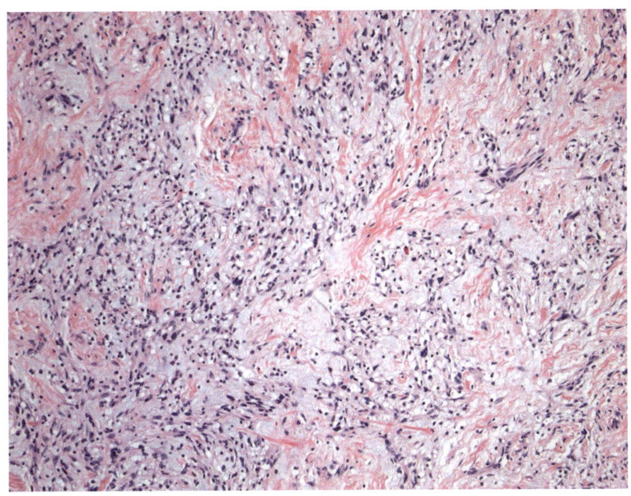

Fig. 27.16 Like schwannomas in other sites, gastric examples have more cellular ("Antoni A") and less cellular ("Antoni B") areas. Much of the right half of this photomicrograph has the hypocellular appearance. Degenerative atypia ("ancient change") is less common in gastric schwannomas than in conventional soft tissue tumors. Mitotic activity is rare

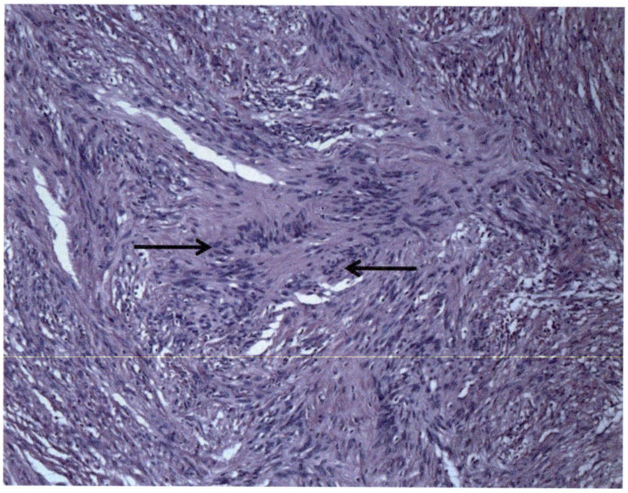

Fig. 27.17 This gastric schwannoma has classic areas of nuclear palisading with intervening fibrillar projections, producing Verocay-like bodies (*arrows*)

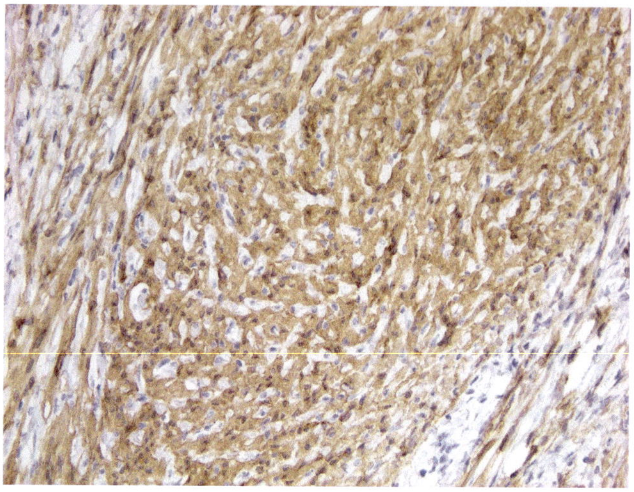

Fig. 27.18 Strong nuclear and cytoplasmic S100 staining characterizes gastric schwannomas. CD117 (c-kit) is negative

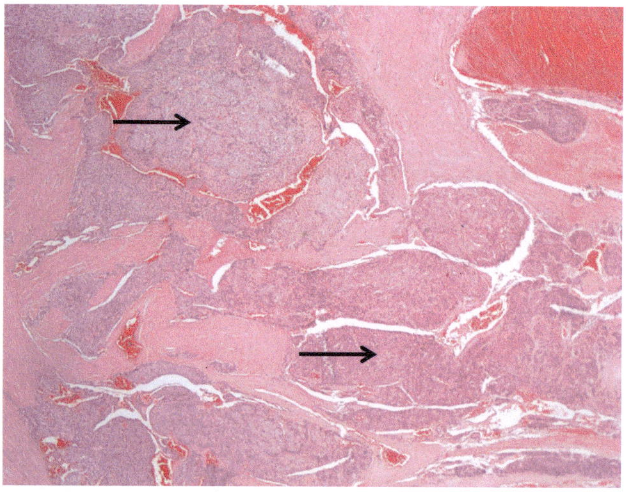

Fig. 27.19 While very rare overall, glomus tumors arising in the GI tract most frequently affect the stomach. Like the other tumors in this chapter, they can lead to upper gastrointestinal bleeding and may be superficially sampled in endoscopic biopsies. At low magnification, the lobulated architecture of this gastric glomus tumor is apparent. The nodules of tumor cells (*arrows*) are separated by eosinophilic bundles of collagen and/or fibers of the muscularis propria

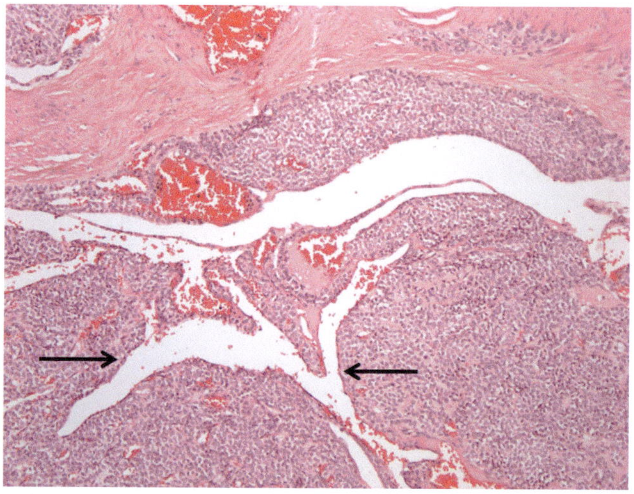

Fig. 27.20 The nodules of tumor cells in this glomus tumor are quite densely cellular, and are arranged around staghorn or "hemangiopericytoma-like" blood vessels (*arrows*). The tumor cell nodules tend to push or bulge into these vascular spaces

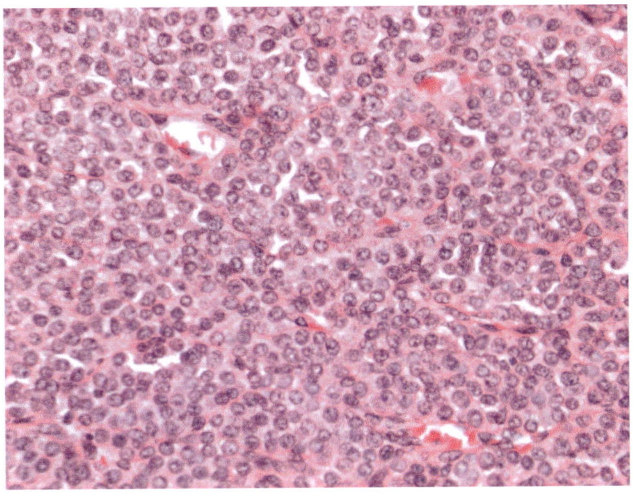

Fig. 27.21 At high magnification, the characteristic, round, monotonous tumor cells are visible. Their cytoplasm may be lightly eosinophilic or clear. Mitotic activity is rare. The tumor cells express smooth muscle actin, calponin, and laminin. They are negative for c-kit

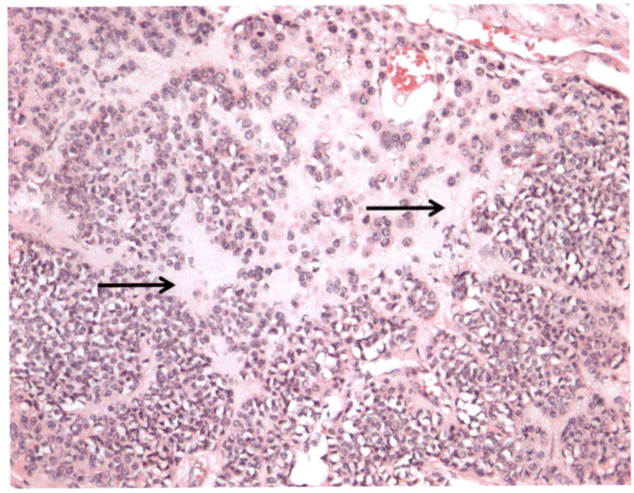

Fig. 27.22 This gastric glomus tumor has small nodules of tumor cells and some areas of hyaline change (*arrows*). The tumor cells are identical to those seen in Fig. 27.21. Areas of myxoid change are possible as well

28 Hematolymphoid Neoplasms

The gastrointestinal (GI) tract is the most common extranodal site of involvement by non-Hodgkin lymphomas, and these entities can be diagnostically challenging, in our experience. The most common of these is diffuse large B-cell lymphoma, but mucosa-associated lymphoid tissue (MALT) lymphoma is frequent in the stomach as well, and is associated with underlying *Helicobacter pylori* gastritis. Large cell lymphomas can mimic epithelial neoplasms, and the overlap between MALT lymphoma and *H. pylori* gastritis can cause diagnostic headaches. Because *H. pylori*-related MALT lymphomas can often be treated simply be eradication of the causative organism, it is important to recognize this entity and differentiate it from other lymphomas affecting the stomach.

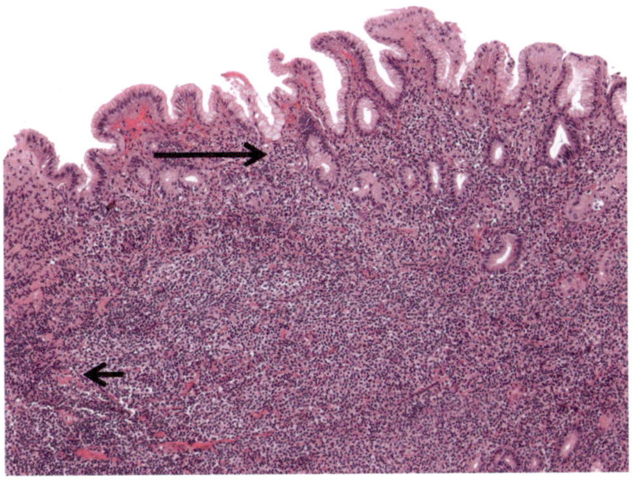

Fig. 28.1 MALT lymphoma (correctly classified as "extranodal marginal zone lymphoma of mucosa-associated lymphoid tissue") is a low-grade B-cell lymphoma, composed predominantly of small B lymphocytes, that is usually associated with underlying *H. pylori* gastritis when it occurs in the stomach. In this case, the background gastritis appears as a band-like superficial inflammatory infiltrate among the gastric pits (*long arrow*) whereas the lymphoma infiltrates the deeper mucosa, disrupting the normal mucosal structures and the muscularis mucosae (*short arrow*)

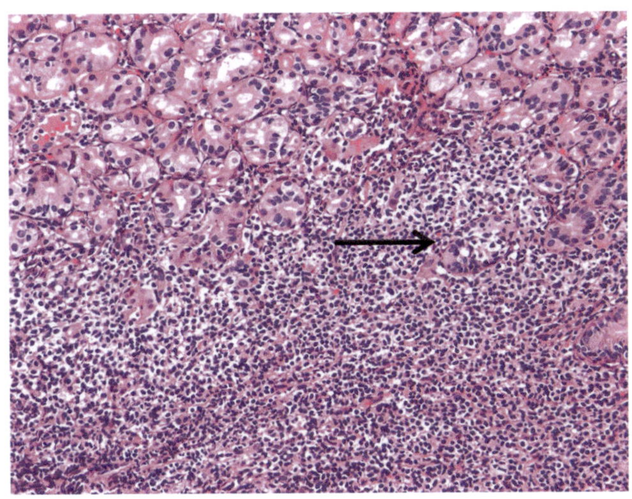

Fig. 28.2 At higher magnification, the dense lymphoid infiltrate of this MALT lymphoma destroys the basal glands. In a few places, the lymphocytes can be seen infiltrating the epithelium of the glands (*arrow*). Many of the lymphocytes have abundant, pale or clear-appearing cytoplasm, which makes them look like they have a clear "halo" at this mag nification. Because the normal stomach is largely devoid of lymphoid tissue, MALT lymphomas are said to arise from "acquired" mucosa-associated lymphoid tissue (as opposed to native GI lymphoid tissue such as that normally found in the Peyer patches of the terminal ileum)

S.R. Owens, H.D. Appelman, *Atlas of Esophagus and Stomach Pathology*, Atlas of Anatomic Pathology,
DOI 10.1007/978-1-4614-8084-6_28, © Springer Science+Business Media New York 2014

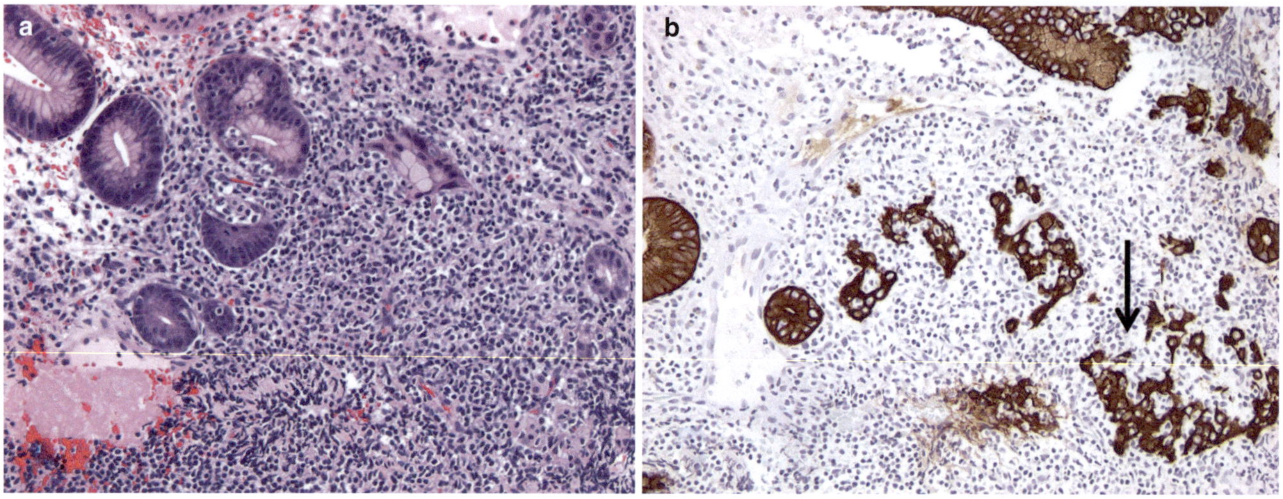

Fig. 28.3 (**a**) Here, numerous lymphocytes disrupt normal gastric glands. (**b**) A cytokeratin immunohistochemical stain further illustrates the disruption of normal epithelial structures, with clusters of neoplastic lymphocytes among the keratin-positive remnants of the gastric glands (*arrow*). This mucosal disruption and expansion of the mucosa can result in endoscopically visible mucosal abnormalities, such as ulcers and thickened gastric folds

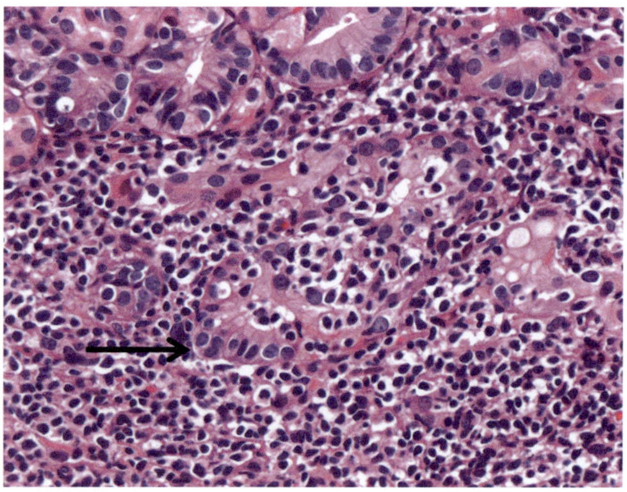

Fig. 28.4 At high magnification, the destructive nature of the lymphoma is clear, with only ragged bits of epithelium visible in this disrupted gland (*arrow*). These so-called "lymphoepithelial lesions" (LELs) are characteristic of MALT lymphoma, but care must be taken not to overinterpret the infiltration of lymphocytes into epithelial structures. In reactive conditions, lymphocytes (especially T cells) can be found among the epithelium, so truly destructive LELs should be found in bona fide MALT lymphoma. Also at this magnification, the cytology of the neoplastic lymphocytes is apparent. Many have indented nuclei and abundant pale cytoplasm, imparting a "monocytoid" appearance. Scattered small cells with scant cytoplasm (centrocyte-like) and large cells (centroblast-like) can also be seen

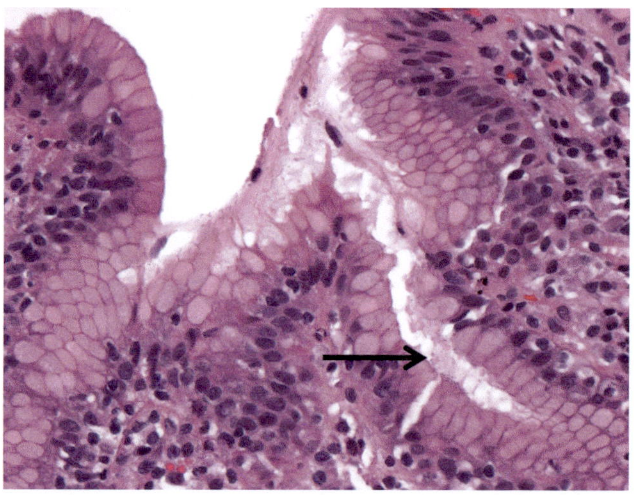

Fig. 28.5 Underlying *H. pylori* gastritis should always be sought when considering the diagnosis of MALT lymphoma. In this case, organisms were found in the superficial mucin of the gastric pits and surface epithelium (*arrow*). Importantly, the vast majority of gastric MALT lymphomas respond to conservative therapy aimed at H. pylori eradication. A small subset of these lymphomas harbors a characteristic genetic translocation [t(11;18)(q21;q21)], which is associated with resistance to *H. pylori* eradication therapy

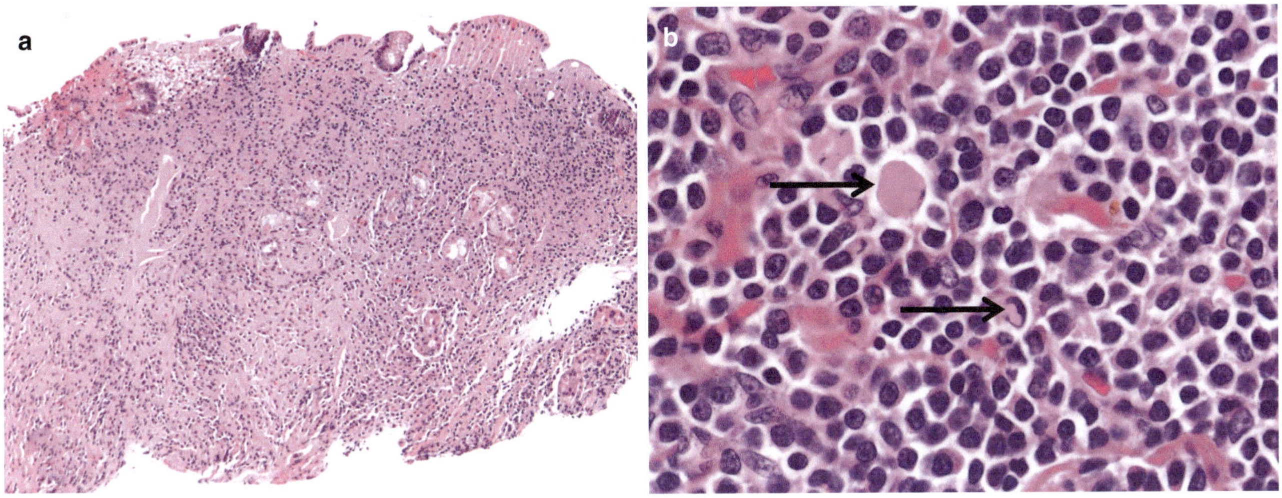

Fig. 28.6 About a third of MALT lymphomas have at least a component of plasmacytic differentiation, which can prove confusing. (**a**) At low magnification, the lymphomatous infiltrate can appear less dense than in conventional cases. Rarely, almost the entire lymphoma can be composed of plasma cells or plasmacytoid cells. In our practice, we have seen such cases misinterpreted as plasma cell myeloma or plasmacytoma. (**b**) At high magnification, intranuclear inclusions composed of immunoglobulin (Dutcher bodies, *arrows*) can be seen, which can raise the differential diagnosis of lymphoplasmacytic lymphoma

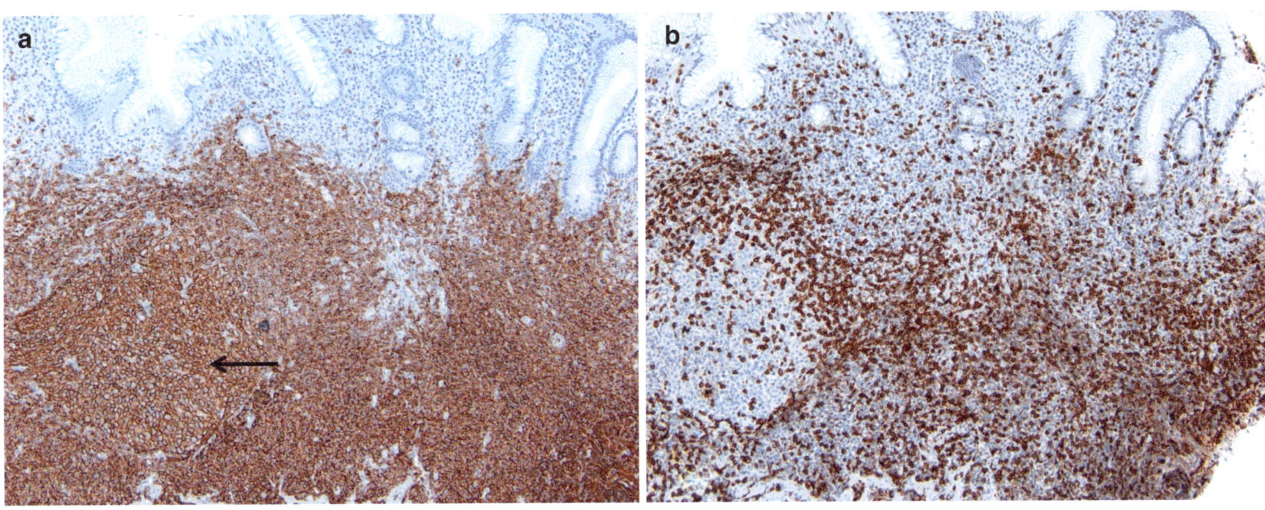

Fig. 28.7 As with other lymphomas, immunohistochemical stains are invaluable in making the diagnosis. (**a**) In this case, CD20 highlighted the majority of the lymphocytes, including a reactive germinal center (*arrow*) related to the underlying *H. pylori* gastritis. (**b**) CD3 stained the non-neoplastic T-cells, which were in the minority, an unusual finding in a reactive condition

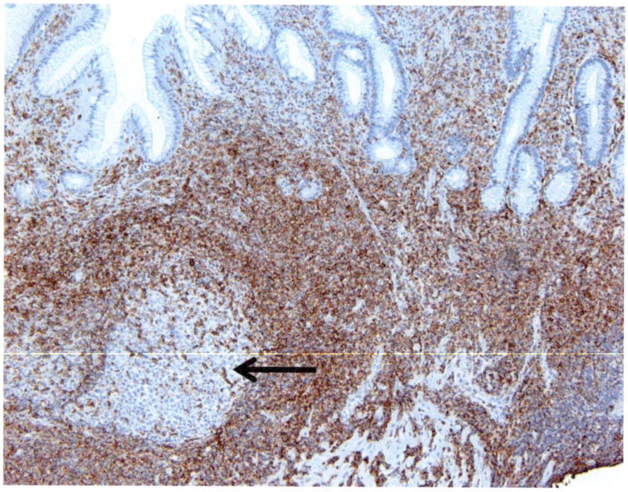

Fig. 28.8 Aberrant co-expression by the neoplastic B-cells of CD43 can be extremely helpful in determining that an infiltrate is truly neoplastic. Compared with the CD20 and CD3 stains in Fig. 28.7, the CD43 expression in this image more closely matches the CD20, apart from the residual germinal center (*arrow*). This helpful feature only occurs in a minority of cases and care must be taken to avoid overinterpreting normal CD43 expression by non-neoplastic plasma cells

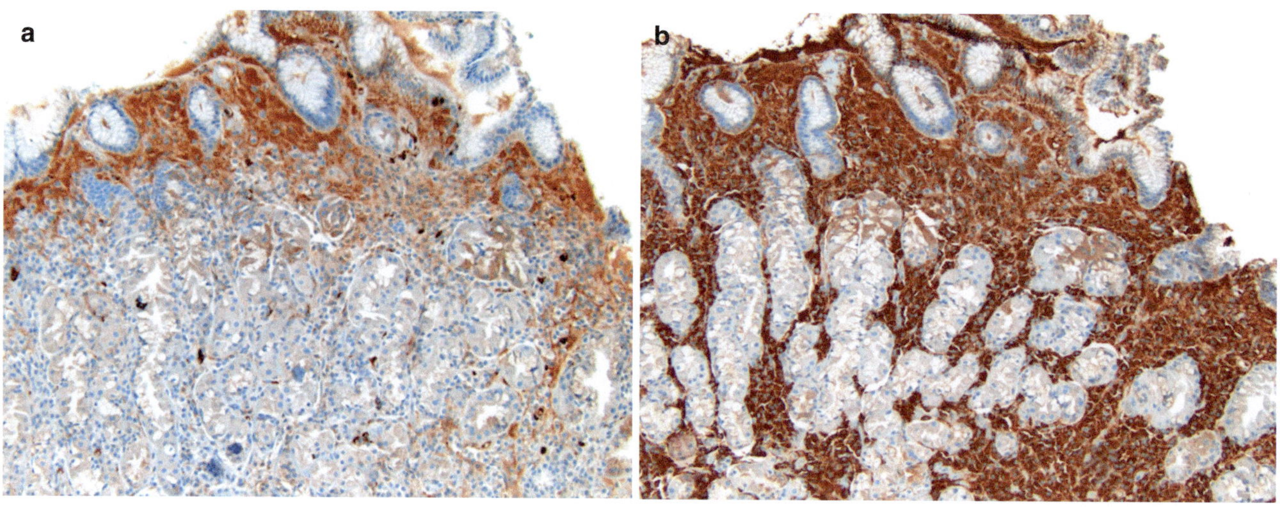

Fig. 28.9 In cases of MALT lymphoma with plasmacytic differentiation, immunohistochemical stains for immunoglobulin light chains can be helpful. In this case, a stain for kappa light chain (**a**) revealed only scattered positive cells, whereas a λ light chain stain (**b**) decorated almost every cell in the lamina propria

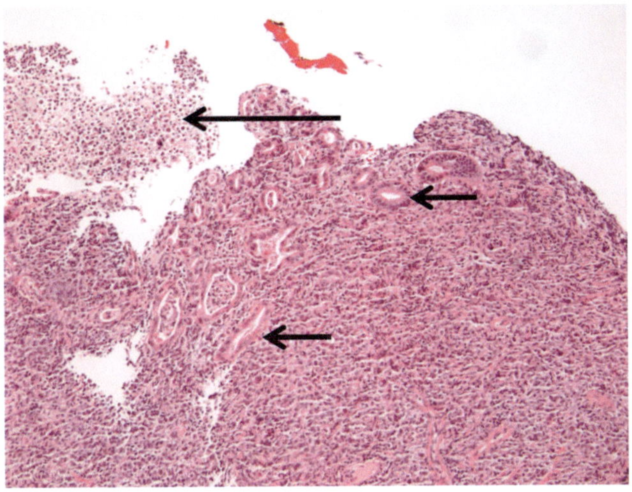

Fig. 28.10 In this example of diffuse large B-cell lymphoma (DLBCL), the mucosa is almost completely replaced by an infiltrate of atypical cells that destroy the normal mucosal components. Only a few glands and pits remain (*short arrows*). In addition, there is an ulcer, as evidenced by the surface exudate (*long arrow*). DLBCL is the most common lymphoma in the gastrointestinal tract, and the gastrointestinal tract is the most common extranodal site of DLBCL. It may evolve from low-grade lymphomas such as MALT lymphoma or follicular lymphoma, or it may occur de novo. At this magnification, it is difficult to know exactly what kind of neoplasm this is without further investigation

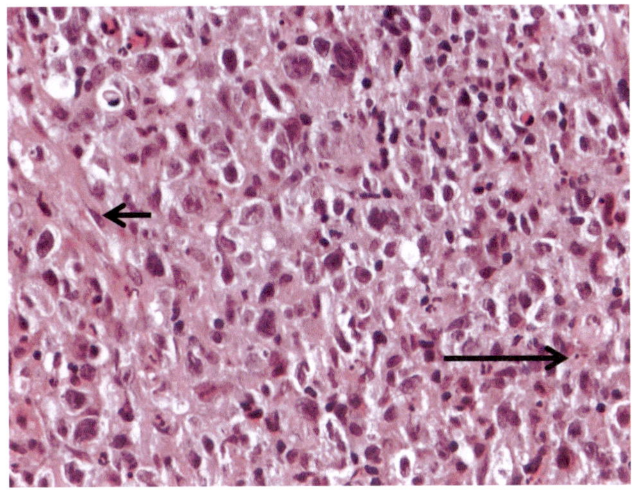

Fig. 28.11 At high magnification, the neoplasm consists of dyscohesive cells that do not make any recognizable structures. Large lymphoid cells are defined as having nuclei that are at least 2× the size of normal lymphocyte nuclei. To judge the size of the cells in a diffuse infiltrate such as this, a convenient comparison can be made to endothelial cells (*short arrow*), which are by definition "medium-to-large." Individual cell necrosis with apoptotic debris (*long arrow*) is evident. DLBCL often causes a large, infiltrative mass that may cause ulceration

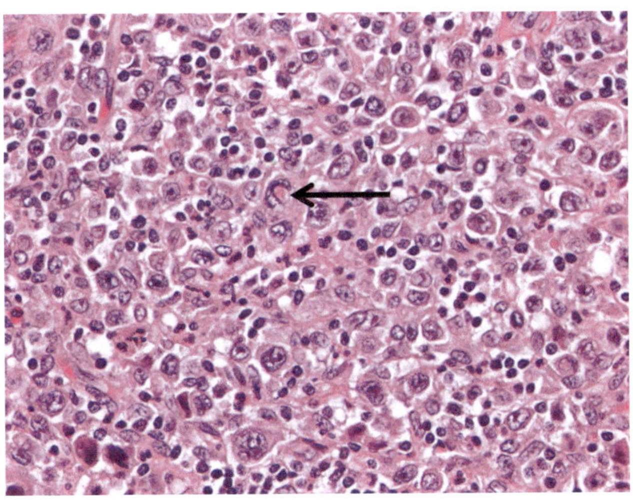

Fig. 28.12 This example of DLBCL has pleomorphic morphology, with large cells that, on occasion (*arrow*), resemble the hallmark cells of anaplastic large cell lymphoma (a T-cell lymphoma), which is rare in the stomach. DLBCL has an aggressive clinical course, but may be curable with appropriate therapy. Usually, chemotherapy is utilized, but surgical approaches may be necessary for cases causing intractable bleeding, perforation, or obstruction. A possible low-grade lymphomatous component from which the DLBCL may have evolved should be kept in mind, as this may be left behind after the large cell component is treated

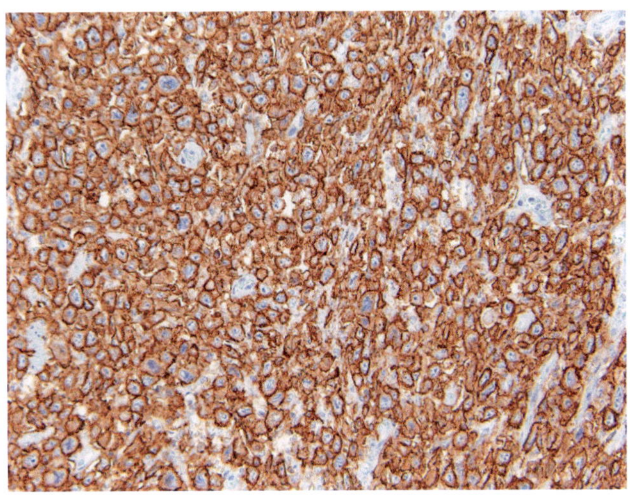

Fig. 28.13 When DLBCL is in the differential diagnosis, a positive CD20 immunohistochemical stain will aid in definitive classification. In this case, the strong membrane positivity is clearly in the large lymphoma cells

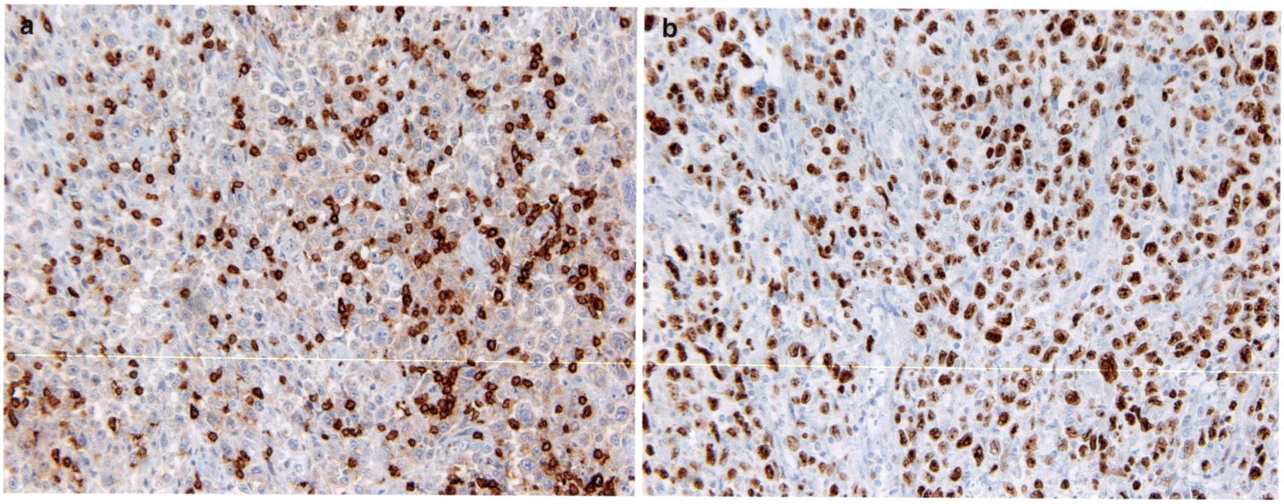

Fig. 28.14 (**a**) A CD3 immunostain will usually highlight admixed, small T cells, but is clearly negative in the large lymphoma cells with pleomorphic nuclei. (**b**) Many DLBCL have a brisk proliferative rate, as highlighted on this Ki-67 immunostain. When the proliferative rate is greater than 90% and the lymphoma co-expresses CD10, one must consider the possibility of a lymphoma harboring genetic abnormalities involving *MYC* along with *BCL2* and/or *BCL6*. Such "double hit" lymphomas (currently classified as "B cell lymphoma, unclassifiable, with features intermediate between DLBCL and Burkitt lymphoma" by the World Health Organization), are thought to have some prognostic differences from conventional DLBCL

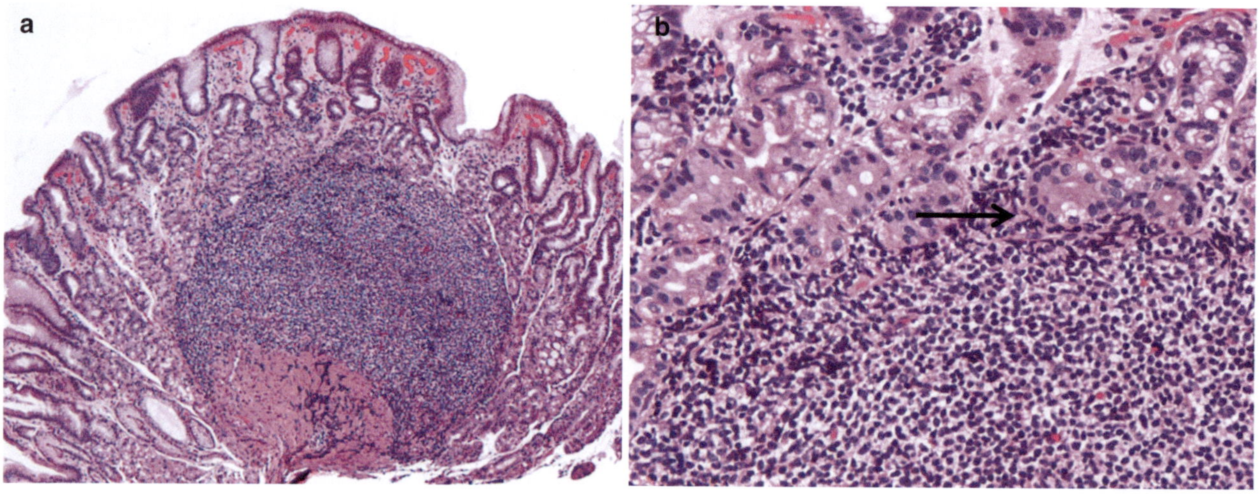

Fig. 28.15 Mantle cell lymphoma (MCL). This lymphoma is a mix of small, innocuous-appearing morphology with relentlessly progressive clinical behavior. MCL can appear as a polyp or polyps in the mucosa of the GI tract, and is the most common cause of so-called "lymphomatous polyposis," which can produce many polyps throughout the GI tract that can mimic an inherited polyposis syndrome when seen endoscopically. (**a**) This gastric nodule of MCL appeared as a polyp, but can be seen at low magnification to consist of a dense collection of small lymphocytes that displace normal mucosal structures. (**b**) At higher magnification, the lymphocytes are monotonous and small. Although well-demarcated, the nodule of lymphocytes truly disrupts the mucosal glands (*arrow*)

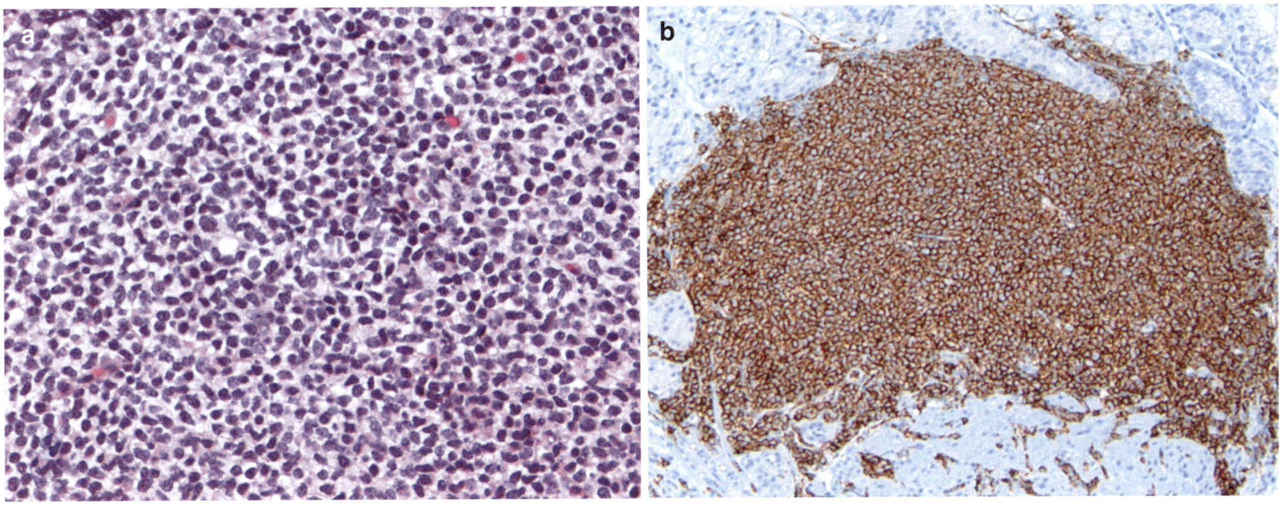

Fig. 28.16 (**a**) At high magnification, the cells of MCL are densely blue and have angulated nuclear contours. The GI tract is the most common extranodal site of involvement, and MCL is associated with a characteristic translocation t(11;14)(q13;q32) that is often demonstrable by classical cytogenetics and essentially always present by more sensitive techniques such as fluorescence in situ hybridization (FISH). (**b**) A CD20 immunostain is positive in the nodule of MCL in this gastric biopsy

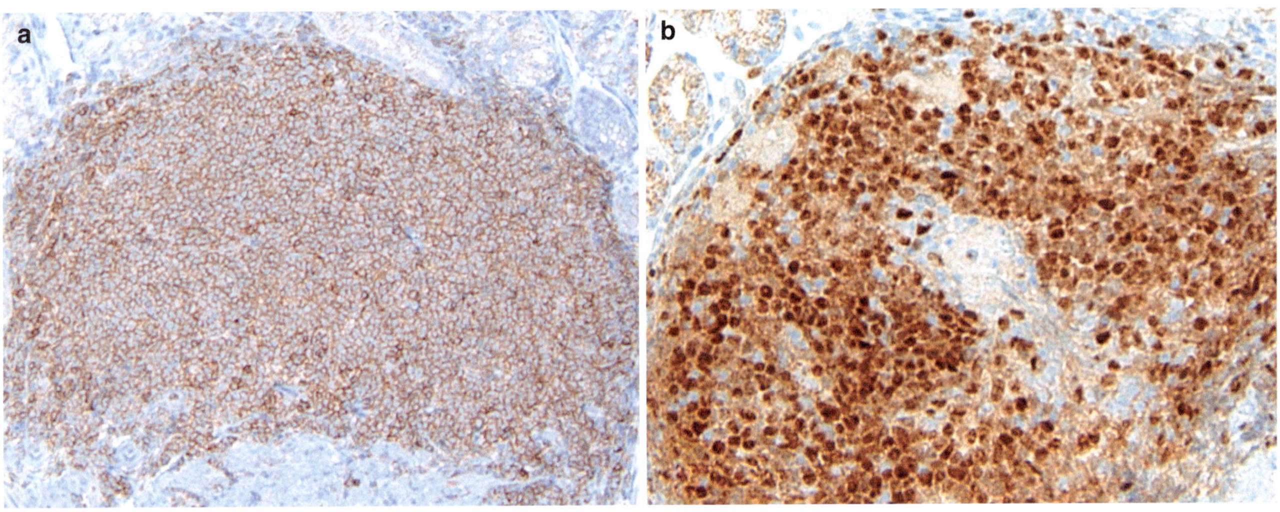

Fig. 28.17 (**a**) Aberrant co-expression of CD5 (a T-cell marker) by the neoplastic B cells in MCL is helpful in the diagnosis. This feature overlaps with chronic lymphocytic leukemia/small lymphocytic lymphoma (CLL/SLL), so it is not specific. (**b**) When accompanied by nuclear expression of cyclin-D1, however, the diagnosis of MCL is made

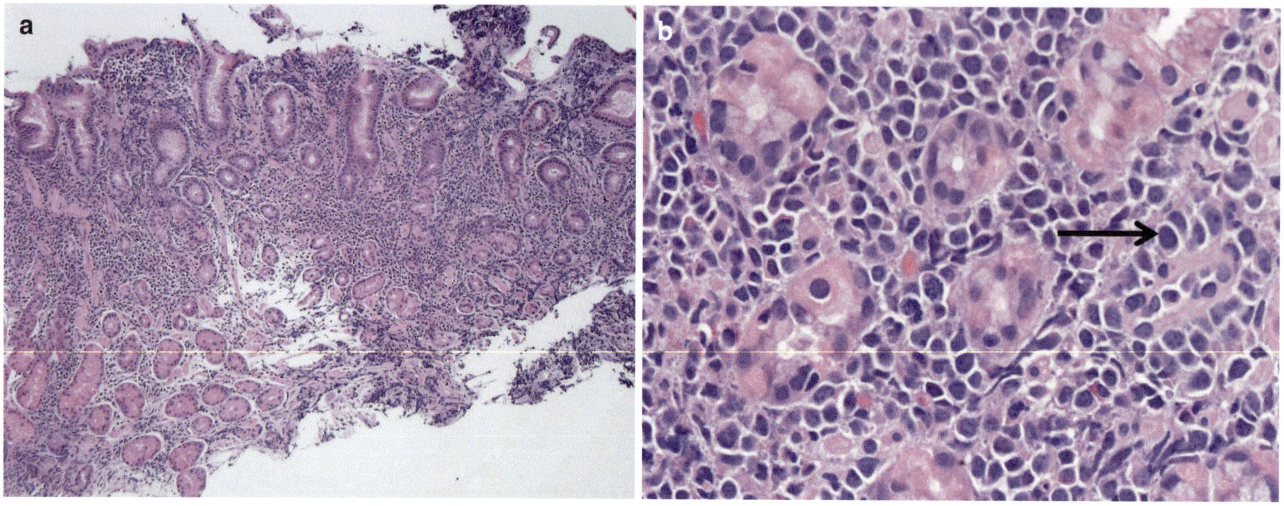

Fig. 28.18 A variety of other hematolymphoid neoplasms occur in the GI tract, but are much more rare. (**a**) In this case, the stomach is involved by acute myeloid leukemia (AML) that disrupts the mucosa in a manner similar to that seen in the lymphomas discussed earlier. (**b**) At high magnification, the neoplastic myeloid blasts have fine nuclear chromatin (*arrow*). The GI tract is a relatively common location for involvement by extramedullary AML, and many cases have a monocytic component

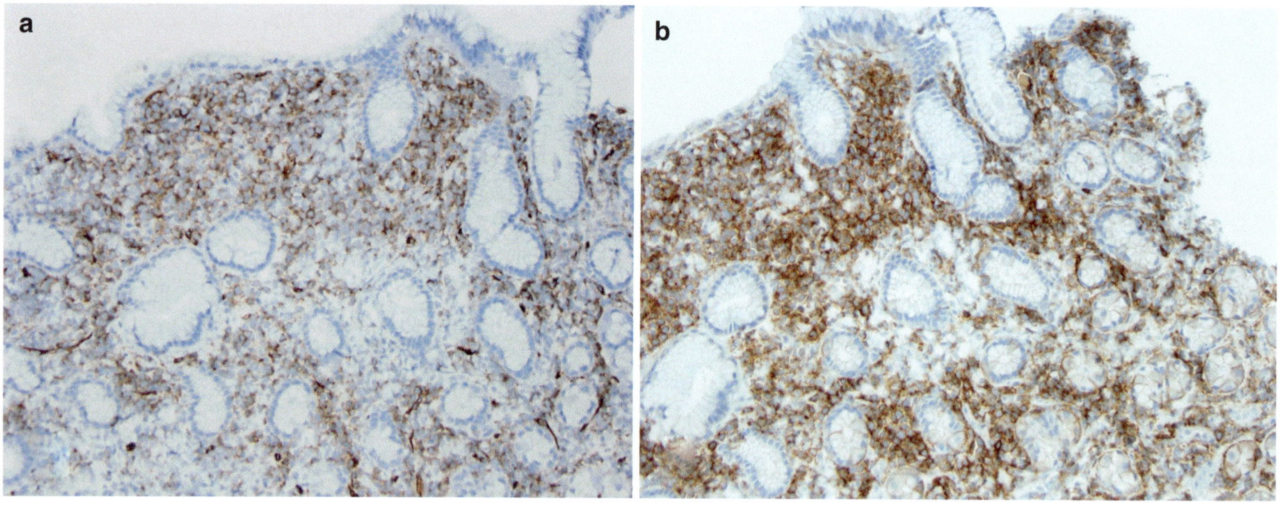

Fig. 28.19 Positive CD34 (**a**) and CD117 (**b**) stains highlight the neoplastic blasts in this case of AML involving the stomach

Gastric Metastases

29

Many, many malignancies can metastasize to the stomach, but this chapter will concentrate on the most common offenders that cause diagnostic difficulty: lobular breast cancer and melanoma. Melanoma is the "great mimicker" and can have a variety of appearances, so a high index of suspicion is important in keeping it in the differential diagnosis of malignancy in the stomach. More troublesome is metastatic lobular carcinoma, for it can spread throughout the mucosa and gastric wall in a way that strongly resembles that of primary diffuse gastric adenocarcinoma. The individual cells of metastatic lobular carcinoma can be nearly indistinguishable from the signet-ring cells of primary gastric cancer, so judicious use of ancillary methods such as immunohistochemistry is warranted to aid in sorting out the issue. Sometimes, unfortunately, it can be nearly impossible to distinguish between primary diffuse gastric carcinoma and metastatic lobular breast carcinoma based on histology alone. Other metastatic carcinomas can mimic primary gastric adenocarcinoma, but clinical correlation and a battery of immunohistochemical stains may prove helpful in sorting out a metastasis from a primary process.

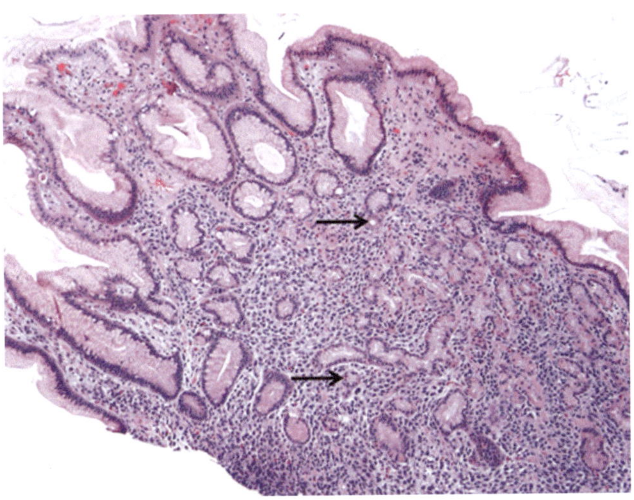

Fig. 29.1 Melanoma can mimic many different tumor types with spindled and epithelioid morphology. In the stomach, it may impersonate lymphoma, diffuse carcinoma, gastrointestinal stromal tumor (GIST), or a variety of other metastatic tumors. In this low-magnification view of a gastric biopsy, the lamina propria is filled with a dense population of atypical cells that spread apart the normal gastric glands (*arrows*). Note the tendency of the cells to be most dense in the base of the mucosa (so-called "bottom-heavy" distribution)

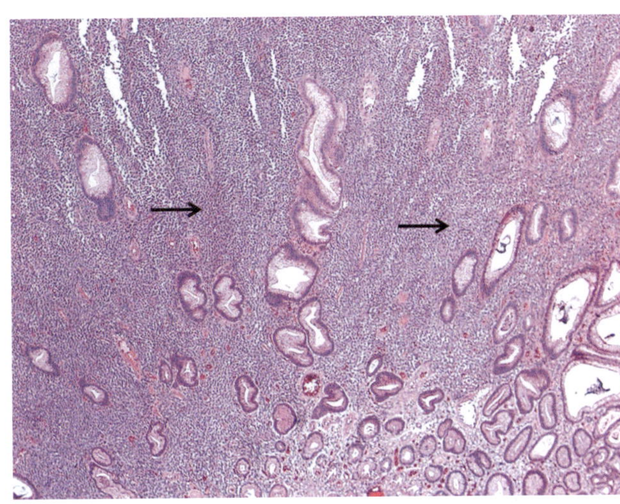

Fig. 29.2 Here, the gastric mucosa is extensively infiltrated by malignant cells (*arrows*), creating a sea of blue between the normal mucosal structures. At this magnification, the appearance is reminiscent of a diffuse lymphoma

S.R. Owens, H.D. Appelman, *Atlas of Esophagus and Stomach Pathology*, Atlas of Anatomic Pathology,
DOI 10.1007/978-1-4614-8084-6_29, © Springer Science+Business Media New York 2014

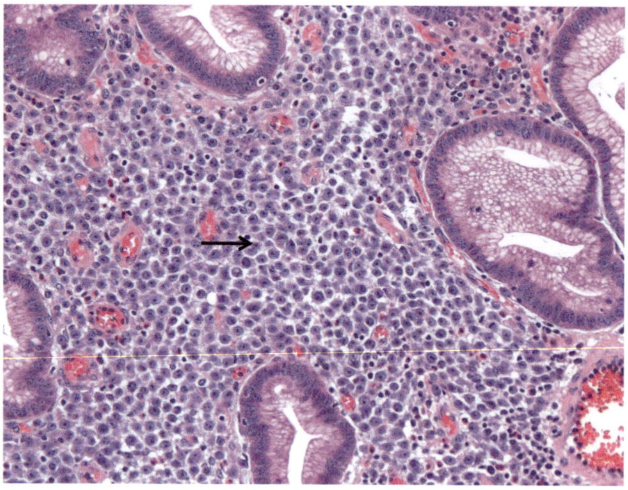

Fig. 29.3 At higher magnification, the cells appear rounded and rather dyscohesive. Some prominent, cherry-red nucleoli are visible (*arrow*). Metastatic melanoma can affect any site in the GI tract, although the colon is most common. Primary melanoma is the stomach is vanishingly rare, and other tumors that can be mistaken for melanoma (including clear cell sarcoma, GIST, schwannoma, and others) are rare as well. Thus, the usual dilemma is distinguishing metastatic melanoma from common primary gastric tumors

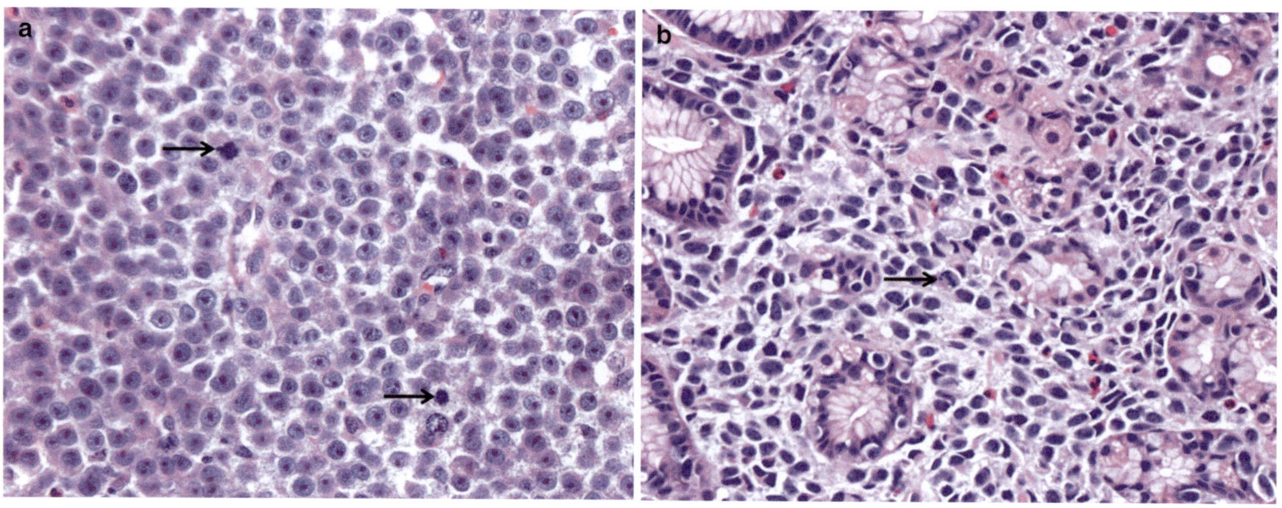

Fig. 29.4 (**a**) At high magnification, the cherry-red macronucleoli are easily seen in this metastatic melanoma with epithelioid morphology. Pigment may be found, but is usually not present. (**b**) This metastatic melanoma has a mixture of epithelioid and spindle cells that infiltrate between the gastric glands. When extensively spindled, melanoma can mimic schwannoma and GIST. Both photomicrographs contain easily identified mitotic figures (*arrows*)

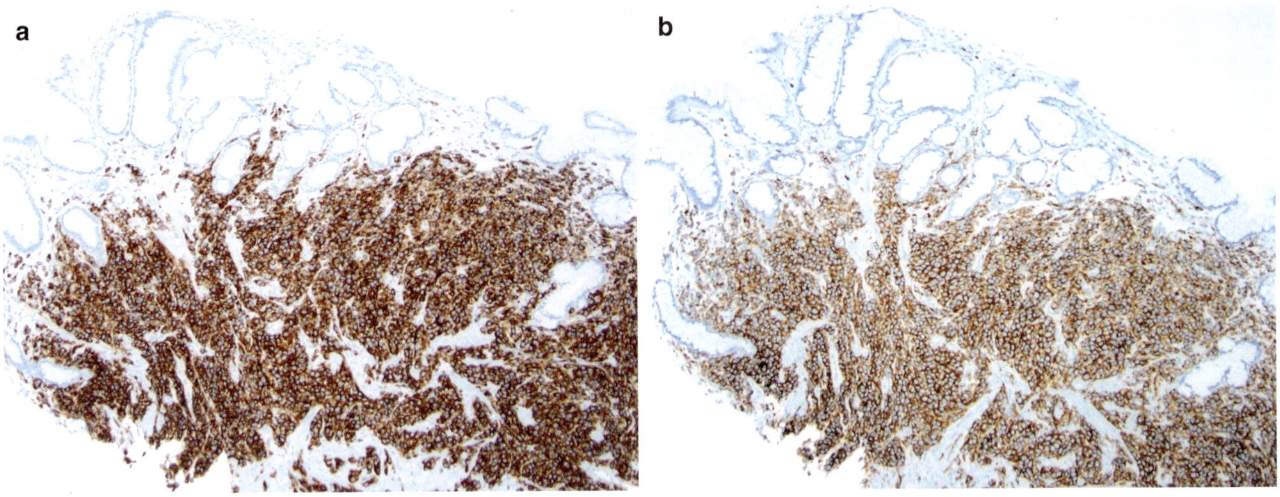

Fig. 29.5 Because of its tendency to masquerade as other neoplasms, metastatic melanoma often requires a battery of immunohistochemical stains to aid in diagnosis. (**a**) Melan-A (MART1) is usually positive and can be very helpful. Melanomas with spindled morphology may be negative, however. Most melanomas of any morphology are positive for S100, although this can potentially cause confusion with other S100-expressing tumors such as schwannoma. The riskiest pitfall, however, is the frequent expression by melanoma of c-kit/CD117 (**b**). This can lead to a misdiagnosis of epithelioid GIST or a hematolymphoid neoplasm such as extramedullary myeloid tumor/granulocytic sarcoma

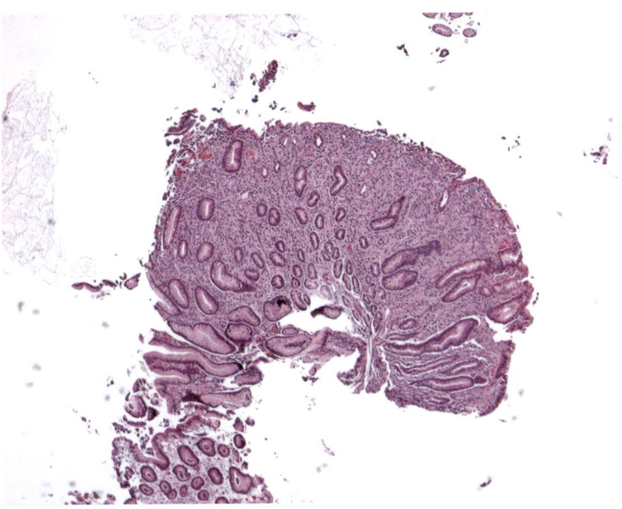

Fig. 29.6 This gastric biopsy clearly contains some type of infiltrate that expands the lamina propria. The epithelium of the pits and glands is hyperchromatic and reactive-appearing

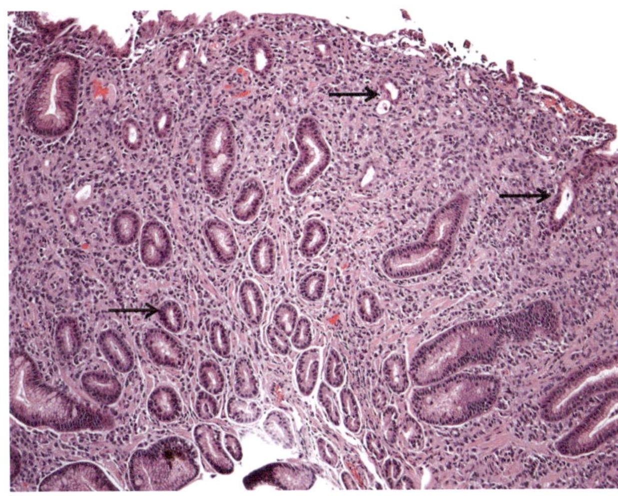

Fig. 29.7 At higher magnification, the individual cells of the infiltrate are better seen, but they do not seem to make any structures. The residual pits and glands (*arrows*) are in various states of injury and regeneration. At this magnification, this could be lymphoma, melanoma, or primary gastric carcinoma, among other things

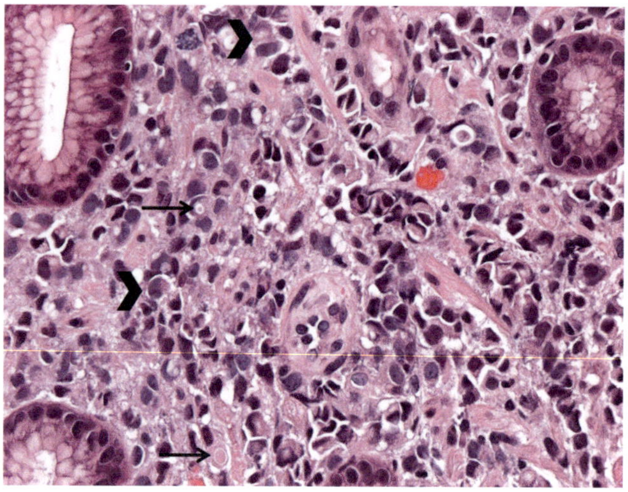

Fig. 29.8 Finally, at high magnification, we can make out the individual cells. Now, however, there is a new problem: many of the cells, which are clearly very pleomorphic and malignant appearing, have eccentric nuclei and a signet ring-like appearance (*arrowhead*). Here is where an index of suspicion is key—one must keep in mind that metastatic lobular breast carcinoma can strongly mimic primary diffuse gastric adenocarcinoma. A helpful feature on hematoxylin and eosin (H&E) stain is the presence of some intracytoplasmic vacuoles with dots of inspissated mucin (*arrows*). Even more helpful is the tendency for lobular breast carcinoma to express estrogen receptor (ER) and lack E-cadherin staining by immunohistochemistry. This is not specific, however, as a handful of gastric adenocarcinomas express ER, and the subset of so-called "hereditary diffuse gastric cancers" are associated with cadherin (*CDH*) gene abnormalities and can be negative for E-cadherin staining (see Chap. 25)

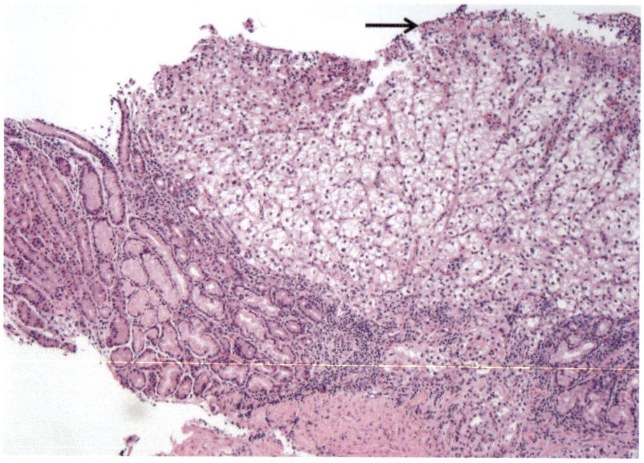

Fig. 29.9 As mentioned earlier, a variety of malignancies can metastasize to the stomach. Here, a cluster of cells with clear cell features and delicate vasculature fills the mucosa and cause surface erosion (*arrow*)

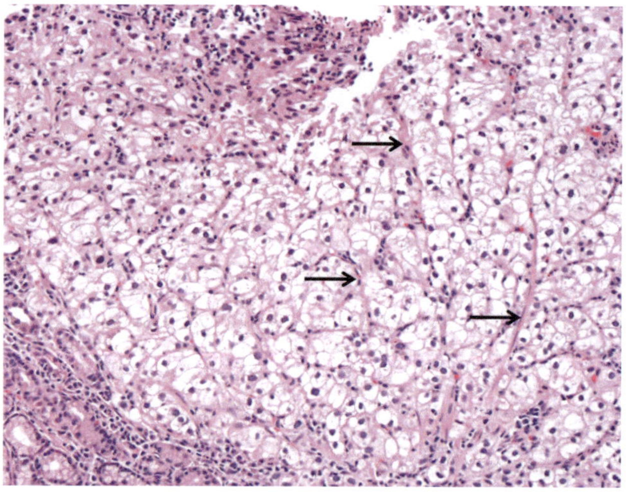

Fig. 29.10 At high magnification, the cells are seen to have central nuclei with occasional prominent nucleoli. The delicate vascular network (*arrows*) is characteristic of this metastatic, classic, clear-cell, renal cell carcinoma. We have seen a number of such cases. We have also encountered metastatic lung carcinoma, leiomyosarcoma, and many others, although these are fairly rare and relatively easy to decipher based on morphology, immunohistochemistry, and clinical history

Index

S.R. Owens, H.D. Appelman, *Atlas of Esophagus and Stomach Pathology*, Atlas of Anatomic Pathology,
DOI 10.1007/978-1-4614-8084-6, © Springer Science+Business Media New York 2014

H

MIX
Papier aus verantwortungsvollen Quellen
Paper from responsible sources
FSC® C105338

If you have any concerns about our products,
you can contact us on
ProductSafety@springernature.com

In case Publisher is established outside the EU,
the EU authorized representative is:
Springer Nature Customer Service Center GmbH
Europaplatz 3, 69115 Heidelberg, Germany

Printed by Libri Plureos GmbH
in Hamburg, Germany